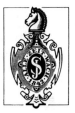

Josef S. Smolen   Christoph C. Zielinski

Systemic Lupus Erythematosus

Clinical and Experimental Aspects

Foreword by G. Geyer

With 60 Figures and 44 Tables

Springer-Verlag Berlin Heidelberg New York
London Paris Tokyo

Univ.-Doz. Dr. Josef S. Smolen
Univ.-Doz. Dr. Christoph C. Zielinski

II. Medizinische Universitätsklinik,
Allgemeines Krankenhaus der Stadt Wien
Garnisongasse 13, A-1090 Wien

ISBN-13:978-3-642-71644-7   e-ISBN-13:978-3-642-71642-3
DOI: 10.1007/978-3-642-71642-3

Library of Congress Cataloging in Publication Data.
Systemic lupus erythematosus. Includes index. 1. Lupus erythematosus, Systemic.
I. Smolen, Josef S., 1950 –. II. Zielinski, Christoph C., 1952 –. [DNLM: 1. Lupus
Erythematosus, Systemic. WR 152 S9952] RC924.5.L85S97 1987 616.7'7 86-31382
ISBN-13:978-3-642-71644-7 (U. S.)

This work is subject to copyright. All rights are reserved, whether the whole or part
of the material is concerned, specifically the rights of translation, reprinting, re-use of
illustrations, recitation, broadcasting, reproduction on microfilms or in other ways,
and storage in data banks. Duplication of this publication or parts thereof is only permitted under the provisions of the German Copyright Law of September 9, 1965, in its
version of June 24, 1985, and a copyright fee must always be paid. Violations fall under the prosecution act of the German Copyright Law.

© Springer-Verlag Berlin Heidelberg 1987
Softcover reprint of the hardcover 1st edition 1987

The use of registered names, trademarks, etc. in this publication does not imply, even
in the absence of a specific statement, that such names are exempt from the relevant
protective laws and regulations and therefore free for general use.

2127/3145-543210

*We dedicate
this book
to our families*

THE EDITORS

Foreword

More than 140 years ago, lupus erythematosus (LE) was recognized as a disease entity by clinicians working in the field of dermatology, which had only recently become an independent medical discipline. Soon after cutaneous lupus was first reported, it was realized that, apart from the skin, the disease could involve other organs and thus be systemic in nature. The latter observations were first made by MORITZ KAPOSI [1], whose work has attracted renewed attention recently and who succeeded FERDINAND VON HEBRA to the chair of dermatology at the Medical Faculty in Vienna. The early description of lupus erythematosus in both its cutaneous and systemic manifestations was thus intimately associated with Vienna and its Medical School.

The next phase in the study of lupus was characterized by an increase in knowledge of the type and extent of organ involvement. The work by OSLER [2], LIBMANN and SACKS [3], and KLEMPERER [4] best represents these advances. The increase in clinical knowledge of LE finally led to DUBOIS' famous monograph [5], which was published at a time of renewed interest in SLE, elicited by the description by HARGRAVES et al. [6] of the LE-cell phenomenon. A more detailed analysis of this finding revealed that the disease was characterized by an abnormal immune response, although its pathogenetic implications were still unclear. Finally, the description of antinuclear antibodies (ANA) and, later, antibodies to double-stranded DNA indicated that these autoantibodies were universally and uniformly present in patients with LE: it thus seemed that the disease was an entity with considerable clinical variability. Later investigations into the nature and composition of ANA subsets led, however, to the conclusion that certain ANA subsets could be associated with certain clinical courses of SLE and thus be important with regard to its prognosis. Over the past two decades attention has focused upon the function of B and T cells, and the belief has prevailed that a dysfunction of either or both of these lymphocyte populations or of their subsets could be responsible for dysregulation of the immune system in LE, which would culminate in B-cell hyperactivity. The application of modern biotechnologic techniques to lupus research may lead to further enlightenment.

Thus, current knowledge indicates that SLE represents a complex syndrome with varying clinical, immunologic and genetic characteristics. Although we have not come to a complete understanding of the etiology and pathogenesis of the disease, the area has become so complex and so many different paths have been followed that it seemed justified to suggest publication of a book on LE presenting the current state of knowledge of scientific and clinical aspects of the disease. I would like to congratulate the editors and the contributors to the book on the fulfillment of this proposal in a very informative monograph. The various papers, written by some of the most knowledgeable scientists in the field, provide every physician and scientist dealing with LE with insights into modern conceptions of this interesting disorder which still represents the prototype "autoimmune disease." Let us all hope that these insights will form a basis upon which our knowledge of LE and autoimmunity in general can build, and that a further elucidation of the pathogenesis of this disease, with which we have been confronted for more than a century, will soon be forthcoming.

Vienna, March 1987

GEORG GEYER
Professor of Medicine and Head,
2nd Department of Medicine,
University Hospital
Vienna, Austria

References

1. Kaposi M (1872) Arch Dermatol Syphil (Prag) 4:36
2. Holubar K (1980) Am J Dermatopathol 2:239
3. Libmann E, Sacks B (1924) Arch Int Med 33:701
4. Klemperer P (1952) Pathology of SLE. In: Progress in Fundamental Medicine, Lea and Fibiger, Philadelphia
5. Dubois EL (1974) Lupus Erythematosus. University of Southern California Press
6. Hargraves MM, Richmond H, Morton R (1948) Proc Staff Meet Mayo Clin 23:25

Table of Contents

Foreword VII
G. GEYER

Part I:
General Considerations

Description of Systemic Lupus Erythematosus:
A Historical Perspective 2
W. GRANINGER, J. S. SMOLEN, and C. C. ZIELINSKI

Etiologic and Pathogenetic Aspects of Systemic Lupus
Erythematosus: A Critical Approach 6
W. GRANINGER, C. C. ZIELINSKI, and J. S. SMOLEN

Part II:
Animal Models of Systemic Lupus Erythematosus:
Genetic, Viral and Immunologic Aspects

Genetic Aspects of Murine Lupus 22
M. F. SELDIN, J. D. MOUNTZ, and A. D. STEINBERG

Autoimmune Disease in New Zealand Mice 50
T. M. CHUSED, K. L. MCCOY, R. B. LAL, TH. R. MALEK,
E. M. BROWN, L. J. EDISON, and P. J. BAKER

The NZB × SWR Model: Insights into
Viral, Immunologic, and Genetic Factors 60
S. K. DATTA

Relevance of the Murine Models of
Systemic Lupus Erythematosus to Human Disease 73
C. A. LASKIN and H. R. SMITH

X Table of Contents

Part III:
Immunologic and Genetic Aspects of Human SLE

The Importance of the Study of Monoclonal Antibodies . . 88
D. ISENBERG, Y. SHOENFELD, and R. S. SCHWARTZ

ANA Subsets in Systemic Lupus Erythematosus 105
M. REICHLIN and J. B. HARLEY

Complement and Complement Deficiencies 124
G. TAPPEINER

The Role of Lymphokines in the Pathogenesis of
Systemic Lupus Erythematosus 145
T. A. LUGER and J. S. SMOLEN

Part IV:
Clinical Aspects of Human SLE

Clinical and Serologic Features:
Incidence and Diagnostic Approach 170
J. S. SMOLEN

Immunologic Similarities and Differences Between
Systemic Lupus Erythematosus and Sjögren's Syndrome . 197
H. M. MOUTSOPOULOS

Pathology 204
W. ULRICH and G. SYRÉ

Cutaneous Manifestations 227
T. A. LUGER and D. BENESCH

Neurological Manifestations 251
E. MAIDA and E. HORVATITS

Radiographic Features 270
G. SEIDL

The Lupus Subset Idea 290
J. S. SMOLEN, A. D. STEINBERG, and T. M. CHUSED

Part V:
Therapeutic Aspects of SLE

An Experimental Therapeutic Approach: Clinical
and Immunological Aspects of Plasmapheresis 300
C. C. ZIELINSKI

Future Immunotherapeutic Possibilities
in Autoimmunity 345
N. TALAL

Subject Index 355

List of Contributors

P. J. BAKER
Laboratory of Microbial Immunity
National Institute of Allergy and Infectious Diseases
National Institutes of Health
Bethesda, Maryland 20205, USA

D. BENESCH
2nd Department of Dermatology
University of Vienna
Alserstraße 4
1090 Vienna, Austria

E. M. BROWN
Laboratory of Microbial Immunity
National Institute of Allergy and Infectious Diseases
National Institutes of Health
Bethesda, Maryland 20205, USA

T. M. CHUSED
Laboratory of Microbial Immunity
National Institute of Allergy and Infectious Diseases
National Institutes of Health
Bethesda, Maryland 20205, USA

S. K. DATTA
Department of Medicine (Hematology/Oncology Division)
Cancer Research Center
New England Medical Center
and Tufts University School of Medicine
171 Harrison Avenue
Boston, Massachusetts 02111, USA

L. J. EDISON
Laboratory of Microbial Immunity
National Institute of Allergy and Infectious Diseases
National Institutes of Health
Bethesda, Maryland 20205, USA

G. GEYER
2nd Department of Medicine, University Hospital
University of Vienna, Garnisongasse 13
1090 Vienna, Austria

W. GRANINGER
2nd Department of Medicine, University Hospital
University of Vienna, Garnisongasse 13
1090 Vienna, Austria

J. B. HARLEY
Arthritis and Immunology Program
Oklahoma Medical Research Foundation
825 Northeast 13th Street
Oklahoma City, OK 73104, USA

E. HORVATITS
Department of Neurology, University Hospital
University of Vienna, Lazarettgasse 17
1090 Vienna, Austria

D. ISENBERG
Department of Rheumatology and Rehabilitation
University College Hospital, Gower Street
London WC 1 E 6 AU, Great Britain

R. B. LAL
Laboratory of Microbial Immunity
National Institute of Allergy and Infectious Diseases
National Institutes of Health
Bethesda, Maryland 20205, USA

C. A. LASKIN
Mt. Sinai Research Institute
Toronto General Hospital and Mt. Sinai Hospital
Toronto, Ontario, Canada

T. A. LUGER
2nd Department of Dermatology, University Hospital
University of Vienna, Alserstraße 4
1090 Vienna, Austria

E. MAIDA
Department of Neurology, University Hospital
University of Vienna, Lazarettgasse 17
1090 Vienna, Austria

T. R. MALEK
Laboratory of Microbial Immunity
National Institute of Allergy and Infectious Diseases
National Institutes of Health
Bethesda, Maryland 20205, USA

K. L. McCoy
Laboratory of Microbial Immunity
National Institute of Allergy and Infectious Diseases
National Institutes of Health
Bethesda, Maryland 20205, USA

J. D. MOUNTZ
Cellular Immunology Section
Arthritis and Rheumatism Branch
Natl. Institute of Arthritis,
Diabetes, Digestive and Kidney Diseases
National Institutes of Health
Bethesda, Maryland 20205, USA

H. M. MOUTSOPOULOS
Department of Medicine, Medical School
University of Ioannina
45332 Ioannina, Greece

M. REICHLIN
Arthritis and Immunology Program
Oklahoma Medical Research Foundation
825 Northeast 13th Street
Oklahoma City, Oklahoma 73104, USA

G. SEIDL
2nd Department of Medicine, University Hospital
University of Vienna, Garnisongasse 13
1090 Vienna, Austria

M. F. SELDIN
Cellular Immunology Section
Arthritis and Rheumatism Branch
Natl. Institute of Arthritis,
Diabetes, Digestive and Kidney Diseases
National Institutes of Health
Bethesda, Maryland 20205, USA

Y. SHOENFELD
Department of Medicine 'D'
Beilinson Medical Centre
Petach Tikva, Israel

H. R. Smith
Medical Service
Boston Veterans Administration Medical Center
and Arthritis Center
Boston University
Boston, Massachusetts, USA

J. S. Smolen
2nd Department of Medicine, University Hospital
University of Vienna, Garnisongasse 13
1090 Vienna, Austria

G. Syre
Department of Pathology, General Hospital
4040 Linz, Austria

R. S. Schwartz
Department of Medicine (Haematology-Oncology Division)
New England Medical Center, 171 Harrison Avenue
Boston, Massachusetts 02111, USA

A. D. Steinberg
Cellular Immunology Section
Arthritis and Rheumatism Branch
Natl. Institute of Arthritis,
Diabetes, Digestive and Kidney Diseases
National Institutes of Health
Bethesda, Maryland 20205, USA

N. Talal
Department of Medicine
The University of Texas Health Science Center at San Antonio
San Antonio, Texas 78284, USA

G. Tappeiner
1st Department of Dermatology, University Hospital,
University of Vienna, Alserstraße 4
1090 Vienna, Austria

W. Ulrich
Institute of Pathology
University of Vienna, Spitalgasse 2
1090 Vienna, Austria

C. C. Zielinski
2nd Department of Medicine, University Hospital
University of Vienna, Garnisongasse 13
1090 Vienna, Austria

Part I:
General Considerations

Description of Systemic Lupus Erythematosus: A Historical Perspective

W. Graninger, J. S. Smolen, and C. C. Zielinski

Ferdinand von Hebra first described a typical skin lesion with aggressive and tissue destructive characteristics in 1845 [1], which — due to its appearance — was named by Pierre Louis Cazanave "lupus [latin *wolf*] erythematosus" in 1851 [2]. Although the term "lupus" was not confined to a single disorder at that time [3], the peculiarity of the skin lesion was fully recognized, resulting in a variety of descriptive terms (e.g., "butterfly rash" [4]) which are in use until today. It was, however, not until Moritz Kaposi succeeded Hebra to the Chair of the Department of Dermatology at the Vienna University Hospital that the systemic nature of lupus was recognized: Kaposi reported in 1872 that certain patients suffering from lupus presented with a syndrome consisting of fever. arthritis, lymphadenopathy, and anemia [5]. It was this report which led to a clear separation of systemic or disseminated lupus erythemntosus (SLE) from the forms definitely limited to the skin. Publications by Jadassohn from Vienna [6] and by William Osler from Baltimore, Maryland, who discussed visceral complications of "erythema exsudativum multiforme" [7] — which rather would be recognized as SLE today [8] — gave additional evidence for the disseminated nature of the disease, while reports on idiopathic thrombotic thrombocytopenic purpura [9], endocarditis [10], and changes in renal histology [11], culminating in the classic study by Klemperer, Pollack, and Baehr on the pathomorphology of SLE in different organs [12], illustrated its puzzling variety of clinical manifestations.

Many hypotheses have been put forward about the etiology of SLE. At first regarded as cancer, it was later believed to represent some form of tuberculosis. The latter hypothesis being disproven by Keil in 1933 [13], various other microorganisms including streptococci [14] mycoplasms, and viruses [15] were implicated in the pathogenesis of the disorder. Based on morphological findings of degenerative alterations of collagen, Klemperer et al. put forward the hypothesis of SLE's being a disorder of the connective tissue [16]. This assumption gave rise to a category of diseases today referred to — misleading as it may be — as (dys-)collagenoses or, rather, connective tissue disorders. Hyperreactivity and allergy to environmental agents and drugs (e.g., penicillin [17]) have also emerged in the discussion on the etiology of SLE, with an observation by Dustan et al. reporting an SLE-like syndrome after exposure to hydralazine [18].

All of these hypotheses vanished, however, in face of the overwhelming evidence of SLE's being an autoimmune disorder. The beginning of these observations can be traced back as far as 1910, when Hauck reported a high incidence of false-positive results in the Wassermann reagin test in lupus patients [19]. Although recognized fairly early, it took 70 years of scientific efforts before the underlying mechanism was clarified by the pioneering an elegant studies of Robert S. Schwartz and his group in Boston [20]. An essential step in the direction of a modern interpretation of SLE was made by Hargraves, who described the "LE cell phenomenon" in 1948 [21]. This was followed by the introduction of the LE cell test by Haserick et al. in 1949 [22]. After Miescher et al. in 1953 had identified the factor responsible for the destruction of white blood cells as an antinuclear antibody [23], further studies by Friou et al. [24] and Holborow et al. [25] demonstrated the affinity of this antibody for cell nuclei. Finally, Holman et al. presented evidence that the LE cell factor was an antibody reacting with deoxyribonucleic acid [26]. These reports led to the clinical use of antinuclear antibody (ANA) assays in routine diagnostic measures in the late 1950s. Over the course of time, the sensitivity and specificity of the immunofluorescence tests for ANA were improved by the use of different substrates [25, 27], and more sophisticated assays for the detection of antibodies against single-stranded and double-stranded DNA became available [28, 29]. Final achievements in this field were initiated by Tan and Kunkel, who described the occurrence of antibodies directed against an acidic nuclear glycoprotein referred to as Sm antigen [30], followed by the discovery of a vast number of antibodies specific for nuclear and ribosomal antigens (reviewed in [31]). These observations coincided in time with Burnet's hypotheses on autoimmunity and the body's ability to discriminate between self and non-self [32, 33] which still intrigue us today.

The scientific community studying SLE soon started to understand the devastating effect of autoantibodies, resulting in the emergence of circulating immune complexes leading to tissue damage mainly of the kidneys and their structures [34], with hypocomplementemia as indirect evidence of immune complex formation having been described as early as 1953 [35]. Springing from these insights, therapeutic strategies were developed to decrease or suppress autoantibody and immune complex formation. With the introduction of glucocorticoids [36], and Dameshek and Schwartz's visionary proposition made as early as 1960, of using antimetabolites for the treatment of SLE [37], the initial foundations of modern treatment were laid. Thus, the history of the description of SLE — long as it might have taken — and the incipient understanding of its underlying disorders at which we have arrived today, stands as an excellent example of how constant research on an immune-mediated disorder starts with simple clinical observations, leads to the description of serological (epi)phenomena, results in mainly effective treatment and, finally — through the use of modern technology — may now be approaching a resolution of the etiology of the disease. Many of the recent insights leading to this conclusion are presented in this book.

References

1. Hebra F (1845) Versuch einer auf pathologischer Anatomie gegründeten Einteilung der Hautkrankheiten. K.k. Gesellschaft der Ärzte in Wien 1:43—52
2. Cazanave PL, Chausit M (1851) Annales des maladies de la peau et de la syphilis, conference du 4 Juin 1851, Paris. 3:297—299
3. Holubar K (1980) Terminology and iconography of lupus erythematosus. Am J Dermatopathol. 2:239—242
4. Hebra F (1846) Bericht über die Leistungen in der Dermatologie. In: Constatt, Eisenmann (eds) Jahresbericht über die Fortschritte der gesamten Medizin, 1845. Enke, Erlangen
5. Kaposi M (1872) Neue Beiträge zur Kenntnis des Lupus erythematosus. Arch Dermatol and Syphilol 4:36—78
6. Jadassohn J (1940) Handbuch der Hautkrankheiten. Mraeck, Berlin
7. Osler W (1900) The visceral lesions of the erythema group of diseases. Br J Dermatol 12:227—245
8. Talbott J (1974) Historical background of discoid and systemic lupus erythematosus. In: Duboid EL (ed) Lupus erythematosus, 2nd ed. University of Southern California Press, Los Angeles
9. Gitlow S, Goldmark C (1939) Generalized capillary and arteriolar thrombosis: report of two cases with a discussion of the literature. Ann Intern Med 13:1046—1067
10. Libman E, Sacks B (1924) A hitherto undescribed form of valvular and mural endocarditis. Arch Intern Med 33:701—737
11. Keith N, Rowntree L (1922) Study of renal complications of disseminated SLE: a report of 4 cases. Trans Assoc Am Physicians 37:487—502
12. Klemperer P, Pollack A, Baehr G (1941) Pathology of disseminated lupus erythematosus. Arch Pathol Lab Med 32:569—631
13. Keil F (1933) Relationship between lupus erythematosus and tuberculosis: critical review based on observations at necropsy. Arch Dermatol 28:765—779
14. Welsh A (1948) Specificity of streptococci isolated from patients with skin diseases: III. Lupus erythematodes. J Invest Dermatol 10:305—326
15. Yoshiki T, Mellors RC, Strand M, August JT (1974) The viral envelope glycoprotein of murine leukemia virus and the pathogenesis of immune-complex glomerulonephritis of New Zealand mice. J Exp Med 140:1011—1027
16. Klemperer P, Pollack A, Baehr G (1942) Diffuse collagen disease: acute disseminated lupus erythematosus and diffuse scleroderma. JAMA 119:331—332
17. Walsh J, Zimmermann G (1953) Demonstration of the LE phenomenon in patients with penicillin hypersensitivity. Blood 8:65—71
18. Dustan H, Taylor R, Corcoran A, Page I (1954) A rheumatic and febrile syndrome during prolonged hydralazine treatment. JAMA 154:23—29
19. Hauck L (1910) The positive reaction of the Wassermann-Neisser-Bruck-Test in acute lupus erythematosus. Münchner Medizinische Wochenschrift 57:17—31
20. Schwartz RS, Stollar BD (1985) Origins of anti-DNA autoantibodies. J Clin Invest 75:321—327
21. Hargraves M, Richmond H, Morton R (1948) Presentation of two bone-marrow elements: "Tart cell" and L.E. cell. Proceedings of the Staff Meetings of the Mayo Clinic 23:25—28
22. Haserick J, Bortz D (1949) A new diagnostic test for acute disseminated lupus erythematosus. Cleve Clin Q 16:158—161
23. Miescher P, Fauconet M, Berand T (1953) Immune-nucleo-phagocytose experimentale et phenomene L.E. Experimental Medicine and Surgery 11:173—179
24. Friou G (1957) Communication to the 9th International Congress of Rheumatic Diseases, Toronto, Ont.
25. Holborow E, Weir D, Johnson G (1957) A serum factor in L.E. with affinity for tissue nuclei. Br Med J 1:732—734
26. Holman H, Deicher H, Kunkel H (1959) The LE cell and LE serum factor. Bull NY Acad Med 35:409—418

27. Clevemaet J, Nakamura R (1972) Indirect immune fluorescence ANA tests: comparison of sensitivity and specificity of different substrates. Am J Clin Pathol 58:383—393
28. Aarden L, deGroot E, Feltkamp T (1975) Immunology of DNA: Crithidia luciliae. Ann NY Acad Sci 254:505—515
29. Pincus T, Schur P, Rose J, Decker J, Talal N (1969) Measurement of serum DNA binding activity in SLE. N Engl J Med 281:701—705
30. Tan E, Kunkel H (1966) Characteristics of a soluble nuclear antigen precipitating with sera of patients with SLE. J Immunol 96:464—471
31. Reichlin M (1981) Current perspectives on serological reactions in SLE patients. Clin Exp Immunol 44:1—10
32. Burnet F (1959) Autoimmune disease: II. Pathology of the immune response. Br Med J 2:720—725
33. Mackay I, Burnet F (1963) Autoimmune diseases. Thomas, Springfield
34. Koffler D, Schur P, Kunkel H (1967) Immunochemical studies on the nephritis of lupus erythematosus. J Exp Med 126:607—619
35. Elliott V, Mathieson D (1953) Complement in disseminated lupus erythematosus. Archives of Dermatology and Syphilology 68:119—128
36. Hench P, Kendall E, Stocumb C, Polley M (1949) Effect of the hormone of adrenal cortex (Compound E) and of pituitary adrenocorticotropic hormone on rheumatoid arthritis. Proceedings of the Staff Meetings of Mayo Clinic 24:181—197
37. Dameshek W, Schwartz RS (1960) Treatment of certain autoimmune diseases with antimetabolites. A preliminary report. Trans Assoc Am Phys 73:113—127

Etiologic and Pathogenetic Aspects of Systemic Lupus Erythematosus: A Critical Approach

W. Graninger, C. C. Zielinski, and J. S. Smolen

It is the fate of review articles and books that their conclusions run the risk of being outdated within a short period after (and sometimes even at the time of) their publication. They do, however, have the advantage that one can dare to raise slightly more critical, speculative, and philosophical views than would be advisable in an original, data-describing scientific paper. Thus, in the following pages, rather than review old and new data on the etiology and pathogenesis of human SLE, it will be our aim to point out the very few highlights of human lupus research, to discuss its conflicting matters, and to speculate on how we might be able to understand the disease better in the future.

The Role of Immune Complexes in SLE

The demonstration of tissue deposition of immunoglobulin and complement components [1, 2] has made possible the resolution of the final pathogenetic steps in SLE. The antibodies may belong to different immunoglobulin classes, and some have been characterized as directed against DNA or other nuclear proteins ([3—5] and pages 88ff. and 105ff.); moreover, their respective antigens can also be detected in the tissue [6—8]. Finally, immune complexes (ICs) may circulate in large quantities [9—11], consist partly of DNA/anti-DNA complexes [12], and may cause hypocomplementemia, characteristically associated with flares of the disease [13]. Further details on immune complex-mediated tissue injury can be obtained from a number of excellent reviews [14—16].

Formation of immune complexes per se is generally neither abnormal nor pathogenic, as every individual is probably constantly coping with immune complex production. Thus, the pathogenicity of ICs in SLE must be based on one or more of the following factors: (a) general overproduction of ICs; (b) production of large amounts of very pathogenic ICs; (c) increased tissue localization of pathogenic ICs; (d) deficient elimination of ICs. In support of these assumptions, we have learned in recent years that (a) large amounts of partly unidentified ICs circulate in SLE patients, especially in the course of flares [9—11]; (b) deposited ICs may be especially pathogenic (immunoglobulin class, IC avidity) [17—23]; (c) certain agents — especially DNA — tend to bind to the glomerular basement membrane, ready to be "attacked" by specific circulating antibodies [24, 25]; moreover, certain tissues contain receptors for complement and may thus "attract" ICs with or without accessible antigenic epitopes [26 a and b]; and (d) clearance of circulating ICs, be it via the reticuloendothelial system [27] or via C3b receptors of erythrocytes [28], may be severely deficient in SLE [29, 30].

The vast, complex actuality behind these simplified notions includes the genetic determination of qualitative and quantitative antigen reactivity [31—35], the finite but nevertheless immense number of autoantibody specificities (see below and pages 88ff. and 105ff.), the possible (but not undisputed) genetic transmission of IC-clearance defects [36—41], and the probability that in any individual patient several of these factors may coincide.

Autoantibodies

As has been mentioned, a large fraction of circulating and tissue-deposited immune complexes in SLE consists of complexes composed of antibodies directed against autoantigens and their antigenic counterpart. Moreover, the description of a vast number of autoantibodies has permitted the understanding of the occurrence of several clinical features, e.g., the cytopenias, clotting defects, etc. The mechanisms involved in target cell/tissue destruction can be complement-mediated, they can be due to trapping by the spleen, and, finally, they can even be cell-mediated [42]. The diversity of these autoantibodies appeared to be unlimited for several decades, although there were occasional reports of cross-reactivity of such autoantibodies [43—46], and it was not until recently that the restriction of this diversity was recognized, and the heterogeneity of the occurring autoantibodies explained by the identity of antigenic epitopes on different substrates (see pages 88ff.).

The genes coding for the variable region of such autoantibodies do not appear to differ generally from genes coding for "normal" immunoglobulins [47]. However, there may still be some genetic abnormalitity in the very fine specificity e.g., of the hypervariable region, since there is evidence for cross-reactivity of idiotypes of anti-DNA antibodies between individual SLE patients as well as for cross-reactivity between idiotypes of anti-DNA antibodies from lupus patients and idiotypes of non-DNA antibodies from their relatives [48—50].

The occurrence of autoantibodies does not per se represent a pathologic event: normal B cells produce autoantibodies in vitro [51, 52], and autoantibodies may occur in patients with a variety of nonautoimmune disorders as well as in healthy individuals [53—56]. Nevertheless, the concept of "healthy autoantibody carriers" is somewhat shaky and appears to be dependent upon the type of autoantibody: thus, healthy anti-Ro positive women may give birth to children with severe congenital cardiac conduction defects [53], and up to 85% of apparently healthy individuals with antibodies to ds-DNA develop SLE within few years [56]. The reason for this delayed onset of the disease is unclear, but it may be related to a gradual increase in pathogenic autoantibody clonotypes as described in lupus mice [57].

The work cited thus far indicates that over the past decades we have learned quite a lot about the vast extent and the limitation of SLE autoantibody specificities, and that investigations into the molecular biology of these autoantibodies have begun. We still do not understand completely the features that make an autoantibody more or less pathogenic, and, in particular, we still do not understand which mechanisms trigger autoantibody production. In this latter respect there are at least three candidate models: (a) autoantibody production is triggered by "liberated" DNA which by itself is not highly immunogenic [60b]); (b) autoantibody production is the consequence of idiotypic cross-reactivity of antibodies directed against environmental antigens with autoantigens via use of particular immunoglobulin variable regions present in susceptible individuals ([48, 61] and this volume, pages 60ff., 88ff.); (c) autoantibodies represent the side effect of a network of interactions between idiotypes, anti-idiotypes, and normal cellular components in the context of environmental insults (such as infections) ([62a and b] and this volume, pages 60ff., 88ff.).

Genetic Susceptibility

Before going on with the discussion of immunologic abnormalities, we would like to allude briefly to the matter of "genetic susceptibility" in the autoimmunologic labyrinth of SLE. Obviously, not every human will (or can) develop SLE, just as not every mouse strain is lupus-prone. However, SLE has not been determined a disorder in which we can precisely define the genetic anomaly: numerous studies in human as well as murine lupus have failed to find "the autoimmunity gene"; rather, there are indications for a polygenic basis of the disorder ([63—65] and this volume, pages 22ff., 60ff. and 74ff.). Moreover, different clinical features might be the consequence of differences in genetic background, and disease severity might be enhanced by genes from innocent, i.e., healthy partners ([65—67] and this volume, pages 60ff.).

Although the majority of such genetic associations have been studied in inbred animals, investigations in human SLE have revealed two types of associations: one is familial SLE, which does not appear to be major histocompatibility complex (MHC-) linked, and the other is "spontaneous" SLE, which appears to be linked to genes coding for HLA-DR2 and DR3 [68—73]. This linkage of a nonorgan-specific, polyautoimmune disorder with the MHC has led to some confusion; however, recent evidence suggests that the genes coding for HLA-DR antigens are not associated with the disease itself, but rather with the expression of particular autoantibodies characteristic for the disease [74—76]. Thus, one would speculate that multiple non-MHC genes are responsible for disease susceptibility and that some characteristics of the autoantibody response are under the influence of the MHC, a notion consistent with observations in lupus-prone mice [66] as well as with observations in familial SLE. It is these complex genetic interactions which we mean in the first place when speaking of "genetic susceptibility".

The complexity is increased by the recent detection of an MHC association of genes (class 3 MHC genes on human chromosome 6 or mouse chromosome 17) coding for several complement components (C2, C4, and factor B; in mice also for C3, and C3b receptor, CR1) [77]. In fact, initial studies of class 3 MHC genes have revealed some associations of SLE with C4 genes [78]. Bearing in mind that (a) SLE is a disorder in which complement is consumed, (b) several inherited complement deficiencies are associated with the occurrence of SLE-like disorders (see pages 124ff.), and (c) SLE patients as well as patients with C2 deficiency have a high frequency of HLA-DR2 [79], one can see links between HLA-B, HLA-DR, and complement genes, suggesting that they have a major influence upon the etiology of SLE.

Finally, it should be mentioned that at least one enzyme important for proper steroid hormone synthesis is also encoded by genes linked to the MHC [80]; whether or not this finding is related to potential endocrine abnormalities in SLE (see below) is as yet unknown.

Endocrine Factors

One of the most puzzling aspects of SLE, namely its predominance in females, has been elucidated over the past decade by the demonstration that the manifestation of SLE is sex hormone-mediated to a large extent: usually, estrogens enhance and androgens retard the disease [81, 82]. In addition, abnormalities of estrogen metabolism have been described in SLE patients [83, 84]. Moreover, there is a predisposition of patients with Klinefelter's syndrome to develop SLE [85]. Nevertheless, there are exceptions to the rule: one mouse strain (BXSB) has a male preponderance; furthermore, SLE may occur in otherwise "normal" men sporadically and familially. Further details on this subject are discussed on pages 74ff. and 347ff., and are reviewed in [87—89].

B Cell Hyperactivity

"The enhanced autoantibody production in SLE is the consequence of B cell hyperactivity." Superficial as this statement may be, it is the reduction of the complex pathogenetic riddle of the disease to its real kernel. The most important question in our struggles to understand the pathogenesis of SLE regards the mechanisms responsible for this B cell hyperactivity. Is it an inherited abnormality? Is it due to the loss of some intracellular regulatory mechanism? Is it due to polyclonal B cell stimulation (which even in normal subjects can induce autoantibody production) [90, 91]? Is it a consequence of abnormal immune regulation (and if so, of what type)? How is it triggered? How perpetuated? And how many different pathways to B cell hyperactivity may there be?

B cell hyperactivity is not only reflected by hypergammaglobulinemia and circulation of autoantibodies; it can also be demonstrated in vitro via increased spontaneous secretion of immunoglobulins [92—94]; this indicates that in an ex vivo situation the cells are already activated. On the other hand, SLE B cells respond normally (i.e., neither in an enhanced nor a diminished fashion) to polyclonal activators, such as Epstein-Barr virus [95]. Stimulation with the T cell-dependent pokeweed mitogen leads to reduced in vitro B cell immunoglobulin secretion [96—98], which may in part be due to a regulatory T cell abnormality [97] and partly unrelated to regulatory abnormalities [98]. Thus the issue of B cell hyperactivity is complex and unresolved even when it comes to its in vitro analysis, and is further complicated by the potential influence of soluble regulatory products (see pages 145ff.). Interestingly, at least in mice, a particular B cell subset, the Lyb 5 subset, is responsible for spontaneous synthesis of the vast majority of autoantibodies [64, 99, 100]. In fact, lupus-prone mice which bear a gene associated with the lack of this B cell subset have only minimal autoantibody production and do not develop SLE [64, 100, 101].

Abnormal Immunoregulation

With the recognition of interaction between different cell types of the immune system and the understanding of the concept of immunoregulation [102—104], SLE has become a major target disease for analyses of immunoregulatory abnormalities. In the late 1970s, the main pathogenic step in human SLE appeared resolved, since many of its features, especially B cell hyperactivity, could be explained by the finding of a defective suppressor cell system [105—107]. This concept was further substantiated by demonstration of anti-suppressor cell antibodies [109—111] and initial findings of numerical deficiencies of T cells with a suppressor phenotype [105—108, 112]. But it soon became clear that the postulated defect could not be upheld against additional evidence. First, different suppressor cell assays revealed discrepant results in the same individual [113]; second, the same type of suppressor cell analysis revealed discrepant results in different study populations (e.g., [107] as against [114]); third, in some test systems excessive suppression was even observed [97]; fourth, helper T cell abnormalities were also described, which included deficient helper cell activity [114, 115]; fifth, autoantibodies against helper T cells were detected [116, 117]; sixth, the T cell phenotype in SLE was revealed to be quite heterogeneous [118—120]; and seventh, no global suppressor cell abnormalities were found in lupus-prone mice [121, 122]. Finally, with the description of defective feedback inhibition and deficient contrasuppression in autoimmune mice [123—125], and the demonstration of a deficient autologous mixed lymphocyte reaction (AMLR) and lymphokine abnormalities in both human and murine SLE ([126—130] and this volume, pages 145ff.), the issue has become only more confusing. Even approaching the issue with purified T cell subpopulations, although helpful for understanding additional new aspects, has not led to elucidation of major pathogenetic pathways [131, 132].

Human lupus research suffers from several major limitations: (a) Whereas conclusions obtained from experimental animals have been mainly drawn from in vivo manipulations, such as cell transfer or breeding experiments, we rely almost exclusively upon in vitro tests in analyses of human SLE; (b) in vitro test systems do not necessarily reflect what is going on in vivo; and (c) murine lupus research has always differentiated between the various affected mouse strains individually, but human lupus reasearch has generally regarded individual patients as well as groups of patients with SLE as unconditionally comparable.

Thus the question arises which mechanisms "really" lead to B cell hyperactivity in SLE. The simple answer appears to be that there is no single truth, since (a) several immunoregulatory abnormalities may be operative in the development of human SLE, just as the cellular bases of murine SLE differ between different strains; (b) SLE as defined by its serologic and clinical abnormalities is tremendously heterogeneous, a notion that appears compatible with different pathogenetic fine specificities (see pages 74ff., 170ff. and 290ff.); and (c) it is currently extremely difficult to differentiate between primary and secondary abnormalities, since several immunoregulatory anomalies may be the consequence of the occurrence of certain autoantibodies [116, 117, 133—135] and may theoretically even coincide in time. First attempts to cope with this problem have been made in lupus-prone animals by sequentially analysing genetic abnormalities on a molecular basis and cell population disturbances on a phenotypic and functional basis (see pages 22ff. and 290ff.).

Some of the findings mentioned deserve special attention. It has already been stated that — despite in vivo and spontaneous in vitro B cell hyperactivity — mitogenic stimulation of lupus B cells gives abnormally deficient responses, which may be partly due to regulatory aberrations [97], but could also be associated with B cell exhaustion [94, 96, 98]. Similarly, the Interleukin 2 (IL2) deficiency in SLE (see pages 145ff.) might be also at least partly due to increased suppressor cell activity of SLE T cells [136]; but refractoriness to secrete sufficient amounts of IL2 upon appropriate stimulation could, again, be related to some in vivo preexhaustion in the context of a hyperactivated immune system. Similar mechanisms have been implicated for the deficient in vitro response of SLE lymphocytes to secrete gamma-Interferon (see pages 145ff.). Finally, the deficient AMLR responses in active SLE patients could also be explained by in vivo exhaustion; SLE patients have a large number of Ia-positive T cells in their circulation [133, 137], indicating T cell activation; it is conceivable that the activated SLE B cells might trigger T cell activation [138] in vivo, like an in vivo AMLR; the preactivated T cells could then be refractory to their physiologic stimuli in vitro or, alternatively, a T-T-AMLR might occur, which has been shown to preferentially induce suppressor T cells [139]. Thus several different abnormalities of immunoregulation, on both the cellular level and that of soluble mediators of immunoregulation, could be explained via one mechanism: preactivation of T cells with the emergence of (specific?) suppressor T cells and deficiency of subsequent immune responses in in vitro assays.

Environmental Insults

It has been postulated that SLE may be initiated and that flares are often precipitated by infections, sun exposure, operations, and pregnancy [140—142]. In addition, several drugs have been implicated in causing SLE, while other drugs may induce the so-called drug-induced lupus syndrome [143]. Taken together, the reported evidence indicates that environmental influences may be important in the pathogenesis of SLE. The mechanisms could operate by directly initiating production of (auto)antibodies and subsequent (cross-)reactivity, as discussed above; alternatively, the hypothesis of the induction of some type of chronic "graft versus host disease," which under certain circumstances can lead to autoantibody production and an SLE-like disease [144, 145], is very challenging. Although, among other environmental insults, viral infections may trigger SLE, the disease does not appear to be viral in origin ([146, 147] and this volume, pages 60 ff.), although this is still a matter of controversy [148, 149].

SLE Does Not Constitute a Disease Entity — Does It Constitute an Etiologic Entity?

The issues discussed above indicate that we are far from approaching the "bellevue-point" of understanding SLE. This is partly due to the intrinsic heterogeneity of SLE (see Chap. 17), partly due to the insufficiency of in vitro techniques in analysis of in vivo anomalies, and may, finally, be partly due to misleading approaches. Whether we look at SLE as a spectrum of disorders manifested by various clinical courses or as the disease of a single individual, we must acknowledge that it is induced by a variety of cooperating mechanisms, genetic, environmental, and immunologic. With repeated, severe environmental insults, SLE might occur even where susceptibility is low. On the other hand, relatively little might be necessary to trigger the disease when genes coding for susceptibility are present. The immune response will be further modified by its own products, and finally by our therapeutic interventions. With the rapid advance of molecular biologic techniques we will hopefully soon be able to discover the meaning of "susceptibility" to SLE, the effects of being "environmentally insulted"; to discover whether autoantibodies may modify immune responses, and if so, how, and what approaches can be chosen for appropriate lupus therapy.

References

1. Mellors RC, Ortega LG, Holman HR (1957) Role of gamma-globulins in the pathogenesis of renal lesions in systemic lupus erythematosus and chronic membraneous glomerulonephritis, with an observation on lupus erythematosus cell reaction. J Exp Med 106:191—203
2. Paronetto F, Koffler D (1965) Immunofluorescent localization of immunoglobulins, complement and fibrinogen in human diseases: I. Systemic lupus erythematosus. J Clin Invest 44:1657—1664
3. Lewis EJ, Busch GJ, Schur PH (1970) Gamma G globulin subgroup composition of the glomerular deposits in renal diseases. J Clin Invest 49:1103—1113
4. Krishnan C, Kaplan MH (1967) Immunopathologic studies of systemic lupus erythematosus: II. Antinuclear reaction of gamma-globulin eluted from homogenates and isolated glomeruli of kidneys from patients with lupus nephritis. J Clin Invest 46:569—579
5. Andres GA, Accinni L, Beiser SMN, Christian CL, Cinotti GA, Erlanger BF, Hsu KC, Segal BC (1970) Localization of fluorescein labelled antinucleotide antibodies in glomeruli of patients with active systemic lupus erythematosus and nephritis. J Clin Invest 49:2106—2118
6. Koffler D, Agnello V, Kunkel HG (1974) Polynucleotide immune complexes in serum and glomeruli of patients with systemic lupus erythematosus. Am J Pathol 74:109—122
7. Maddison PJ, Reichlin M (1979) Deposition of antibodies to a soluble cytoplasmic antigen in the kidneys of patients with systemic lupus erythematosus. Arthritis Rheum 22:858—863
8. Yoshiki T, Mellors RC, Strand M, August JT (1974) The viral envelope glycoprotein of murine leukemia virus and the pathogenesis of immune-complex glomerulonephritis of New Zealand mice. J Exp Med 140:1011—1027
9. Agnello V, Koffler D, Eisenberg JW, Winchester RJ, Kunkel HG (1971) C1q precipitins in the sera of patients with systemic lupus erythematosus and other hypocomplementemic states: characterization of high and low molecular weight types. J Exp Med 134:228s—241s
10. Lambert PH et al (1978) A WHO collaborative study of the evaluation of eighteen methods for detecting immune complexes in serum. J Clin Lab Immunol 1:1—16
11. Menzel EJ, Smolen JS, Knapp W, Scherak O, Steffen C (1979) Klinische Relevanz zirkulierender Immunkomplexe bei Patienten mit systemischem Lupus erythematodes und chronischer Polyarthritis. Acta Med Austriaca 6:212—214
12. Bruneau C, Benveniste J (1979) Circulating DNA: anti-DNA complexes in systemic lupus erythematosus. J Clin Invest 64:191—198
13. Schur PH, Sandson J (1968) Immunologic factors and clinical activity in systemic lupus erythematosus. N Engl J Med 278:533—538
14. Johnson KJ, Ward PA (1982) Biology of disease: newer concepts in the pathogenesis of immune-complex-induced tissue injury. Lab Invest 17:218—226
15. Koffler D, Agnello V, Kunkel HG (1974) Polynucleotide inmune complexes in serum and glomeruli of patients with systemic lupus erythematosus. Am J Pathol 74:109—124
16. Barnett EV (1979) Circulating immune conplexes: their immunochemistry, detection and importance. Ann Intern Med 91:430—440
17. Leon SA, Green A, Ehrlich GC, Poland M, Shapiro B (1977) Avidity of antibodies in SLE: relationship of severity of renal involvement. Arthritis Rheum 20:23—29
18. Gershwin ME, Steinberg AD (1975) Qualitative characteristics of anti-DNA antibodies in lupus nephritis. Arthritis Rheum 17:947—954
19. Clough JD, Valenzuela R (1980) Relationship of renal histopathology in SLE nephritis to immunoglobulin class of anti-DNA. Am J Med 68:80—85
20. Winfield JB, Faiferman I, Koffler D (1977 Avidity of anti-DNA antibodies in serum and IgG glomerular eluates from patients with systemic lupus erythematosus: association of high avidity anti-native DNA antibody with glomerulonephritis. J Clin Invest 59:90—96

21. Cochrane CG, Hawkins DJ (1968) Studies on circulating immune complexes: III. Factors governing the circulating complexes to localize in blood vessels. J Exp Med 127:137—146

22. Soothill JF, Steward MW (1971) The immunopathologic significance of the heterogeneity of antibody affinity. Clin Exp Immunol 9:193—202

23. Eblin F, Hahn BH (1980) Restricted subpopulations of DNA antibodies in kidneys of mice with systemic lupus: comparison of antibodies in serum and renal eluates. Arthritis Rheum 23:392—403

24. Izui S, Lambert PH, Miescher PA (1976) In vitro demonstration of a particular affinity of glomerular basement membrane and collagen for DNA: a possible basis for a local formation of DNA-anti-DNA complexes in systemic lupus erythematosus. J Exp Med 144:428—436

25. Izui S, Lambert PH, Fournie GJ, Turler H, Miescher PA (1977) Features of systemic lupus erythematosus in mice injected with bacterial lipopolysaccharides: identification of circulating DNA and renal localization of DNA-anti-DNA complexes. J Exp Med 145:1115—1130

26a. Gelfand MC, Frank MM, Green I (1975) A receptor for the third component of complement in the human renal glomerulus. J Exp Med 142:1029—1034

26b. Kazatchkine MD, Fearon DT, Appay MD, Mandet C, Bariety J (1982) Immunohistochemical study of the human glomerular C3b receptor in normal kidney and in seventy-five cases of renal diseases. J Clin Invest 69:900—912

27. Finbloom DS, Plotz PH (1977) Studies of reticuloendothelial function in the mouse with model immune complexes: II. Serum clearance, tissue uptake and reticuloendothelial saturation in NZB/W mice. J Immunol 123:1600—1603

28. Siegel I, Liu TL, Gleicher N (1981) The red cell immune system. Lancet 2:556—558

29. Frank MM, Hamburger MI, Lawley TJ, Kimberly RP, Plotz PH (1979) Defective reticuloendothelial system Fc receptor function in systemic lupus erythemaosus. N Engl J Med 300:518—523

30. Iida K, Mornaghi R, Nussenzweig V (1982) Complement receptor (CR1) deficiency in erythrocytes from patients with systemic lupus erythematosus. J Exp Med 155:1427—1438

31. Dixon FJ, Feldman JD, Vazquez JJ (1961) Experimental glomerulonephritis: the pathogenesis of a laboratory model resembling the spectrum of glomerulonephritis. J Exp Med 113:899—920

32. Kappler JW, Marrack P (1978) The role of H-2 linked genes in helper T cell function: IV. Importance of T-cell genotype and host environment in I-region and Ir gene expression. J Exp Med 148:1510—1522

33. Singer A, Hathcock KS, Hodes RJ (1979) Cellular and genetic control of antibody responses: V. Helper T-cell recognition of H-2 determinants on accessory but not B cells. J Exp Med 149:1208—1226

34. Soothill JF, Steward MW (1971) The immunopathological significance of the heterogeneity of antibody affinity. Clin Exp Immunol 9:193—202

35. Germain RN, Benacerraf B (1981) A single major pathway of T-lymphocyte interactions in antigen-specific immune suppression. Scand J Immunol 13:1—10

36. Lawley TJ, Hall RP, Fauci AS, Katz SI, Hamburger MI, Frank MM (1981) Defective Fc receptor functions associated with the HLA B8 DR3 haplotype. N Engl J Med 304:185—192

37. Williams BD, O'Sullivan MM, Ratanachaiyavong S (1985) Reticuloendothelial Fc function in normal individuals and its relationship to the HLA antigen DR3. Clin exp Immunol 60:532—538

38. Miyakawa Y, Yamada A, Kosaka K, Tsuda F, Kosugi E, Mayumi M (1981) Defective immune adherence (C3b) receptors on erythrocytes from patients with systemic lupus erythematosus. Lancet 2:493

39. Wilson JG, Wong WW, Schur PH, Fearon DT (1982) Mode of inheritance of decreased C3b receptors on erythrocytes of patients with systemic lupus erythematosus. N Engl J Med 307:981

40. Wilson JG, Fearon DT (1984) Altered expression of complement receptors as a pathogenetic factor in systemic lupus erythematosus. Arthritis Rheum 27:1321—1328

41. Walport MJ, Ross DG, Mackworth-Young C, Watson JV, Hogg N, Lachmann PJ (1985) Family studies of erythrocyte complement receptor type 1 levels: reduced levels in patients with SLE are acquired, not inherited. Clin Exp Immunol 59:547—554
42. Steinberg AD, Smolen JS, Sakane T, Kumagai S, Morimoto C, Chused TM, Green I, Hirata F, Siminovitch KA, Steinberg RT (1982) Immune regulatory abnormalities in systemic lupus erythematosus. In: Cummings, Michael, Wilson, (eds) Immune mechanisms in renal disease. Plenum, New York, pp 529—548
43. Rekvig OP, Hannestad K (1979) Certain polyclonal antinuclear antibodies crossreact with the surface membrane of human lymphocytes and granulocytes. Scand J Immunol 6:1042—1049
44. Searles RP, Messner RP, Bankhurst AD (1979) Cross reactivity of antilymphocyte and antinuclear antibodies in systemic lupus erythematosus. Clin Immunol Immunopathol 14:292—299
45. Hannestad K, Stollar BD (1978) Certain rheumatoid factors react with nucleosomes. Nature 275:671—673
46. Rekvig OP, Hannestad K (1980) Human autoantibodies that react with both cell nuclei and plasma membranes display specificity for the octamer of histones H2A, H2B, H3, and H4 in high salt. J Exp Med 152:1720—1733
47. Kofler R, Perlmutter RM, Noonan DJ, Dixon FJ, Theofilopoulos AN (1985) Ig heavy chain variable region gene complex of lupus mice exhibits normal restriction fragment length polymorphism. J Exp Med 162:346—351
48. Halpern R, Schiffenbauer J, Solomon G, Diamond B (1984) Detection of masked anti-DNA antibodies in lupus sera by a monoclonal anti-idiotype. J Immunol 133:1852—1856
49. Isenberg DA, Shoenfeld Y, Madaio MP, Rauch J, Reichlin M, Stollar BD, Schwartz RS (1984) Anti-DNA antibody idiotypes in systemic lupus erythematosus. Lancet 2:417—422
50. Jacob L, Lety MA, Louvard D, Bach JF (1985) Binding of a monoclonal anti-DNA autoantibody to identical protein(s) present at the surface of several human cell types involved in lupus pathogenesis. J Clin Invest 75:315—317
51. Koopman WJ, Schrohenloher RE (1980) In vitro synthesis of IgM rheumatoid factor by lymphocytes from healthy adults. J Immunol 125:934—939
52. Cairns E, Block J, Bell DA (1984) Anti-DNA autoantibody producing hybridomas of normal human lymphoid cell origin. J Clin Invest 74:880—887
53. Harley JB, Kaine JL, Fox OF, Reichlin M, Gruber B (1985) Ro/SSA antibody and antigen in congenital complete heart block. Arthritis Rheum 28:1321—1325
54. Maddison PJ, Skinner RP, Vlachoyiannopoulos P, Brennand DM, Hough D (1985) Antibodies to nRNP, Sm, Ro (SSA) and La (SSB) detected by ELISA: their specificity and inter-relations in connective tissue disease. Clin Exp Immunol 62:337—345
55. Seelig HP (1983) Antikörper gegen Zellkernantigene. Fischer, Stuttgart, pp 43 and 60
56. Swaak T, Smeenk R (1985) Detection of anti-dsDNA as a diagnostic tool: a prospective study in 441 non-systemic lupus erythematosus patients with anti-dsDNA antibody (anti-dsDNA). Ann Rheum Dis 44:245—251
57. Yoshida H, Yoshida M, Izui S, Lambert PH (1985) Distinct clonotypes of anti-DNA antibodies in mice with lupus nephritis. J Clin Invest 76:685—694
58. Sano H, Morimoto C (1982) DNA isolated from DNA/anti-DNA antibody immune complexes in systemic lupus erythematosus is rich in guanine-cytosine content. J Immunol 128:1341—1345
59. Steinman CR (1984) Circulating DNA in systemic lupus erythematosus: isolation and characterization. J Clin Invest 73:832—841
60a. Seelig HP (1983) Antikörper gegen Zellkernantigene. Fischer, Stuttgart, pp 8—11
60b. Schwartz RS, Stollar BD (1985) Origins of anti-DNA autoantibodies. J Clin Invest 75:321—327
61. Diamond B, Scharff MD (1984) Somatic mutation of the T15 heavy chain gives rise to an antibody with autoantibody specificity. Proc Natl Acad Sci USA 81:5841—5844
62a. Datta SK, Stollar BD, Schwartz RS (1983) Normal mice express idiotypes related to autoantibody idiotypes of lupus mice. Proc Natl Acad Sci USA 80:2723—2727

62b. Halpern R, Davidson A, Lazo A, Solomon G, Lahita R, Diamond B (1985) Familial systemic lupus erythematosus: presence of a cross-reactive idiotype in healthy family members. J Clin Invest 76:731—736

63. Arnett FC, Reveille JD, Wilson RW, Provost TT, Bias WB (1984) Systemic lupus erythematosus: current state of the genetic hypothesis. Semin Arthritis Rheum 14:24—35

64. Raveche ES, Novotny EA, Hansen CT, Tjio JH, Steinberg AD (1981) Genetic studies in NZB mice: V. Recombinant inbred lines demonstrate that separate genes control autoimmune phenotype. J Exp Med 153:1187—1197

65. Taurog JD, Raveche ES, Smathers PA, Glimcher LH, Huston DP, Hansen CT, Steinberg AD (1981) T cell abnormalities in NZB mice occur independently of autoantibody production. J Exp Med 153:221—234

66. Yoshida H, Kohno A, Ohta K, Hirose S, Maruyama N, Shirai T (1981) Genetic studies of autoimmunity in New Zealand mice: III. Associations among anti-DNA antibodies, NTA, and renal disease in (NZB x NZW) F1 X NZW backcross mice. J Immunol 127:433—337

67. Eastcott JW, Schwartz RS, Datta SK (1983) Genetic analysis of the inheritance of B cell hyperactivity in relation to the development of autoantibodies and glomerulonephritis in NZBxSWR crosses. J Immunol 131:2232—2239

68. Cleland LG, Bell DA, Williams M, Saurino BC (1978) Familial lupus: family studies of HLA and serologic findings. Arthritis Rheum 21:183—191

69. Reinertsen JL, Klippel JH, Johnson AH, Steinberg AD, Decker JL, Mann DL (1982) Family studies of B lymphocyte alloantigens in systemic lupus erythematosus. J Rheumatol 9:253—262

70. Reinertsen JL, Klippel JH, Johnson AH, Decker JL, Steinberg AD, Mann DL (1978) B lymphocyte alloantigens associated with systemic lupus erythematosus. N Engl J Med 299:515—518

71. Gibosky A, Winchester RJ, Patarroyo M, Kunkel HG (1978) Disease associations of the Ia-like human alloantigens: contrasting patterns in rheumatoid arthritis and systemic lupus erythematosus. J Exp Med 148:1728—1732

72. Scherak O, Smolen JS, Mayr WR (1980) HLA-DRw3 and systemic lupus erythematosus. Arthritis Rheum 23:954—957

73. Celada A, Barras C, Benzonana G, Jeannet M (1979) Increased frequency of HLA-DRw3 in systemic lupus erythematosus. N Engl J Med 301:1398 (Letter)

74. Schur PH, Meyer I, Garovoy M, Carpenter CB (1982) Associations between systemic lupus erythematosus and the major histocompatibility complex: clinical and immunological considerations. Clin Immunol Immunopathol 24:263—275

75. Smolen JS, Klippel JH, Penner E, Reichlin M, Steinberg AD, Chused TM, Zielinski CC, Scherak O, Hartter E, Wolf A, Davie R, Mann DL, Mayr WR (1986) HLA-DR antigens in specificity of autoantibody responses to nuclear antigens (submitted for publication)

76. Ahearn JM, Provost TT, Dorsch CA, Stevens MB, Bias WB, Arnett FC (1982) Interrelationships of HLA-DR. MB and MT phenotypes, autoantibody expression, and clinical features in systemic lupus erythematosus. Arthritis Rheum 25:1031—1040

77. Porter RR (1985) The complement components coded in the major histocompatibility complexes and their biological activities. Immunol Rev 87:7—17

78. Fielder AHL, Walport MJ, Batchelor JR, Rynes RI, Black CM, Dodi IA, Hughes GRV (1983) Family studies of the major histocompatibility complex in patients with systemic lupus erythematosus: importance of null alleles of C4A and C4B in determining disease susceptibility. Br Med J 286:425—428

79. Fu SM, Stern R, Kunkel HG, Dupont B, Hansen JA, Day NK, Good RA, Jersild C, Fontino M (1975) Mixed lymphocyte culture determinants and C2 deficiency: LD7a associated with C2 deficiency in four families. J Exp Med 142: 495

80. Carroll MC, Belt KT, Palsdottir A, Yu Y (1985) Molecular genetics of the fourth component of human complement and steroid 21-hydroxylase. Immunol Rev 87:39—60

81. Roubinian JR, Talal N, Greenspan JS, Goodman JR, Siiteri PK (1978) Effect of castration and sex hormone treatment on survival, anti-nucleic acid antibodies, and glomerulonephritis in NZB/NZW F1 mice. J Exp Med 147:1568—1583

82. Steinberg AD, Melez KA, Raveche ES, Reeves JP, Boegel WA, Smathers PA, Taurog JD, Weinlein L, Duvic M (1979) Approach to the study of the role of sex hormones in autoimmunity. Arthritis Rheum 22:1170—1176
83. Lahita RG, Bradlow HL, Kunkel HG, Fishman J (1981) Increased 16alpha-hydroxylation of estradiol in systemic lupus erythematosus. J Clin Endocrinol Metab 53:174—178
84. Lahita RG, Bradlow HL, Fishman J, Kunkel HG (1982) Estrogen metabolism in systemic lupus erythematosus: patients and family members. Arthritis Rheum 25:843—846
85. Stern R, Fishman J, Brudman H, Kunkel HG (1977) Systemic lupus erythematosus associated with Klinefelter's syndrome. Arthritis Rheum 20:18—22
86. Lahita RG, Chiorazzi N, Gibofsky A, Winchester RJ, Kunkel HG (1983) Familial systemic lupus erythematosus in males. Arthritis Rheum 26:39—44
87. Steinberg AD, Melez KA, Raveche ES, Reeves JP, Boegel W (1979) Approach to the study of the role of sex hormones in autoimmunity. Arthritis Rheum 22:1170—1175
88. Smolen JS, Steinberg AD (1981) Systemic lupus erythematosus and pregnancy: clinical, immunological, and theoretical aspects. In: Gleicher N (Ed) Reproductive immunology. Liss, New York pp 283—302 (Progress in biological research, vol 67)
89. Talal N (1982) Sex hormones and modulation of immune response in SLE. Clin Rheum Dis 8:23—28
90. Izui S, Lambert PH, Fournie PH, Turler H, Miescher PA (1977) Features of systemic lupus erythematosus in mice injected with bacterial lipopolysaccharides. J Exp Med 145:1115—1130
91. Smith HR, Green DR, Raveche ES, Smathers PK, Gershon RK, Steinberg AD (1982) Studies of the induction of anti-DNA in normal mice. J Immunol 129:2332—2237
92. Jasin HE, Ziff M (1975) Immunoglobulin synthesis by peripheral blood cells in systemic lupus erythematosus. Arthritis Rheum 18:218—228
93. Budman DR, Merchant EB, Steinberg AD (1977) Increased spontaneous activity of antibody forming cells in the peripheral blood of patients with active systemic lupus erythematosus. Arthritis Rheum 20:829—833
94. Nies KM, Louie JS (1978) Impaired immunoglobulin synthesis by peripheral blood cells in systemic lupus erythematosus. Arthritis Rheum 21:51—58
95. Tsokos GC, Magrath IT, Balow JE (1983) Epstein-Barr virus induces normal B-cell responses but defective suppressor T cell responses in patients with systemic lupus erythematosus. J Immunol 131:1797—1801
96. Ginsburg WW, Finkelman FD, Lipsky PE (1979) Circulating and pokeweed mitogen induced immunoglobulin-secreting cells in systemic lupus erythematosus. Clin Exp Immunol 35:76—88
97. Beale MG, Nash GS, Bertovich MJ, McDermott P (1982) Similar disturbance in B cell activity and regulatory T cell function in Henoch-Schönlein purpura and systemic lupus erythematosus. J Immunol 128:486—491
98. Saiki O, Saeki Y, Kishimoto S (1985) Spontaneous immunoglobulin A secretion and lack of mitogen-responsive B cells in systemic lupus erythematosus. J Clin Invest 76:1865—1870
99. Scher I, Steinberg AD, Berning AK, Paul WE (1975) X-linked B-lymphocyte immune defect in CBA/N mice: II. Studies of mechanisms underlying the immune defect. J Exp Med 142:637—650
100. Smathers PA, Steinberg BJ, Reeves JP, Steinberg AD (1982) Effect of polyclonal immune stimulators upon NZB.xid congenic mice. J Immunol 128:1414—1419
101. Smith HR, Chused TM, Steinberg AD (1983) The effect of the X-linked immune deficiency gene (xid) upon the Y chromosome-related disease of BXSB mice. J Immunol 131:1257—1260
102. Gershon RK (1980) Immunoregulation circa 1980. J Allergy Clin Immunol 66:18—22
103. Green DR, Flood PM, Gershon RK (1983) Immunoregulatory T cell pathways. Annual Review of Immunology 1:439
104. Dorf ME, Benacerraf B (1984) Suppressor cells and immunoregulation. Annual Review of Immunology 2:127

105. Abdou NI, Sagawa A, Pascal E, Hevert J, Sadeghee S (1976) Suppressor T cell abnormality in idiopathic systemic lupus erythematosus. Clin Immunol Immunopathol 6:192—199

106. Bresnihan B, Jasin HE (1977) Suppressor function of peripheral blood mononuclear cells in normal individuals and in patients with systemic lupus erythematosus. J Clin Invest 59:106—116

107. Sakane T, Steinberg AD, Green I (1978) Studies of immune function of patients with SLE: I. Dysfunction of suppressor T cells related to impaired generation of, rather than response to, suppressor cells. Arthritis Rheum 21:657—664

108. Tsokos GC, Balow JE (1983) Phenotypes of T lymphocytes in systemic lupus erythematosus: decreased cytotoxic/suppressor subpopulation is associated with deficient allogeneic cytotoxic responses rather than with concanavalin A-induced suppressor cells. Clin Immunol Immunopathol 26:267—275

109. Sagawa A, Abdou NI (1979) Suppressor cell antibody in systemic lupus erythematosus: possible mechanism for suppressor cell dysfunction. J Clin Invest 63:536—539

110. Sakane T, Steinberg AD, Reeves JP, Green I (1979) Studies of immune functions in systemic lupus erythematosus. Complement-dependent immunoglobulin M anti-thymus-derived cell antibodies preferentially inactivate suppressor cells. J Clin Invest 63:954—965

111. Morimoto C, Reinherz EL, Abe T, Homma M, Schlossman SF (1980) Characteristics of anti-T cell antibodies in SLE: evidence for selective reactivity with normal suppressor cells defined by monoclonal antibodies. Clin Immunol Immunopathol 16:474—484

112. Morimoto C, Reinherz EL, Schlossmann SF, Schur PH, Mills JA, Steinberg AD (1980) Alterations in immunoregulatory T cell subsets in active systemic lupus erythematosus. J Clin Invest 66:1171—1174

113. Steinberg AD, Smolen JS, Sakane T, Kumagai S, Morimoto C, Chused TM, Green I, Hirata F, Siminovitch KA, Steinberg RT (1982) Immune regulatory abnormalities in systemic lupus erythematosus. In: Cummings, Michael, Wilson (Eds) Immune mechanisms in renal disease. Lenum New York, pp 529—548

114. Delfraissy JE, Segond P, Gelanaud P, Wallon C, Massias P, Dormont J (1980) Deprived primary in vitro antibody response in untreated systemic lupus erythematosus. T helper cell defect and lack of defective suppressor cell function. J Clin Invest 66:141—148

115. Kumagai S, Sredni B, House S, Steinberg AD, Green I (1982) Defective regulation of B lymphocyte colony formation in patients with systemic lupus erythematosus. J Immunol 128:258—262

116. Edelson R, Finkelman F, Steinberg AD, et al (1978) Reactivity of lupus erythematosus antibodies with leukemic helper T cells. J Invest Dermatol 70:42—50

117. Morimoto C, Reinherz EL, Distaso JA, Steinberg AD, Schlossman SF (1984) Relationship between systemic lupus erythematosus T cell subsets, anti-T cell antibodies, and T cell functions. J Clin Invest 73:689

118. Smolen JS, Chused TM, Leiserson WM, Reeves JP, Alling D, Steinberg AD (1982) Heterogeneity of immunoregulatory T correlation with clinical features. Am J Med 72:783—790

119. Smolen JS, Morimoto Ch, Steinberg AD, Wolf A, Schlossman SF, Steinberg RT, Penner E, Reinherz E, Reichlin M, Chused TM (1985) Systemic lupus erythematosus: delineation of subpopulations by clinical, serologic, and T cell subset analysis. Am J Med Sci 289:139—147

120. Bakke AC, Kirkland PA, Kitridou RC, Horwitz DA (1983) T lymphocyte subsets in systemic lupus erythematosus. Arthritis Rheum 26:745—750

121. Taurog JD, Raveche ES, Smathers PA, Steinberg AD (1981) T cell abnormalities in NZB mice occur independently of autoantibody production. J Exp Med 153:221—234

122. Primi D, Hammarstrom L, Smith CIE (1978) Genetic control of lymphocyte suppression: I. Lack of suppression in aged NZB mice is due to B cell defect. J Immunol 121:2241—2243

123. Cantor H, McVay-Boudreau L, Hugenberger J, Naidorf K, Shen FW, Gershon RK (1978) Immunoregulatory circuits among T-cell subsets: II. Physiologic role of feedback inhibition in vivo: absence in NZB mice. J Exp Med 147:1116—1125

124. Gershon RK, Horowitz M, Kemp JD, Murphy DB, Murphy ED (1978) The cellular site of immunoregulatory breakdown in the lpr mutant mouse. In: Rose NR, Bigazzi PE, Warner NL (Eds) Genetic control of autoimmune disease. Elsevier North Holland, New York, pp 223—227
125. Sakane TA, Steinberg AD, Green I (1978) Failure of autologous mixed lymphocyte reactions between T and non-T cells in patients with systemic lupus erythematosus. Proc Natl Acad Sci USA 75:135—142
126. Kuntz MM, Innes JB, Weksler ME (1979) The cellular basis of the impaired autologous mixed lymphocyte reaction in patients with systemic lupus erythematosus. J Clin Invest 63:151—154
127. Smith JB, De Horatius RJ (1982) Deficient autologous mixed lymphocyte reaction correlates with disease activity in systemic lupus erythematosus and rheumatoid arthritis. Clin Exp Immunol 47:155—162.
128. Smolen JS, Siminovich K, Luger TA, Steinberg AD (1983) Responder cells in the human autologous mixed lymphocyte reaction (AMLR). Characterization and interactions in healthy individuals and patients with systemic lupus erythematosus. Behring Institute Mitteilungen 72:135—142
129. Smith JB, Pasternak PD (1978) Syngeneic mixed lymphocyte reaction in mice: strain distribution, kinetics, participating cells, and absence in NZB mice. J Immunol 121:1889—1893
130. Glimcher LH, Steinberg AD, House SB, Green I (1980) The autologous mixed lymphocyte reaction in strains of mice with autoimmune disease. J Immunol 125:1832—1837
131. Sakane T, Kotani H, Takada S, Murakawa Y, Ueda Y (1983) A defect in suppressor circuits among OKT4+ cell populations in patients independently of a defect in the OKT8+ suppressor T cell function. J Immunol 131:753—761
132. Murakawa Y, Takada S, Ueda Y, Suzuki N, Hoshino T, Sakane T (1985) Characterization of T lymphocyte subpopulations responsible for deficient interleukin 2 activity in patients with systemic lupus erythematosus. J Immunol 134:187—195
133. Okudaira K, Searles RP, Ceuppens JL, Williams RC (1982) Anti-Ia reactivity in sera from patients with systemic lupus erythematosus. J Clin Invest 69:17—24
134. Litvin DA, Cohen PL, Winfield JB (1983) Characterization of warm-reactive IgG antilymphocyte antibodies in systemic lupus erythematosus: relative specificity for mitogen-activated T cells and their soluble products. J Immunol 130:181—186
135. Shirai T, Hayakawa K, Okumura KO, Tada T (1978) Differential cytotoxic effect of natural thymocytotoxic autoantibody of NZB mice on functional subsets of T cells. J Immunol 120:1924—1929
136. Linker-Israeli M, Bakke AC, Quismorio FP, Horwitz D (1985) Correction of Interleukin-2 production in patients with systemic lupus erythematosus by removal of spontaneously activated suppressor cells. J Clin Invest 75:762—768
137. Yu DTY, Winchester RJ, Fu SM, Kunkel HG (1980) Peripheral blood Ia positive T cells: increases in certain diseases and after immunization. J Exp Med 151:91—100
138. James SP, Yenokida GG, Graeff AS, Elson CO, Strober W (1981) Immunoregulatory function of T cells activated in the autologous mixed lymphocyte reaction. J Immunol 127:2605—2609
139. Smith JB, Knowlton RP (1979) Activation of suppressor T-cells in human autologous mixed lymphocyte culture. J Immunol 123:419—422
140. Dubois EL, Tuffanelli DL (1964) Clinical manifestations of systemic lupus erythematosus: computer analysis of 520 cases. JAMA 190:104—111
141. Ropes MW (1976) Systemic lupus erythematosus. Harvard University Press, Cambridge
142. Louis PA, Lambert PH (1979) Lipopolysaccharides: from immune stimulation to autoimmunity. Springer Semin Immunopathol 2:215—228
143. Alarcon-Segovia D (1975) Drug-induced systemic lupus erythematosus and related syndromes. Clin Rheum Dis 1:573—582
144. Gleichmann E, Gleichmann H (1976) Graft-versus-host reaction: a pathogenetic principle for the development of drug allergy, autoimmunity, and malignant lymphoma in non-chimeric individuals. Hypothesis. Zeitschrift für Krebsforschung 85:91—109

145. Gleichmann E, Issa P, Elven EHV, Lamers MC (1978) The chronic graft versus host reaction: a lupus like syndrome caused by abnormal T — B cell interaction. Clin Rheum Dis 4:587—602
146. Kimura M, Andoh T, Kai K (1980) Failure to detect type-C virus p30-related antigen in systemic lupus erythematosus: false positive reaction due to protease activity. Arthritis Rheum 23:111—113
147. Kurata M, Katamine S, Fukuda T, Mine M, Ikari N, Kanazawa H, Matsunaga M, Eguchi K, Nagataki S (1985) Production of a monoclonal antibody to a membrane antigen of human T-cell leukemia virus (HTLV/ATLV)-infected cell lines from a systemic lupus erythematosus (SLE) patient: serologic analyses for HTLV infections in SLE patients. Clin Exp Immunol 62:65—74
148. Panem S, Ordonez NG, Kirstein WH, Katz AI, Spargo BH (1976) C-type virus expression in systemic lupus erythematosus. N Engl J Med 295:470—475
149. Maeda S, Yonezawa K, Yachi A (1985) Serum antibody reacting with placental syncytiotrophoblast in sera of patients with autoimmune diseases — a possible relation to type C RNA retrovirus. Clin Exp Immunol 60:645—553

Part II:
Animal Models of Systemic Lupus Erythematosus: Genetic, Viral and Immunologic Aspects

Genetic Aspects of Murine Lupus

M. F. Seldin, J. D. Mountz, and A. D. Steinberg

Introduction

A number of inbred strains of mice and various crosses and recombinant inbred lines spontaneously develop manifestations of autoimmune disease which resemble those of patients with systemic lupus erythematosus and, to some extent, Sjögren's syndrome, rheumatoid arthritis, and other autoimmune diseases. These mice have provided substantial insights into the bases for human disease. One conclusion of the mouse studies is that there are critical genetic factors underlying disease and that those factors are different in different mice (Table 1). More recently, our laboratory and others have started to address the question of abnormal gene expression in autoimmunity at a molecular level. In this chapter, we will discuss genetic aspects of murine lupus with emphasis on the most widely studied mice and suggest new approaches to elucidate the genetic mechanisms by which autoimmunity results.

New Zealand Mice

Several inbred strains of New Zealand mice have been developed, some of which are unrelated (such as NZB and NZW) and others derived from very closely related stock (such as NZB and NZO). The first reported spontaneously occurring autoimmune disease was described in the New Zealand black (NZB) strain 30 years ago [1]. These mice spontaneously develop an illness characterized by early onset of antibodies reactive with thymocytes and certain T-lymphocytes [2, 3], progressive increase in antierythrocyte autoantibodies between 4 and 12 months of age terminating in severe hemolytic anemia [4], and late-life glomerulonephritis which morphologically has features of membranous and mesangial disease as well as interstitial nephritis [5]. The females have a median survival of approximately 15 months and the males 17 months, with considerable variation from colony to colony as well as within a given colony. These mice lack the fifth component of complement [6] which has been suggested to be a protection against more severe renal disease. NZB mice manifest much less sex difference in disease than do the F_1 hybrids of NZB mice with other strains, in part due to a single recessive gene for androgen insensitivity [7].

Table 1. Features of lupus in different mice

Feature	NZB	(NZB × NZW) F₁	MRL-Mp-*lpr/lpr*	BXSB
Genetic	At least 6 autosomal genes	Multiple genes, some from NZW	Multiple background genes, *lpr* major accelerator	Multiple background Y chromosome gene major accelerator
Major histocompatibility	d/d	d/z	k/k	b/b
Sex	Little effect Recessive gene for androgen insensitivity	Marked effect Androgens protect, estrogens worsen	Androgens protect slightly	Marked acceleration in males, not hormonal, but androgens retard
Immunoglobulins	↑IgM	↑IgM, ↑IgG₁	↑IgG₁, ↑IgG2a	↑IgG₁, ↑IgG2b
Lymphoid organs	Lymphoid hyperplasia	Lymphoid hyperplasia	Marked↑T cells	Moderate↑B cells
Effects of *xid*	Prevents disease	Prevents disease	Retards disease	Prevents disease
Disease manifestations	Anti-T cell antibodies, Coombs-positive hemolytic anemia, Late-life renal disease, Splenic hyperdiploidy, Death occurs after 1 year	Anti-DNA, LE cells, Membranoproliferative glomerulonephritis, Sjögren's syndrome, Females die in first year of life	Marked lymphadenopathy, Anti-DNA, anti-Sm, Arthritis and anti-Ig Membranoproliferative glomerulonephritis, Vasculitis, Males and females die in first year of life	Immune complex glomerulonephritis, Degenerative coronary artery disease, Serologically less abnormal than others, Moderate adenopathy, Males die in first year of life

A number of breeding studies have been conducted in an attempt to determine the number of genes required for individual traits of NZB mice and also the number required for the entire syndrome of the mice. The earliest studies investigated the possible influence of the NZB parent on F_1 offspring after matings with a variety of non-NZB parents. Such studies demonstrated that (NZB × NZW)F_1 and (NZB × NZY)F_1 mice developed more rapidly fatal autoimmune disease than did either parent, and that a rapidly progressive glomerulonephritis was responsible [8]. In contrast, matings with such mice as C3H led to offspring with minimal autoimmune features [9]. Thus, the full syndrome of NZB mice is not dominant; however, the expression of disease can be markedly altered in matings with the appropriate non-NZB strain, even to the extent of worse disease in some instances. This latter observation has more recently been extended to matings of NZB with SWR and inbred NIH Swiss mice [10, 11]. In an attempt to determine the relative contributions of each parent, mating studies have led to the conclusion that each parent contributes one or more genes to the accelerated disease of the offspring [12—14].

A series of backcross studies were carried out over the years in an attempt to determine the number of genes responsible for individual traits. One interesting study was of NZB mice with New Zealand Chocolate (NZC). First, the NZC mouse, although not autoimmune by itself, did provide a genetic contribution to autoimmune hemolytic anemia [15]. Moreover, the severity of disease was found to be linked to coat color [15]. Similar backcross studies suggested that anti-ssDNA required a single co-dominant gene, as did naturally occurring thymocytotoxic antibodies (NTA) [16]. These latter studies uncovered a problem facing previous genetic studies: the role of sex hormones in modifying disease expression. Thus, it was necessary to study only females or to castrate all offspring at an early age to determine the true expression of a gene without the confounding modifying variable of sex hormones [16].

Although the major histocompatibility (MHC) type of the NZB (H2-d) has not been emphasized over the years, recent matings have produced NZB mice with MHC genes from the NZW (H-2^z), which have accelerated disease. This finding led to the conclusion that either a part of the H-2^z MHC itself or a gene linked to this MHC on chromosome 17 of the mouse is critical to accelerated disease expression [13].

Perhaps one of the most enlightening, and at the same time most humbling, approaches has been that adopted in a series of studies of recombinant inbred mice. In these studies NZB parents were mated with non-NZB parents, and the $F_1 × F_1$ mating used to generate F_2 mice which were then brother—sister mated in isolation. In other words, each $F_2 × F_2$ cross from single parents was highly inbred separately from a large number of others. In this way a number of distinct inbred lines were generated, each carrying different genes from the original NZB parent. These various recombinant inbred lines were then studied for a variety of phenotypes. The humbling aspect of these studies was that there were large numbers of phenotypes which appeared to bear no relationships to each other [17, 18] although the numbers of genes contributing to each could be estimated [19]. The enlightenment was the recognition that there was no single "autoimmunity gene" in NZB mice, but that a number of genes conspired together to produce

Genetic Aspects of Murine Lupus **25**

disease [19, 20]. Moreover, such studies have demonstrated that there are two families of unlinked genes, one dealing with stem cell and B cell maturation abnormalities and the other with autoantibodies [11].

A number of additional genetic studies with NZB mice are notable. Consistent with the minimal sex differences, NZB mice, in common with LG/J mice (the major contributor to the MRL strain, see below), have *Slp* production by both males and females [19], and this is a single recessive trait [21]. This is of special interest because the *Slp* locus resides within the MHC. In addition, NZB mice have a single recessive gene which dramatically predisposes to the development of hyperdiploidy in spleen cells [22]. A more complicated issue is that of the ability of NZB mice to recognize and mount a primary cytotoxic cellular response against non-MHC determinants [20], including a maternally transmitted antigen [23, 24]. Table 2 summarises some of the results of the extensive studies in NZB mice.

The New Zealand white (NZW) strain arose quite remotely from the NZB. It is thought to be relatively nonautoimmune, although it is somwhat more resistant to experimental tolerance than many other nonautoimmune strains [25]. As noted above, it produces an F_1 offspring with NZB which has accelerated renal disease. This (NZB × NZW)F_1 mouse has been widely studied as a model of lupus nephritis. The females have earlier onset of disease than do male littermates as a consequence of their sex hormone differences: androgens retard and estrogens accelerate disease [26—28]. Essentially all the females develop positive LE cell preparations and antibodies reactive with native and heat-denatured single-stranded DNA. They die of renal disease between 9 and 12 months of age. The NZW mouse also appears to have genes which conspire with the BXSB Y chromosome accelerator (see below) to produce accelerated disease in (NZW × BXSB)F_1 males [29] and also in congenic NZW.BXSB-Y males [30]. Thus, although the NZW mouse carries many genes which can interact with those of autoimmune mice to lead to offspring with severe autoimmune disease,

Table 2. Number of genes necessary for NZB autoimmune traits[a]

Trait	Number of genes	Minimum number of unique genes[b]
Anti-T-cell antibodies	1	1
Hypergammaglobulinemia	1	0
Anti-DNA	1	1
Antierythrocytes	2 or 3	1
Splenomegaly	2	1
Hyperdiploidy	2	0
Hyperproliferation	3	1
Abnormal tolerance	2	1
Total		≥6

[a] Based on an analysis of recombinant inbred lines
[b] Not linked to preceding traits

the NZW mouse itself is relatively unaffected, apparently because it lacks some critical gene(s).

The New Zealand obese mouse (NZO) was derived after three generations from the NZB. It develops obesity, mild hyperglycemia, glucose intolerance, hyperinsulinemia, and insulin resistance [31, 32]. As a result, it has been regarded as a model of human adult-onset insulin-resistant diabetes. Since these mice were derived from the same stock as the NZB [33], they were studied for features of disease seen in NZB mice. It was found that such mice develop antibodies to native and ssDNA and deposit immune complexes in their kidney [34]. Such mice are apparently protected against severe renal disease because of a failure to deposit much IgG and also a decline with age in the production of anti-DNA.

NZB mice carry a xenotropic murine leukemia virus [35] and not only express large amounts of viral products, but make antibodies to them which contribute to disease [36—38]. The same is true of (NZB × NZW)F_1 mice [39, 40]. Two loci have been described for the regulation of this virus, one quantitatively more important than the other [41, 42]. Breeding studies have been able to separate virus expression from glomerulonephritis [11, 43] and from other autoimmune traits [44, 45]. Thus, although virus product-antibody complexes may contribute to the renal immunopathology [39, 46], virus expression does not appear to be necessary for disease, suggesting that a variety of different kinds of complexes can lead to the renal immunopathology.

Although the studies discussed above are largely directed at genes which increase disease, we did mention that brown coat color is associated with decreased hemolytic anemia in (NZB × NZC) backcrosses and inbreeding [15]. A more profound suppression of NZB disease was discovered when the *xid* gene was bred onto the NZB background [47]. The *xid* gene stands for X chromosome-linked immune deficiency and was derived originally from the X chromosome of the CBA/N mouse. This gene causes the NZB mice to produce little in the way of anti-T cell, anti-RBC, or anti-DNA autoantibodies [47]; in addition, it prevents renal pathology and allows the NZB mice to live a normal lifespan. The same result obtains when the *xid* gene is bred onto the (NZB × NZW)F_1 mice [48]. The ability to overcome the effects of the *xid* gene by manipulation is somewhat different in the two cases. Whereas (NZB × NZW)F_1 *xid/xid* mice do not produce anti-DNA or develop renal disease even when chronically stimulated with polyclonal immune activators [48], the NZB.*xid* mice do produce autoantibodies when stimulated chronically or if they are neonatally thymectomized [49]. The reasons for these differences are unclear, and other workers have reported some production of autoantibodies by (NZB × NZW)F_1 mice with the *xid* defect [50], suggesting that the differences may be quantitative. Recent advances in the molecular biology of the X-linked gene family to which *xid* belongs [51, 52] suggest that *xid* most probably slows the maturation of mature B cells, thereby reducing autoantibody production. It is likely that NZB mice produce growth factors in greater quantity or that their B cells are intrinsically more susceptible to such factors so that they can more easily overcome the defect. Nevertheless, such studies of *xid* demonstrate that disease can be prevented or greatly retarded by a single gene, providing hope that future studies will allow more directed efforts at understanding the details of disease induction and retardation.

Genetic Aspects of Murine Lupus 27

BXSB Mice

The availability of single genes, such as *lpr, gld,* and the BXSB-Y factor, which induce or accelerate autoimmune disease [52—58] provide new and powerful tools for dissecting the genetic basis for autoimmune phenomena and ultimately the mechanisms by which the genes operate to induce or accelerate disease. The BXSB mouse is a recombinant inbred mouse (B = C57BL/6; SB = satin beige; X = recombinant inbred) of somewhat complex origin, in which the Y chromosome of the SB/Le mouse carries an unusual genetic factor. The studies of Murphy and Roths and of the Scripps group have demonstrated that the Y chromosome of the BXSB mouse induces accelerated autoimmune and immunopathologic abnormalities [53—57]. Those studies further show that the BXSB Y chromosome can induce accelerated cardiac disease in (NZW × BXSB)F$_1$ mice [29, 59]. The accelerated autoimmune disease of BXSB males is indepedent of sex hormones [60] and depends upon stem cells present in males [61]. Impaired tolerance to heterologous gamma globulins characteristic of BXSB males [62, 63] is also dependent upon stem cells in the males [63]. However, recent studies of (NZW × BXSB)F$_1$ female mice show disease without a tolerance defect [64]. The *xid* gene can suppress the acceleration due to the BXSB Y chromosome in BXSB mice and in (NZB × BXSB)F$_1$ mice [65]. This is consistent with studies suggesting that abnormal B cells in BXSB males are critical for disease expression [61—63, 65, 66] and that such B cells do not develop in *xid* mice [65, 67, 68].

The genetic interactions which underlie the phenotypic changes induced by the BXSB-Y have not yet been elucidated. To further address this problem, consomic CBA/J.BXSB-Y, NZB.BXSB-Y, and NZW.BXSB-Y mice have been extensively studied in our laboratory [30] for possible interactions of the BXSB-Y chromosome with genes of a non-autoimmune prone mouse (CBA/J), an autoimmune prone mouse (NZB), and a mouse which by itself expresses little autoimmunity (NZW) but which upon breeding with autoimmune-prone strains (BXSB and NZB) can give rise to offspring with severe disease [29, 57, 65]. The consomic mice had the autosomal genes of the parent strain but the Y chromosome of the BXSB strain.

CBA/J.BXSB-Y males develop very few autoimmune phenomena. The CBA/J.BXSB-Y males did not produce abnormal quantities of antibodies to autologous erythrocytes or single-stranded DNA. The CBA/J.BXSB-Y mice did not develop splenomegaly or significant cardiac or kidney disease and they lived a normal life span. Thus, the BXSB-Y chromosome had minimal effects on the CBA/J "background" genes. This result suggested that the BXSB-Y chromosome might accelerate disease when there is a predisposition to autoimmunity, but might not actually, by itself, induce disease. This concept is consistent with the results of other studies, which have revealed much milder disease in (CBA/J × BXSB)F$_1$ males than in BXSB males [69, 70] and the development of late life autoimmune abnormalities in BXSB females and the female offspring of BXSB males and NZB or NZW females [29, 53—57, 59, 60].

NZW males without BXSB-Y chromosomes did not develop accelerated splenomegaly, renal disease, or cardiac disease, whereas all of these abnormalities were observed in NZW.BXSB-Y consomic mice. Just as BXSB males produce very little high-affinity anti-DNA detectable by the ammonium sulfate precipitation assay (which dissociates low-affinity antibody-DNA interactions because of the high salt concentration), the sick NZW.BXSB-Y males did not have acceleration of anti-DNA production. The histological abnormalities observed in the NZW.BXSB-Y congenic males were almost as severe as those in the (BXSB × NZW)F$_1$ males, previously described as contracting severe disease [29, 60]. Consistent with the histologic disease, the NZW.BXSB-Y consomic males have markedly reduced survival. Reduced survival has also been observed in (NZB × NZW.BXSB-Y)F$_1$ males and (NZW × NZB.BXSB-Y)F$_1$ males relative to consomic males. A further reduction in survival was seen in castrated consomic males with BXSB-Y chromosomes. Thus, androgens may provide partial protection against BXSB-Y chromosome-accelerated disease in these mice.

NZB.BXSB-Y consomic males, like CBA/J.BXSB-Y and NZW-BXSB-Y males, did not have major acceleration of anti-ssDNA production. They did, however, have markedly accelerated anti-erythrocyte autoantibody production. Moreover, the capacity of the Y chromosome of the NZB.BXSB-Y consomic mice to accelerate anti-DNA was demonstrated in (BXSB × NZB.BXSB-Y)F$_1$ males. Thus, although NZB.BXSB-Y males have a gene from the BXSB-Y chromosome which causes marked acceleration of anti-ssDNA in (BXSB × NZB.Y)F$_1$ males, such acceleration of anti-ssDNA was not seen in NZB.BXSB-Y males. These results suggest that one or more non-Y genes from the BXSB mouse interacts in some way with the BXSB-Y to accelerate anti-ssDNA in (NZB × BXSB)F$_1$ and (BXSB × NZB.BXSB-Y)F$_1$ mice. The acceleration was largely of IgG anti-ssDNA; since NZB mice make largely IgM anti-DNA [71, 47], it is possible that genes contributing to the capacity to make IgG autoantibodies are affected by the BXSB-Y to accelerate anti-ssDNA.

Unlike the NZW.BXSB-Y consomic mice, the NZB.BXSB-Y mice did not show accelerated splenomegaly, renal disease, cardiac disease, or mortality. Thus, whereas NZW mice have genes upon which the BXSB-Y can work, NZB mice appeared to lack some of the genes required for the full action of the BXSB-Y chromosome. It is likely that some of the relevant genes upon which the BXSB-Y might operate are present in (NZB × BXSB)F$_1$ males by virtue of the presence of BXSB non-Y genes. However, the breeding of the NZB.BXSB-Y mice was very difficult, and it is possible that the least autoimmune NZB.BXSB-Y males were the only ones able to produce offspring, thereby giving rise to offspring with minimal disease. This possibility is strengthened by more recent observations that NZB.SB/Le-Y males have accelerated death (A.D. Steinberg, unpublished observation). Table 3 dramatizes the profound effects of introducing this Y chromosome gene.

Taken together, the studies provide support for the view that the BXSB-Y accelerating factor is an accelerator of autoimmune disease rather than an inducer of disease [57, 72]. The factor does not induce severe autoimmune disease or autoantibodies in CBA/J.BXSB-Y males, although it does induce mild coronary disease. Thus, it appears that the BXSB-Y chromosome accelerating factor operates on other genes. Further work will be necessary to determine exactly how the BXSB-Y works. It is possible that it acts like certain oncogenes [73, 74]

Table 3. Survival of mice with the BXSB Y chromosome

Strain or cross	Sex	Median survival (months)
BXSB	M	7
BXSB	F	16
(NZW × BXSB)F₁	M	7
(NZW × BXSB)F₁	F	12
(BXSB × NZW)F₁	M	19
(NZW.BXSB-Y consomic	M	7
CBA/J.BXSB-Y consomic	M	24
NZB.BXSB-Y consomic	M	14
NZB.SB/Le-Y consomic	M	6
NZB	M	18
NZW	M	24
CBA/J	M	27

to regulate gene expression within the nucleus. This may be a general strategy for certain sex chromosome genes.

Mice with the lpr Genotype

The *lpr/lpr* genotype was originally discovered when the MRL strain was produced, a strain which consists of LG/J (75.0%), AKR (12.6%), C3H (12.1%), and C57BL/6 (0.3%), and which by itself develops late-life autoimmune disease including the production of large amounts of antinuclear antibodies such as anti-DNA and anti-Sm [53, 55, 75—81]. Although the majority of studies are of MRL-*lpr/lpr* mice, more recently C3H/HeJ-*lpr/lpr,* AKR-*lpr/lpr,* and C57BL/6-*lpr/lpr* mice have been studied in detail and even NZB-*lpr/lpr* mice have been produced [81—84]. The *lpr/lpr* genotype is associated with the expansion of an unusual population of T cells (dull Lyt 1^+, Thy 1^+) which bear cell surface markers usually not found on T cells (6B2, 9F3). Such cells expand first in mesenteric lymph nodes and then in peripheral lymph nodes. Neonatal thymectomy markedly retards both the lymphadenopathy and the autoimmune syndrome [84]. Such adenopathy occurs on all genetic backgrounds studied to date, but varies somewhat in degree [83]. Moreover, some mice actually manifest a reduction in adenopathy late in life. This occurs especially in mice which live substantially longer than their littermates, and is perhaps most evident in MRL-*lpr/lpr.xid* congenic mice [85]. In addition to the uniform manifestation of lymphadenopathy (*lpr* = lymphoproliferation), all strains of mice bearing *lpr/lpr* develop anti-DNA antibodies [82, 83], although the magnitude is substantially reduced by the *xid* gene [85]. Moreover, they all die prematurely [83]; however, the development of severe renal disease is not uniform. It appears that *lpr/lpr* induces severe renal disease only when introduced into a genetic background

30   M. F. Seldin et al.

which is already characterized by a predisposition to autoimmunity, such as MRL or NZB [81—84]. Thus, the "background genes" are critical to the details of expression of *lpr/lpr*. The *lpr* gene is recessive in that MRL-*lpr/*+ mice do not develop adenopathy. This may not be strictly true, however, since some *lpr/*+ mice develop more anti-DNA than do +/+ mice (A.D. Steinberg, unpublished observations), and SJL-*lpr/*+ mice are different from SJL +/+ mice (H.C. Morse III, personal communication). Until the nature of the gene product is elucidated, these observations will be difficult to reconcile.

One interesting and disturbing finding is H-2d$^+$ cells (Ia—d) derived from the MRL-*lpr/lpr* (H-2k) peritoneal cavity [86]. This is difficult to explain on the grounds of ordinary genetic mechanisms, and if the d+ cells exist in the intact mouse, they must make up an extremely small percentage of all the cells, since the genes for cannot be found in the DNA from spleen (D. Klinman, A.D. Steinberg, and R. Germain, unpublished observations). Perhaps this represents a vertically transmitted agent derived originally from the LG/J parent, or more probably, unusual genetic deregulation resulting from the *lpr/lpr* genotype and serologic cross-reactivity.

The *lpr* gene has not yet been mapped; however, another mutation, *gld,* gives rise to lymphadenopathy and similar unusual subpopulations of T cells [87]. This *gld* gene (*gld* = generalized lymphoproliferative disease) is also recessive and has been mapped to chromosome 1 of the mouse [87]. Moreover, it is not allelic to *lpr* [87]. Thus, it is possible that more than one kind of genetic defect can give rise to similar abnormalities characterized by lymphadenopathy and antinuclear antibody production.

Molecular Genetic Studies

Although the Mendelian genetic studies have been quite informative, a much more definitive understanding of the genetic bases of autoimmune disease will require an understanding of the gene products and the mechanisms of their effects. It will be necessary to isolate specific genes and determine their products and how they influence other genes or otherwise manifest their effects before better understanding of the autoimmune processes is possible. Such are still in their infancy. To date, there is some information regarding differential expression of certain genes critical to lymphocyte growth and differentiation. Since lymphocytes appear to be very important in the expression of murine lupus, such information provides the first molecular approach to a genetic understanding of disease. The study of proto-oncogene expression in the lymphoid tissues of the various strains and crosses of autoimmune mice is of particular import, since oncogenes are now known to code for growth factors and receptors for growth factors.

We will now describe the recent work performed in our laboratory on oncogene expression in autoimmune mice [88—90]. Initially, oncogenes were found to be genetic sequences in acute transforming retroviruses, which mediated rapid neoplastic transformation. Sequences homologous to viral oncogenes (v-*onc*) have been found as genes in normal cells (c-*onc*) [91]. The function of the c-*onc* genes in normal cells became clearer when one *(sis)* was found to be structurally related to platelet derived growth factor [92] and another *(erb-B)* was found to be homologous to the gene for epidermal cell growth factor receptor [93]. More recently, possible growth factor functions have been ascribed to other oncogenes [94, 95]. Another clue to the function of c-*onc* genes in normal cells has come from functional studies. Stimulation of lymphoid cells by Con A or lipopolysaccharide (LPS) in vitro results in 1—2 hrs. in high expression of the c-*myc* oncogene, which then returns to baseline levels [96]. Further information regarding the role of c-*onc* genes can be gained by examining the cellular location of their products or the biochemistry of their interaction with substrates. The oncogenes c-*myc* and c-*myb* probably act in the nucleus [97, 98], but other oncogenes *(abl, bas, raf)* act at the cell surface [91]. There is good evidence that *myc* protein binds to DNA [98]. *Abl* is a member of the tyrosine kinase family [91] and has been associated with malignancies of the T and B cell lineage. *Raf* is believed to be related to the *src* family of oncogenes [99] and was originally associated with oat cell carcinoma [100], but is elevated in normal mouse thymus and autoimmune mouse spleen cells (see below). *Bas* is homologous to the *ras* gene, which codes for proteins thought to be associated with cell surface receptors involved in growth control. Furthermore, the presence of a point mutation in this cellular oncogene has been linked with tumorogenesis [101, 102]. Thus, oncogenes appear critical to both normal and abnormal growth/differentiation of eukaryotic cells.

High c-*myb* expression in *lpr/lpr* Lymph Node Cells

The most striking association between oncogene expression and autoimmunity is a marked elevation of a normal size *myb* RNA in peripheral lymph nodes (30—fold) and mesenteric lymph nodes (60—fold) in the MRL-*lpr/lpr* mouse, compared with peripheral lymph nodes of the MRL-+/+ mouse. The *lpr* gene is implicated because these strains are co-isogenic except for this locus. Also, high *myb* RNA expression occurred in the lymph nodes of two other strains which had been inbred for the *lpr* gene, AKR-*lpr/lpr* and C57BL/6-*lpr/lpr*, but not +/+ controls. *Myb* expression required the *lpr* gene to be present in homozygous form, as normal myb expression was observed in the (+/+ × *lpr/lpr*)F$_1$ mouse. Lymph nodes from *lpr/lpr* mice are massively enlarged; over 90% of the cells are T cells with one cell type predominating, the abnormal Thy 1$^+$, dull Ly 1$^+$, 6B2$^+$ T cell. Early in their illness, C57BL/6 *lpr/lpr* mice are heterogeneous with regard to massive splenic enlargement. Moderately enlarged spleens from C57BL/6-*lpr/lpr*, with fewer abnormal T cells, had less *myb* RNA expression per microgram of messenger RNA than did large spleens with more abnormal T cells. Further studies of the MRL-*lpr/lpr* mice, which will be discussed below, using in vivo T cell depletion studies with cytoxan therapy, or studies of the effects of the X-linked immunodeficiency gene *(xid)* on MRL-*lpr/lpr* mice implied that only the abnormal peripheral T cells have high *myb* RNA. High *myb* expression is also observed in T cell lines from MRL-*lpr/lpr* mice [103]. Together these results indicate that the abnormal T cells in MRL-*lpr/lpr* mice express high *myb* RNA, and that *myb* may be an important differentiation gene associated with the arrested development of this cell.

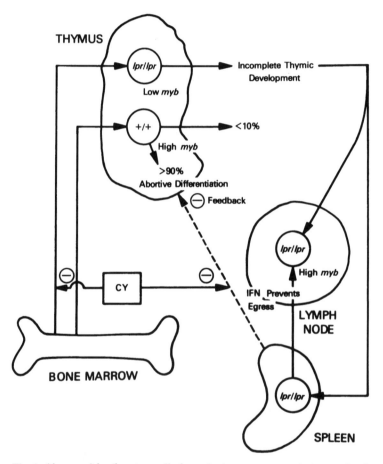

Fig. 1. Abnormal *lpr/lpr* stem cells from the bone marrow migrate to the thymus and undergo partial development. They leave the thymus prematurely before the stage of high *myb* RNA expression and migrate to the spleen and lymph nodes. The accumulation of immature Thy 1[+], dull Ly 1[+] T cells in these organs results in high levels of interferon, which prevent egression of cells from lymph nodes, and production of factors that inhibit thymic activity. Cyclophosphamide therapy acts directly on abnormal stem cells in the bone marrow to allow dominance of normal stem cells which undergo full maturation in the thymus and express high *myb*, as found in the MRL-+/+ mouse. CY therapy may also indirectly affect thymus activity, because it results in a decrease in abnormal T cell traffic to the spleen and lymph node and a decrease in negative feedback to the thymus

Thymuses Provide a Clue to lpr/lpr Cells

The thymuses of MRL-*lpr/lpr* mice had markedly reduced quantities of *myb* RNA, but thymic tissue from other autoimmune (e.g., NZB, BXSB) and several nonautoimmune strains had abundant *myb* expression. This is exactly the opposite of the peripheral lymphoid organs and suggests that in the *lpr/lpr* mouse the underdeveloped pre-T cells do not express *myb* in the thymus, but leave prematurely and accumulate in the lymph nodes. The accumulation in lymph nodes may be facilitated by the presence of high levels of interferon in these mice [85, 104]. Some aspect of development similar to that associated with high *myb* in a normal thymus may occur in the *lpr/lpr* lymph nodes (Fig. 1).

Cyclophosphamide Corrects the Defect of lpr/lpr Mice

Cyclophosphamide (CY) therapy is known to cause regression of lymphadenopathy and return of normal T cell function in *lpr/lpr* mice [105]. However, CY preferentially affects rapidly proliferating cells such as those found in the bone marrow. Moreover, only 4%—6% of the *lpr/lpr* lymph node cells are in S + G2 + M phases of the cell cycle [106, 107]. Therefore, it was postulated that CY acted on the marrow pre-T stem cell to prevent migration of abnormal lymph node precursors cells to the node. It was predicted on the basis of this model for CY action that lymph node *myb* RNA expression would be lost after therapy and this, indeed, is what was found. This result demonstrated that decreased expression of *myb* RNA in the lymph node correlated with clinical benefit of CY therapy.

A second interesting observation was that thymic *myb* expression increased to normal after CY therapy. This finding was initially surprising, because previous experiments using hydrocortisone treatment of Balb/c mice to deplete the thmus of cortical thymocytes also decreased thymic *myb* RNA [108]. The return of thymic *myb* RNA to normal in *lpr/lpr* mice after CY therapy can be explained by consideration of the regulation and traffic involved in T cell development, as shown in Fig. 1. Normally, pre-T cells enter the thymus, where 90% are found to be immature PNA$^-$ cortical thymocytes and 10% are more mature, PNA$^+$ medullary thymocytes. For MRL-+/+ mice, T cell development continues through all stages of development, resulting in a high-*myb* RNA stage; 96% are eliminated by the thymus, presumably because they would develop into autoreactive T cells. In the thymus of MRL-*lpr/lpr* mice, abnormal pre-T cells from the bone marrow do not develop completely, and do not reach the stage for high *myb* RNA expression. The abnormal cells leave the thymus in high numbers and enter the lymph node or spleen. It is possible that enlarged lymph nodes or enlarged spleens packed with the abnormal T cells inhibit the development of pre-T cells in the thymus. Previous evidence has suggested the presence of such a feedback loop from the spleen to the thymus, shown as a dashed line in Fig. 1.

Table 4. *Myb* expression in thymus and lymph nodes of *lpr/lpr* mice with and without cyclophosphamide (CY)

Strain	Organ	Treatment	*Myb* expression
Nonautoimmune[a]	Thymus	0	+ + + +
	Lymph Node	0	+
lpr/lpr[b]	Thymus	0	+
	Lymph Node	0	+ + + +
lpr/lpr	Thymus	CY	+ + +
	Lymph Node	CY	+
NZB, BXSB[c]	Thymus	0	+ + +
	Lymph Node	0	+

[a] Balb/C, CBA/J, C57BL/6, DBA/2 (MRL-+/+ did not differ)
[b] Most studies were done with MRL-*lpr/lpr* mice, but similar results were obtained with C57BL/6-*lpr/lpr* mice and also other strains with the *lpr/lpr* genotype. In the latter mice, thymic myb was normal and a single dose of cyclophosphamide was sufficient to cause regression of lymphadenopathy.
[c] Autoimmune mice without the *lpr/lpr* genotype

CY therapy results in regression of splenomegaly and lymphadenopathy, and may interrupt this negative feedback. CY therapy probably also interferes with abnormal pre-T cell development in the bone marrow. When CY therapy was discontinued, lymphadenopathy recurred in most cases after many months, indicating that abnormal *lpr/lpr* stem cells were still present and could once again dominate the T cell development pathways. The effect of CY therapy on *myb* expression in the thymus and lymph node of *lpr/lpr* mice is summarized in Table 4.

Studies of Other Oncogenes in *lpr/lpr* Mice

The protein product of the oncogene c-*myc* acts at the nucleus, like *myb* [96, 98]. *Myc* RNA was not increased in the lymph nodes of *lpr/lpr* mice. Also, RNAs homologous with the oncogenes *abl, bas, mos fes, fms, ras,* and *erb* B were not elevated in lymph nodes of the *lpr/lpr* mice. These findings suggest that *myb* plays a rather unique role in the differentiation of normal thymic T cells, and that *myb* is particularly associated with abnormal differentiation of T cells with the *lpr/lpr* genotype. *Myb* expression in T cells appears to be more closely associated with differentiation rather than proliferation, though it may be important for both. Spleen cells stimulated with Con A or LPS express high levels of *myc* in the first few hours after stimulation. However, under the same conditions, only modest amounts of *myb* RNA are produced. Also, *myb* expression is highest in the lymph nodes of *lpr/lpr* mice, but there are only 6% of cells in S + G2 + M phases of the cell cycle [106, 107]. High *myb* in the normal thymus in probably not related primarily to proliferation, but rather to the differentiation of T cells

[108]. In normal mouse strains, over 90% of cells die within the thymus. These cells, which have been allowed to develop and then found unsuitable for emigration, undergo a maturation arrest until their death. It is possible that *myb* RNA expression could be even higher in the T cells of the MRL-*lpr/lpr* mouse which have undergone a cell cycle-specific maturation arrest, because the cells are allowed to synchronize at one point in the cell cycle and at one point along the differentiation pathway. This would explain the extraordinary high *myb* RNA levels in MRL-*lpr/lpr* lymph node cells, which have both a development arrest at a high *myb* RNA expression stage, and a cell cycle arrest in late G_1 stage. One could also speculate that if the *myb* protein product is driving a cell through a particular differentiation step which was blocked by a genetic abnormality, a compensatory increase in *myb* RNA may occur.

Although elevated *myb* expression in *lpr/lpr* mice may be an important clue to the mechanism of control of differentiation in T cells, and may allow a better understanding of the cause of lymphoproliferation in *lpr/lpr* mice, it is not the primary cause of the disease. *Myb* is not a product of the *lpr* gene, because lower but definitely detectable amounts of *myb* RNA are found in non-*lpr* mice. As mentioned above, the *myb* RNA transcript from *lpr/lpr* mice appears normal in size, with electrophoretic properties equal to *myb* RNA from non-*lpr* mice. Furthermore, Southern blot analyses of DNA from *lpr/lpr* and $+/+$ mice fail to demonstrate amplification or rearrangement of the *myb* gene in *lpr/lpr* mice. This result suggests that the *lpr* gene most likely results in abnormal regulation of *myb* expression, as a result of the differentiation defect.

Abnormal T Cells and Increased Lymph Node c-myb *RNA Characterize* gld/gld *Mice*

Another strain, the *gld/gld* mouse (generalized lymphoproliferative disease), also develops massive lymphadenopathy and autoimmune disease. In addition to a relative increase in null cells, this mouse has large numbers of Thy 1^+, dull Ly 1^+, $6B2^+$ cells in its lymph nodes, just as *lpr/lpr* mice do [87]. We predicted that *gld/gld* mice would also have markedly increased quantities of *myb* RNA in lymph nodes, and this is what we in fact found. The *gld* gene has been mapped to chromosome 1 [87] and is not linked either to *lpr*, which is unmapped, or to *myb*, which is on chromosome 10 the mouse. Thus, the *gld* gene acts at a distance, perhaps by *trans*-regulation, to affect the *myb* locus. Taken together, the data suggest the existence of at least one additional gene product, besides the *myb* protein, which participates in regulation of lymphoproliferation of *lpr/lpr* and *gld/gld* mice.

T Cell Dysfunction and Increased *myb* Expression may be Related to IL-2 Independence

It has been suggested that derangements in IL-2 (T cell growth factor) function could lead to the development of autoimmune disease [109]. The inability to synthesize, absorb, and proliferate to IL-2 are most prominently displayed by mice which bear the *lpr* gene [110]. We have recently found that high *myb* expression may be characteristic of IL-2-independent T cells (M.F. Seldin, J.D. Mountz, A.D. Steinberg, unpublished observations). Thus an IL-2-independent T cell line derived from *lpr/lpr* lymphoid tissue [103] and two thymoma-derived cell lines, EL-4 and BW5147, expressed very high levels of *myb,* whereas IL-2-dependent T cell lines HT2 and CTL-L expressed low levels of this RNA transcript. In addition, preliminary experiments indicate that in the absence of IL-2 these IL-2-dependent lines dramatically and specifically increase *myb* RNA transcription. These data suggest that *myb* expression may be linked in some way to IL-2. Although recent studies imply that the autoimmune *lpr/lpr* T cells have the inherent ability to use IL-2 as a growth factor, special conditions were required [111]. Further studies at the molecular level should help clarify this intriguing relationship, which may bear on the development of autoimmunity in the *lpr/lpr* and *gld/gld* mice and intrathymic T cell differentiation in both these and normal mice.

C-raf RNA Expression in Autoimmune Mice

Our survey of the expression of several additional oncogenes in *lpr/lpr* and *gld/gld* mice has demonstrated that *raf* RNA is also abnormally increased in lymph nodes from these mice. The oncogene *raf* was originally associated with small cell carcinoma of the lung and is believed to code for a cell surface molecule with tryosine kinase activity [99]; it has been mapped to chromosome 6 in the mouse [100]. The association of high *raf* RNA with the abnormal lymph node cells in *lpr/lpr* mice was initially not well understood. More recent evidence suggests that small cell carcinoma of the lung expresses surface antigens found on macrophages [112]. It has been postulated that these tumors, and therefore high *raf* expression, originate in hematopoietic precursor cells. Expression of *raf* RNA is high in some B cell lines. We have also found high levels of *raf* expression in normal thymus. These data suggest that *raf* RNA may code for a growth factor receptor on pre-B, pre-T and macrophage precursor cells. Like *myb, raf* RNA was high in *lpr/lpr* and *gld/gld* lymph nodes, and nearly absent in *lpr/lpr* thymus. The *raf* RNA was a normal-sized 3.2-kb transcript. Also, after CY treatment, *raf* expression was lost from *lpr/lpr* lymph nodes, but returned to normal in the thymus. Thus, expression of *myb* and *raf* superficially appeared to be paralleled in *lpr/lpr* mice. One could speculate that abnormal cell surface expression of the *raf* product promotes elevated *myb* expression or vice versa. It may

Genetic Aspects of Murine Lupus   37

be that *raf* expression, like *myb* expression, is associated with the same abnormal T cell in *lpr/lpr* and *gld/gld* mice; however, *raf* is expressed at least as well in *lpr/lpr* spleens as nodes (whereas *myb* is higher in nodes than spleen), suggesting that *raf* expression is possibly associated with a second cell in *lpr/lpr* mice. Moreover, *raf* is strongly expressed in lymph node cells from congenic NZB.BXSB-Y males, which have large numbers of Ly 1^+ B cells. Thus, *raf* expression is probably a feature of autoimmune B cells from many strains as well as the abnormal T cells of *lpr/lpr* and *gld/gld* mice.

Oncogene Expression in NZB and BXSB Mice

The cellular basis of autoimmune disease in two other strains of autoimmune mice, NZB and male BXSB mice, is thought to be due primarily to hyperactivity of B cells [113—116]. NZB mice develop marked splenomegaly and BXSB impressive lymphadenopathy, which, however, is much less remarkable than in *lpr/lpr* or *gld/gld* mice. The large peripheral lymph nodes of the male BXSB mouse are enriched not with T cells but rather with autoantibody-producing B cells. The cells in lymphoid organs of these mice are much more heterogeneous than in the *lpr/lpr* mouse. It is thought that the Ly 1^+ B cell subset is responsible for autoantibody production and may therefore be a result of abnormal growth regulation [114, 118]. Although Ly 1^+ B cells are increased to 10%, compared with 1% in nonautoimmune mice, they still represent a minority cell population. In addition, the cells do not appear to be arrested in any given stage of their cell cycle. If abnormal expression of a growth or differentiation gene causes the B cell abnormalities of BXSB or NZB mice, detection of the gene might be complicated by the further development of the affected cells to a more mature antibody-secreting phenotype. For all these reasons, detection of abnormal gene expression in BXSB and NZB mice may prove to be more difficult than in *lpr/lpr* or *gld/gld* mice.

We have found an association of the oncogenes c-*myc* and c-*bas* with splenic B cells of NZB and BXSB mice. Whole spleens show a modest increase in c-*myc* expression compared with control mice. As *myc* RNA is increased during early stages of proliferation this finding is not surprising, since B cell activation is increased in male BXSB and NZB mice. To study oncogene expression in B cells, spleen cells were depleted of macrophages by adherence and T cells by anti-Thy 1.2 and complement treatment. Elevated levels of c-*myc* RNA were found in the B cell-enriched fraction (increased compared with B cells from nonautoimmune mice). It is possible that some endogenous signal triggers NZB and BXSB B cells, and c-*myc* may increase as an early event after such a signal. Similarly, the oncogene c-*bas* was found to be elevated in spleens from young NZB and male BXSB mice. In unsynchronized spleen cells, expression of *myc* RNA and *bas* RNA would be occurring in different B cell populations at distinct points along the mitogenic pathways. Studies of total B cells allow detection of both elevations.

The *xid* Gene Modifies Oncogene Expression

The X-linked immunodeficiency gene *(xid)* eliminates the Lyb 5$^+$ B cell subset from the spleen and decreases autoantibody production, as previously discussed [48, 119]. Inbred autoimmune mice bearing this gene, congenic NZB.*xid*, MRL-*lpr/lpr.xid*, etc., have smaller spleens and reduced B cell proliferation [48, 65, 85, 113]. Expression of the c-*myc* and c-*bas* oncogenes in spleens from NZB and male BXSB mice are correspondingly reduced to that seen in control nonautoimmune mice, or even lower. This observation suggests that the increased *myc* RNA and *bas* RNA in B cells of NZB and male BXSB mice is predominantely associated with the Lyb 5$^+$ subset, the mature B cell subset responsible for autoantibody production. Moreover, *raf* expression is decreased in MRL-*lpr/lpr.xid* spleens, lending further support to the idea that *raf* is expressed by MRL-*lpr/lpr* splenic B cells. In contrast, *myb* expression, which is associated with the abnormal T cell, is not reduced in spleens or lymph nodes of MRL-*lpr/lpr.xid* mice (which also contain the abnormal T cells). Thus, the effects of *xid* on oncogene expression support the concept that different abnormal cells in autoimmune mice exhibit differential gene expression.

Future Directions

The oncogenes studied thus far may not be the primary genetic triggers which cause expansion of abnormal lymphocyte populations in autoimmune mice. Factors which allow increased expression, such as external triggers [117] and insertions of retroviral promoters [120], would be primary. However, this does not exclude the possibility that an oncogene homologous to the *lpr* gene will be found in the future. The oncogenes described here are, however, influenced by the genes causing autoimmune disease. Furthermore, distinctive patterns of oncogene expression occur in the different organs of various strains of autoimmune mice, as summarized in Table 5. Thus, oncogenes are the first molecular probes to be used to attempt to understand genetically defined abnormalities of lymphocyte development in autoimmune mice. Future work with additional probes should allow a better understanding of the molecular genetics underlying abnormal expansion of cell subpopulations in autoimmunity. The use of eukaryotic gene transfer technology [121, 126] should further clarify the role of specific oncogenes in altering lymphocyte growth and differentiation. To this end, we have recently constructed retroviral vectors containing oncogenes which may prove insightful.

Other approaches will be needed to unravel the complex genetic mechanisms underlying the autoimmune process. The evolution of new molecular technology, such as RNA subtraction, may allow the isolation of autoimmunity genes. Although this is an extremely difficult task at present, the success of recent efforts to isolate the T cell receptor genes [127–129] is encouraging.

Table 5. Oncogene expression in normal and autoimmune mice[a]

	myb	*myc*	*raf*	*bas*
CBA/J SP[b]	+	±	+	±
C57BL/6 SP	±	±	±	0
NZB SP female	+	+ + +	±	+
BXSB SP female	+	+	ND	+ +
BXSB SP male	+	+ + +	+	+ +
BXSB PLN male	+ +	+ +	+ + +	+
MRL-+/+ SP	+	+	+	+
MRL-*lpr/lpr* SP	+ + +	+ + +	+ + +	+ + +
MRL-*lpr/lpr* PLN	+ + + +	+ +	+ + +	+ +
MRL-*lpr/lpr* MLN	+ + + +	ND	+ + +	+ +
BXSB.*xid* SP male	ND	+	0	+
BXSB.*xid* PLN male	ND	ND	0	±
NZB.*xid* SP female	ND	+	0	±
MRL.*lpr/lpr.xid* SP	+ + + +	ND	0	+
MRL.*lpr/lpr.xid* PLN	+ + + +	+	+ +	+
(NZB × BXSB)F$_1$ SP male	ND	+	±	+ +
(NZB × BXSB)F$_1$ PLN male	ND	+	+ + +	+ +
(NZB × BXSB)F$_1$ SP female	ND	±	±	ND
C3H/HeJ SP	+ +	ND	+	ND
C3H/HeJ PLN	+	ND	±	±
C3H/HeJ-*gld/gld* SP	+ +	ND	+	ND
C3H/HeJ-*gld/gld* PLN	+ + + +	ND	+ + +	+ + +
CBA/J THY	+ + +	+ +	+ +	ND
DBA/2 THY	+ + +	+ +	+ +	ND
MRL-+/+ THY	+ +	+	+	ND
MRL-*lpr/lpr* THY	±	±	±	ND
BXSB THY male	+ + +	+	+ +	ND
NZB THY female	+ +	+	+	ND

[a] Summary of data on the expression of four oncogenes in different lymphoid organs of various autoimmune and control mouse strains. Poly (A)$^+$ RNA was isolated from lymphoid organs of over 3500 mice. Expression is denoted as: 0, no expression detected; + to + + + +, low to high levels of expression; ND, not done.

[b] CBA/J, C57BL/6, C3H/HeJ, and DBA/2 strains are not autoimmune mice. Recessive traits are described in Table 1. SP, spleen; PLN, peripheral lymph node; MLN, mesenteric lymph node; THY, thymus.

Utilizing the same concepts as have allowed the isolation of genes that can induce neoplastic events [130—135], we have recently initiated another series of experiments designed to uncover the molecular events in autoimmunity. In general, this approach consists in: (a) isolating high-molecular-weight DNA from abnormal tissue of interest: (b) transfecting this DNA into an indicator cell line [123—125]; and (c) observing changes in the growth characteristics of the indicator cell line upon successful integration of the gene(s) in question. As a first attempt we have used a 3T3 transformation assay similar to that which led to the discovery in many tumors of transforming oncogenes [101, 102, 130—135]. We have reasoned that some of the abnormal lymphocytes involved in autoimmunity may have undergone molecular events similar to those in neoplastic cells, resulting in changes in DNA, which might be able to transfer changes in growth characteristics to 3T3 fibroblasts. High molecular weight DNA was obtained from multiple organs of autoimmune and nonautoimmune strains of mice and transfected into 3T3 cells. In preliminary studies it appears that transforming DNA may be present in appropriate autoimmune tissue. Most striking thus far has been the isolation of one transformed clone from a transfection with NZB spleen DNA (M.F. Seldin, A.D. Steinberg, and D.I. Cohen, unpublished observation). This transformant has the ability to cause very rapidly growing tumors when injected subcutaneously into nude mice. Althought this result is extremely tantalizing it is not yet clear what has caused this phenomenon or whether it will prove to reflect true changes in NZB spleen DNA.

If substantiated, the above finding should allow characterization of at least one gene involved in the autoimmune mechanism. It is quite possible that this gene is also an oncogene similar to those involved in neoplasia, perhaps with a point mutation such as has been found with the *ras* oncogene [101, 102] or alternatively reflecting a gene rearrangement or insertion of genetic elements able to cause gene activation [120]. Good candidates for inducers of gene activation include retroviruses themselves or, alternatively, endogenous retroviral sequences present in the mouse genome as provirus. Further speculation on the possible molecular relationship between events that may cause autoimmunity and those that lead to neoplasia is profound but obviously premature. Experiments are currently under way in an attempt to verify and extend this exciting possibility.

Conclusions

It is clear that there is a genetic basis for autoimmunity in the mice discussed in this paper. However, the genetic basis is both complex and incompletely understood. The data suggest that at least three different kinds of genes are involved in predisposition to or expression of autoimmune disease. The first type is exemplified by the *lpr/lpr* genotype (*gld/gld* is also of this class). This is a gene which, by itself, can induce certain autoimmune features, such as antinuclear antibodies. The second type of gene is the BXSB-Y or the SB/Le-Y, which are presumably the same (but which might have diverged). This gene apparently cannot induce disease in nonautoimmune strains, but can cause acceleration of disease in concert with other genes in autoimmune mice. Thus, *lpr/lpr* and *gld/gld* may be thought of as inducing genes and the BXSB or SB/Le-Y as accelerator genes. Finally, there are a large number of "background" genes upon which those genes can work. These can also be subdivided, an exercise which has little meaning at the moment. Some of the background genes underlie specific traits — such as the predisposition to anti-DNA or to anti-RBC autoantibodies. Others lead to B cell hyperactivity, perhaps by virtue of leading to the production of factors or increased sensitivity of lymphocytes to such factors. In the NZB mouse, such genes have been studied by Mendelian genetics, but little is known about back-

Table 6. Comparison of murine and human SLE

Mouse strain	Murine system	Human SLE
NZB	Inherited autoimmune traits with a lack of sex difference [20]	Familial incidence of SLE [138] Concordance in identical twins [139]
F_1 hybrids with NZB	Androgens suppress and mask genetic mechanisms [16, 140]	Female predominance in SLE [138, 139]
BXSB	Male-linked inheritance [20, 113, 116]	Inheritance of male-predominant SLE [136]
Recombinant inbred lines of NZB × normal	Independent inheritance of many autoimmune traits [19]	Family members of SLE patients develop some autoimmune features without clinical SLE [140, 142]
F_1 and backcross analysis	Dominant and recessive inheritance of autoimmune traits with additional modifying genes; many genes show gene dosage effects [16]	Dominant inheritance of DNA and anti-ssDNA 143; two genes may give greater abnormality than one [142]
Modifying factors *xid* gene retards	Predisposing factors [20, 113] Retarding factors [47, 48, 85, 113, 148]	B cell hyperactivity in SLE [144–147]

ground genes in other mice. Moreover, other genes (e.g., contributed by NZW, NZY, NZC, SWR, NFS) which modify the expression of autoimmune disease are virgin territory. It is likely that the oncogenes tie in with the background genes in terms of regulation of lymphocyte maturation and proliferation, but the exact relationship is unknown.

How does this information help us to understand human SLE? It suggests that there may be more than one genetic mechanism for predisposing to human SLE. This is already suggested by family studies indicating that in addition to the usual female-oriented disease, certain families have Y chromosome-associated disease (like BXSB) [136]. The possibility that different patients might have different bases for disease is supported by recent cluster analyses of patients' signs and symptoms of disease [137] and the many similarities between autoimmune patients and autoimmune mice (Table 6) [16, 19, 47, 48, 85, 136, 140—148]. Moreover, the possibility of different genetic bases leaves open the possibility that somewhat different pathways to illness exist. If so, different approaches to therapy might be indicated in the different situations. Finally, attempts at prevention or prophylaxis would depend upon a fundamental understanding of the molecular genetic basis of disease. Quite different approaches to patient populations would be dictated by more than one genetic mechanism. As a result, the murine genetic studies should point the way to new approaches to the human condition. If two patients differ, we should not throw our hands up in despair. Rather, we should be aware of the possibility that different mechanisms may underlie disease in the two individuals and that appropriate approaches to each may still be devised.

References

1. Bielschowsky M, Helyer BJ, Howie JB (1959) Spontaneous anemia in mice of the NZB/BL strain. Proc Univ Otago Med Sch 37:9—11
2. Shirai T, Mellors RC (1979) Natural thymocytotoxic antibody and reactive antigen in New Zealand Black and other mice. Proc Natl Acad Sci USA 68:1412—1415
3. Klassen LW, Krakauer RS, Steinberg AD (1977) Selective loss of suppressor cell function in New Zealand mice induced by NTA. J Immunol 119:830—837
4. Detteer DH, Edgington TS (1976) Cellular events associated with the immunogenesis of anti-erythocyte autoantibody responses of NZB mice. Transplant. Rev. 31:116—155.
5. Mellors RC (1965) Autoimmune disease in NZB/BL mice. I. Pathology and pathogenesis of a model system of spontaneous glomerulonephritis. J Exp Med 122:25
6. Howie JB, Helyer BJ (1968) The immunology and pathology of NZB mice. Adv Immunol 9:215—266
7. Raveche ES, Tjio JH, Steinberg AD (1980) Genetic studies in NZB mice. IV. The effect of sex hormones on the spontaneous production of anti-T cell autoantibodies. Arthritis Rheum 23:48—56
8. Helyer BJ, Howie JB (1963) Renal disease associated with positive lupus erythematosus tests in a cross-bred strain of mice. Nature 197:197—198
9. Holmes MC, Burnet FM (1964) The inheritance of autoimmune disease in mice. A study of hybrids of the strains NZB and C3H. Heredity (Edinburgh) 19:419—428

Genetic Aspects of Murine Lupus   43

10. Datta SK, Owen FL Womack JE, Riblet RJ (1982) Analysis of recombinant inbred lines derived from "autoimmune" (NZB) and "high leukemia" (C58) strains: independent multigenic systems control B cell hyperactivity, retrovirus expression, and autoimmunity. J Immunol 129:1539

11. Miller ML, Raveche ES, Laskin CA, Klinman DM Steinberg AD (1984) Genetic studies in NZB mice: IV. Association of autoimmune traits in recombinant inbred mice. J Immunol 133:1325—1331

12. Braverman IM (1968) Study of autoimmune disease in New Zealand mice: I. Genetic features and natural history of NZB, NZY and NZW strains and NZB/NZW hybrids. J Invest Dermatol 50:483—499

13. Yoshida H, Kohno A, Ohta K, Hirose S, Maruyama N, Shirai T (1981) Genetic studies of autoimmunity in New Zealand mice: III. Association among anti-DNA antibodies NTA, and renal disease in (NZB × NZW)F₁ × NZW backcross mice. J Immunol 127:433

14. Izui S, McConahey PJ, Clark JP, Hang LM, Hara I, Dixon FJ (1981) Retroviral gp70 immune complexes in NZB × NZW F₂ mice with murine lupus nephritis. J Exp Med 154:517

15. Warner NL (1977) Genetic control of autoimmunity. In: Talal N (ed), Autoimmunity, Academic, New York, p 33

16. Raveche ES, Steinberg AD, Klassen LW, Tjio JH (1978) Genetic studies in NZB mice: I. Spontaneous autoantibody production. J Exp Med 147:1487—1502

17. Riblet R, Claflin L, Gibson DM, Mathieson BJ, Weigert M (1980) Antibody gene linkage studies in (NZB × C58) recombinant-inbred lines. J Immunol 124:787

18. Riblet RJ (1980) Genetic analysis of autoimmune disease NZB × C58 recombinant inbred strains. Presented at the 64th Annual Meeting of the Federation of American Societies for Experimental Biology, April 13—18, 1980, Anaheim, CA, USA

19. Raveche ES, Novotny EA, Hansen CT, Tjio JH, Steinberg AD (1981) Genetic studies in NZB mice. V. Recombinant inbred lines demonstrate that separate genes control autoimmune phenotype. J Exp Med 153:1187—1197

20. Steinberg AD, Huston DP, Taurog JD et al. (1981) The cellular and genetic basis for murine lupus. Immunol Rev 55:121

21. Raveche ES, Tjio JH, Boegal WA, Steinberg AD (1979) Studies of the effects of sex hormones on autosomal and X-linked genetic control of induced and spontaneous antibody production. Arthritis Rheum 22:1177—1187

22. Raveche ES, Tjio JH, Steinberg AD (1979) Genetic studies in NZB mice. II. Hyperdiploidy in the spleen of NZB mice and their hybrids. Cytogenet Cell Genet 23:182—193

23. Fischer-Lindahl K, Burk K (1982) Mta, a maternally inherited cell surface antigen of the mouse, is transmitted in the egg. Proc Natl Acad Sci USA 79:5362

24. Huston MM, Smith R, Huston DP, Rich RR (1983) Differences in maternal lineages of New Zealand Black mice defined by restriction endonuclease analysis of mitochondrial DNA and by expression of maternally transmitted antigen. J Exp Med 157:2154

25. Staples PJ, Steinberg AD, Talal N (1970) Induction of immunologic tolerance in old New Zealand mice repopulated with young spleen, bone marrow, or thymus. J Exp Med 131:1223—1238

26. Melez KA, Reeves JP, Steinberg AD (1978) Regulation of the expression of autoimmunity in NZB × NZW F₁ mice by sex hormones. J Immunopharmacol 1:27

27. Roubinian JR, Talal N, Greenspan JS, Goodman JR, Siiteri PK (1978) Effect of castration and sex hormone treatment on survival, anti-nucleic acid antibodies and glomerulonephritis in NZB × NZW F₁ mice. J Exp Med 147:1568—1583

28. Roubinian JR, Talal N, Greenspan JS, Goodman JR, Siiteri PK (1979) Delayed androgen treatment prolongs survival in murine lupus. J Clin Invest 63:902—911

29. Hang LM, Izui S, Dixon FJ (1981) (NZW × BXSB)F₁ hybrid. A model of acute lupus and coronary vascular disease with myocardial infarction. J Exp Med 154:216

30. Hudgins CC, Steinberg RT, Reeves JP, Steinberg AD (in press) Studies of congenic mice bearing the X chromosome of the BXSB mouse. J Immunol

31. Bielschowsky M, Bielschowsky F (1956) The New Zealand strain of obese mice. Their response to stilboesterol and insulin. Aust J Exp Biol Sci 34:181—198

32. Herberg L, Major E, Hennings U, Gruneklee D, Freytag G, Gries FA (1970) Differences in the development of the obese hyperglycermic syndrome in ob/ob and NZO mice. Diabetelogia 6:292—299
33. Bielschowsky M, Goodall CM (1970) Origin of inbred NZ mouse strain. Cancer Res 30:834—836
34. Melez KA, Harrison CC, Gilliam JN, Steinberg AD (1980) Diabetes 29:835—840
35. Levy JA, Pincus T (1970) Demonstration of biological activity of a murine leukemia virus of New Zealand black mice. Science 170:326—327
36. Mellors RC, Aoki T, Huebner RJ (1969) Further implications of murine leukemia-like virus in the disorder of NZB mice. J Exp Med 129:1045—1061
37. Mellors RC, Shirai T, Aoki T (1971) Wildtype gross leukemia virus and the pathogenesis of the glomerulonephritis of New Zealand mice. J Exp Med 133:113
38. Izui S, McConahey PJ, Theofilopoulos AN, Dixon FJ (1979) Association of circulating retroviral gp70-anti-gp70 immune complexes with murine systemic lupus erythematosus. J Exp Med 149:1099
39. Dixon FJ, Oldstone MBA, Tonietti G (1971) Pathogenesis of immune complex glomerulonephritis of New Zealand mice. J Exp Med 134:65s—71s
40. Maruyama N, Furukawa F, Nakai Y, Sasaki Y, Ohta K, Ozaki S, Hirose S, Shirai T (1983) Genetic studies of autoimmunity in New Zealand mice. IV. Contribution of NZB and NZW genes to the spontaneous occurrence of retroviral gp70 immune complexes in (NZB × NZW)F_1 hybrid and the correlation to renal disease. J Immunol 130:740
41. Levy JA, Johner J, Nayar KT, Kouri RE (1979) Genetics of xenotropic virus expression in mice. I. Evidence for a single locus regulating spontaneous production of infectious virus in crosses involving NZB/BlNJ and 129/J strains of mice. J Virol 30:754
42. Putman DL, Nayar KT, O'Neill B, Premkumar-Reddy E, Levy JA, Kouri RE (1983) Genetics of xenotropic virus expression in mice. II. Expression of major virus structural proteins in crosses involving NZB/BlNJ, SWR/J, and 129/J strains of mice. Proc Soc Exp Biol Med 173:219
43. Datta SK, Schwartz RS (1976) Genetics of expression of xenotropic virus and autoimmunity in NZB mice. Nature 263:412
44. Datta SK, McConahey PJ, Manny N, Theofilopoulos AN, Dixon FJ, Schwartz RS (1978) Genetic studies of autoimmunity and retrovirus expression in crosses of New Zealand Black mice. II. The viral envelope glycoprotein gp70. J Exp Med 147:872
45. Datta SK, Schwartz RS (1978) Genetic, viral and immunologic aspects of autoimmune disease in NZB mice. In: Rose NR, Bigazzi PE, Warner NL (eds) Genetic Control of autoimmune disease. Elsevier/North-Holland, New York, p 193
46. Izui S, McConahey PJ, Clark JP, Hang LM, Hara I, Dixon FJ (1981) Retroviral gp70 immune complexes in NZB × NZW F_2 mice with murine lupus nephritis. J Exp Med 154:517
47. Taurog JD, Raveche ES, Smathers PA, Glimcher LH, Huston DP, Hansen CT, Steinberg AD (1981) T cell abnormalities in NZB mice occur independently of autoantibody production. J Exp Med 153:221
48. Steinberg BJ, Smathers PA, Frederiksen K, Steinberg AD (1982) Ability of the *xid* gene to prevent autoimmunity in (NZB × NZW)F_1 mice during the course of their natural history after polyclonal stimulation or following immunization with DNA. J Clin Invest 70:587—597
49. Smathers PA, Steinberg BJ, Reeves JP, Steinberg AD (1982) Effects of polyclonal immune stimulators upon NZB.*xid* congenic mice. J Immunol 128:1414—1419
50. Ohsugi I, Gershwin ME, Ahmed A, Skelly R, Milich DR (1982) Studies of congenitally immunologic mutant New Zealand mice. IV. Spontaneous and induced autoantibodies to red cells and DNA occur in New Zealand X-linked immunodeficient mice without phenotypic alterations of the *xid* gene or generalized polyclonal B cell activation. J Immunol 128:2220—2227
51. Cohen DI, Steinberg AD, Paul WE, Davis MM (1985) Expression of an X-linked gene family. Nature

Genetic Aspects of Murine Lupus   45

52. Cohen DI, Hedrick, Nielsen EA, D'Eustachio P, Ruddle F, Steinberg AD, Paul WE, Davis MM (in press) Isolation of a cDNA clone corresponding to an X-linked gene family (XLR) closely linked to the murine immunodeficiency gene, *xid*. Nature
53. Murphy ED, Roths JB (1978) New inbred strains. Mouse News Letter 58:51
54. Murphy ED, Roths JB (1979) A Y-chromosome associated factor in strain BXSB producing accelerated autoimmunity and lymphoproliferation. Arthritis Rheum 22:1188
55. Andrews BB, Eisenberg RA, Theofilopoulos AN, Izui S, Wilson CB, McConahey PJ, Murphy ED, Roths JB, Dixon FJ (1978) Spontaneous murine lupus-like syndromes. Clinical and immunopathological manifestations in several strains. J Exp Med 148:1198
56. Theofilopoulos AN, Shawler DL, Eisenberg RA, Dixon FJ (1980) Splenic immunoglobulin-secreting cells and their regulation in autoimmune mice. J Exp Med 151:446
57. Theofilopoulos AN, Dixon FJ (1981) Etiopathogenesis of murine lupus. Immunol Rev 55:179
58. Roths JB, Murphy ED, Eicher EM (1984) A new mutation, *gld,* that produces lymphoproliferation and autoimmunity in C3H/HeJ mice. J Exp Med 159:1
59. Berden JHM, Hang LM, McConahey PJ, Dixon FJ (1983) Analysis of vascular lesions in murine SLE. I. Association with serologic abnormalities. J Immunol 130:1699
60. Eisenberg RA, Dixon FJ (1980) Effect of castration on male-determined acceleration of autoimmune disease in BXSB mice. J Immunol 125:1959
61. Eisenberg RA, Izui S, McConahey PJ et al. (1980) Male determined accelerated autoimmune disease in BXSB mice: transfer by bone marrow and spleen cells. J Immunol. 125:1032
62. Laskin CA, Taurog JD, Smathers PA, Steinberg AD (1981) Studies of defective tolerance in murine lupus. J Immunol 127:1743
63. Hang L, Izui S, Slack JH, Dixon FJ (1982) The cellular basis for resistance to induction of tolerance in BXSB SLE male mice. J Immunol 129:787
64. Izui S, Masuda K (1984) Resistance to tolerance induction is not prerequisite to development of murine SLE. J Immunol 133:3010
65. Smith HR, Chused TM, Steinberg AD (1983) The effect of the X-linked immune deficiency gene *(xid)* upon the Y chromosome-related disease of BXSB mice. J Immunol 131:1257
66. Prud'homme G, Balderas RS, Dixon FJ, Theofilopoulos AN (1983) B cell dependence on the response to accessory signals in murine lupus strains. J Exp Med 157:1815
67. Scher I, Ahmed A, Strong D, Steinberg AD, Paul WE (1975) X-linked B-lymphocyte immune defect in the CBA/hN mice. I. Studies of the function and composition of spleen cells. J Exp Med 141:788
68. Scher I, Steinberg AD, Berning AD, Paul WE (1975) X-linked B-lymphocyte immune defect in CBA/N mice. II. Studies of mechanisms underlying the immune defect. J Exp Med 142:637
69. Cowdery JS Jr, Steinberg AD (1980) Genetic studies in MRL/l and BXSB mice. The effect of the CBA/N *xid* on autoimmunity in F_1 and backcross mice. Fed Proc 39:1129
70. Golding B, Golding H, Foiles PG, Morton JI (1983) CBA/N X-linked defect delays expression of the Y-linked accelerated autoimmune disease in BXSB mice. J Immunol 130:1043.
71. Reeves JP, Taurog JD, Steinberg AD (1981) Polyclonal B-cell activation of autoantibodies in (CBA/N × NZB)F_1 mice by polyinosinic.polycytidylic acid. Clin Immunol Immunopathol 19:170
72. Rosenberg YJ, Steinberg AD (1984) Influence of Y and X chromosomes on B cell responses in autoimmune prone mice. J Immunol 132:1251
73. Kelly K, Cochran BH, Stiles CD, Leder P (1983) Cell-specific regulation of the c-*myc* gene by lymphocyte mitogens and platelet-derived growth factor. Cell 35:603
74. Persson H, Leder P (1984) Nuclear localization and DNA binding properties of a protein expressed by human c-*myc* oncogene. Science 225:718
75. Murphy ED, Roths JB (1978) A single gene model for massive lymphoproliferation with immune complex disease in new mouse strain MRL. Proceedings of the 16th International Conference on Hematology. Excerpta Medica, Amsterdam, p 68
76. Pisetsky DS, McCarty GA, Peters DV (1980) Mechanisms of autoantibody production in autoimmune MRL mice. J Exp Med 152:1302

77. Pisetsky DS, Caster SA, Roths JB, Murphy ED (1982) *lpr* gene control of the anti-DNA antibody response. J Immunol 128:2322
78. Theofilopoulos AN, Balderas RS, Shawler DL, Lee S, Dixon FJ (1981) Influence of thymic genotype on the systemic lupus erythematosus-like disease and T cell proliferation of MRL/Mp-*lpr/lpr* mice. J Exp Med 153:1405
79. Murphy ED, Roths JB (1978) Autoimmunity and lymphoproliferation: induction by mutant gene *lpr,* and acceleration by a male-associated factor in strain BXSB mice. In: Rose NR, Bigazzi PE, Warner NL (eds) Genetic control of autoimmune disease. Elsevier/North Holland, New York, p 207
80. Gershon RR, Horowitz M, Kemp JD, Murphy DB, Murphy ED (1978) The cellular site of immunoregulatory breakdown in the *lpr* mutant mouse. Genetic control of autoimmune disease: developments in immunology, vol 1. Elsevier/North-Holland, New York
81. Murphy ED (1981) Lymphoproliferation *(lpr)* and other single-locus models of murine lupus. In: Gershwin ME, Merchant B (eds) Immunologic defects in laboratory animals, Vol 2. Plenum, New York, pp 143—173
82. Davidson WF, Roths JB, Morse HB (1984) Single gene mutations that cause SLE like autoimmune disease in mice. Clin Immunol News Letter 5:17—20
83. Izui S, Kelly VE, Masuda K, Yoshida H, Roth JB, Murphy ED (1984) Induction of various autoantibodies by mutant gene *lpr* in several strains of mice. J Immunol 133:227
84. Steinberg AD, Roths JB, Murphy ED, Steinberg RT, Raveche ES (1980) Effects of thymectomy or androgen administration upon the autoimmune disease of MRL/Mp-*lpr/lpr* mice. J Immunol 125:871-873
85. Steinberg EB, Santoro TJ, Chused TM, Smathers PA, Steinberg AD (1983) Studies of congenic MRL-*lpr/lpr.xid* mice. J Immunol 131:2789—2795
86. Cronin PS, Sing AP, Glimcher LH, Kelly VE, Reinisch CL (1984) The isolation and functional characterization of autoimmune clones expressing inappropriate Ia. J Immunol 133:822
87. Roths JB, Murphy ED, Eicher EM (1984) A new mutation, *gld* that produces lymphoproliferation and autoimmunity in C3H/HeJ mice. J Exp Med 159:1—20
88. Mountz JD, Steinberg AD, Klinman DM, Smith HR, Mushinski JF (1984) Autoimmunity and increased c-*myb* transcription. Science 1087—1089
89. Mountz JD, Mushinski JF, Steinberg AD (1985) Specific gene products are expressed differentially in lymphoid organs of autoimmune mice. J Mol Cell Immunol (in press)
90. Mountz JD, Mushinski JF, Smith HR, Steinberg AD (1985) Modulation of c-*myb* transcription in autoimmune disease by cyclophosphamide. (submitted)
91. Bishop JM (1983) Cellular oncogenes and retroviruses. Annu Rev Biochem 52:301—354
92. Waterfield MD, Scrace GT, Shittle N, Stroobant P, Johnson A, Wasteson A, Westermails B, Heldin CH, Huang JS, Devels TF (1983) Platelet-derived growth factor is structurally related to the putative transforming protein p28 SIS of simian sarcoma virus. Nature 304:35—39
93. Downward J, Yarden Y, Mayes E, Scrace G. Totty N, Stockwell P, Ullrich A, Schlessinger J, Waterfield MD (1984) Close similitarity of epidermal cell growth factor receptor and v-*erb*-B oncogene protein sequences. Nature 307:521—526
94. Heldin CH, Westermails B (1984) Growth factors: mechanisms of action and relations to oncogenes. Cell 37:9—14
95. Cooper GM (1982) Cellular transforming genes. Science 217:801—806
96. Kelly K, Cochran BH, Stiles CD, Leder P (1983) Cell-specific regulation of the c-*myc* gene by lymphocyte mitogens and platelet-derived growth factor. Cell 35:603—610
97. Klempnauer KH, Symonds G, Evan GI, Bishop JM (1984) Subcellular localization of proteins encoded by oncogenes of avian mycoblastosis virus E26 and by the chicken c-*myb* gene. Cell 37:537—547
98. Persson H, Leder P (1984) Nuclear localization and DNA binding properties of a protein expressed by human c-*myc* oncogene. Science 225:718—721
99. Mark GE, Rapp UR (1984) Primary structure of v-*raf:* relatedness to the *src* family of oncogenes. Science 224:285—289

100. Kozak C, Gunnell MA, Rapp UR (1984) A new oncogene, c-*raf* is located on mouse chromosome 6. J Virol 49:297—299
101. Taparowsky B, Suard Y, Fasano O, Shimizu K, Goldfarb M, Wigler M (1982) Activation of the T24 bladder carconoma transforming gene is linked to a single amino acid change. Nature 300:762—764
102a. Reddy EP, Reynolds RK, Santos E, Barbacid M (1982) A point mutation is responsible for the acquisition of transforming properties by the T24 human bladder carcinoma oncogene. Nature 300:149—152
102b. Tabin CJ, Bradley SM, Bargmann CI, Weinberg RA, Papageorge AG, Scolnick EM, Dhar R, Lowy DR, Chank EH (1982) Mechanism of activation of a human oncogene. Nature 300:143—148
103. Rosenberg YJ, Malek TR, Schaefer DE, Santoro TJ, Mark GE, Steinberg AD, Mountz JD (1985) Unusual expression of IL 2 receptors and both the c-*myb* and c-*raf* oncogenes in T cell lines and clones derived from autoimmune MRL-*lpr/lpr* mice. J Immunol (in press)
104. Greeser I, Guy-Grand D, Maury C, Maunoury M-T (1981) Interferon induces peripheral lymphadenopathy in mice. J Immunol 127:1569—1575
105. Smith HR, Chused TM, Steinberg AD (1984) Cyclophosphamide-induced changes in the MRL/*lpr/lpr* mouse: Effects upon cellular composition, immune function, and disease. Clin Immunol Immunopathol 30:51—61
106. Smathers PA, Santoro TJ, Chused TM, Steinberg AD (1984) Induction of massive extrathymic T cell proliferation in vivo. J Immunol (in press)
107. Raveche ES, Steinberg AD, DeFranco AL, Tijo JH (1982) Cell cycle analysis of lymphocyte activation in normal and autoimmune strains. J Immunol 129:1219—1226
108. Sheiness D, Gardinier M (1984) Expression of a proto-oncogene (Proto-*myb*) in hemopoietic tissues of mice. Mol Cell Biol 4:1206—1212
109. Smith JB, Talal N (1982) Significance of self-recognition and interleukin 2 for immunoregulation, autoimmunity and cancer. Scand J Immunol 16:269
110a. Wofsy D, Murphy ED, Roths JB, Daupinee MJ, Kipper SP, Talal N (1981) Deficient interleukin 2 activity in MRL/Mp and C57BL/6J mice bearing the *lpr* gene. J Exp Med 154:1671
110b. Altman A, Theofilopoulos AN, Weiner R, Katz DH, Dixon FJ (1981) Analysis of T cell function in autoimmune murine strains. Defects in production and responsiveness to interleukin 2. J Exp Med 154:791
111. Santoro TJ, Luger TA, Raveche ES, Smolen JS, Oppenheim JJ, Steinberg AD (1983) In vitro correction of the interleukin 2 defect in autoimmune mice. Eur J Immunol 13:601
112. Ruff MR, Pert CB (1984) Small cell carcinoma of the lung: macrophage-specific antigens suggest hemopoietic stem cell origin. Science 225:1034—1036
113. Smith HR, Steinberg AD (1983) Autoimmunity — A perspective. Ann Rev Immunol 1:175—210
114. Hayakawa K, Hardy RR, Honda M, Herzenberg LA, Steinberg AD, Herzenberg LA (1984) Ly-1 B cells: Functionally distinct lymphocytes that secrete IgM autoantibodies. Proc Natl Acad Sci USA 81:2494—2498
115. Theofilopoulos AN, Shawler DL, Eisenberg RA, Dixon FJ (1980) Splenic immunoglobulin-secreting cells and their regulation in autoimmune mice. J Exp Med 151:446—466
116. Theofilopoulos AN, Dixon FJ (1981) Etiopathogenesis of murine lupus. Immunol Rev 55:179—216
117. Steinberg AD, Raveche ES, Laskin CA, Smith HR, Santoro TJ, Miller ML, Plotz PH (1984) Systemic lupus erythematosus: Insights from animal models. Ann Intern Med 100:714—727
118. Smith HR, Chused TM, Smathers PA, Steinberg AD (1983) Evidence for thymic regulation of autoimmunity in BXSB mice: acceleration of disease by neonatal thymectomy. J Immunol 130:1200—1204
119. Scher I, Steinberg AD, Berning AK, Paul WE (1975) X-linked B-lymphocyte immune defect in CBA/N mice. II. Studies of mechanisms underlying the immune defect. J Exp Med 142:637—650
120. Hayward WS, Neel BG, Astrin SM (1981) Activation of a cellular *onc* gene by promoter insertion in ALV-induced lymphoid leukosis. Nature 290:475—480

121. Graham FL, van der Eb AJ (1973) A new technique for the assay of infectivity of human adenovirus 5 DNA. Virology 52:456—467
122. Parker BA, Stark GR (1979) Regulation of simian virus 40 transcription: Sensitive analysis of the RNA species presents early infections by virus or viral DNA. J Virol 31:360—369
123. Chu G, Sharp PA (1981) SV40 DNA transfection of cells in suspension: analysis of the efficiency of transcription and translation of T antigen gene. Scand J Immunol 13:197—202
124. Mann R, Mulligan RC, Baltimore D (1983) Construction of a retrovirus packaging mutant and its use to produce helper-free defective retrovirus. Cell 33:153—159
125. Mulligan RC (1984) Construction of highly transmissible mammalian cloning vehicles derived from murine retroviruses. In: Inouye M (ed) Academic, Orlando, pp 155—173
126. Williams DA, Lemischka IR, Nathan DG, Mulligan RC (1984) Introduction of new genetic material into pluripotent hematopoietic stem cells of mouse. Nature 310:476—480
127. Hedrick SM, Cohen DI, Nielsin EA, Davis MM (1984) Isolation of cDNA clones encoding T cell-specific membrane-associated proteins. Nature 308:149—153.
128. Yanagi Y, Yoshikai Y, Leggett K, Clark SP, Aleksander I, Mak TW (1984) A human T cell-specific cDNA clone encodes a protein having extensive homology to immunoglobulin chains. Nature 308:145—149
129. Saito H, Kranz DM, Takagaki Y, Hayday AC, Eisen HN, Tonegawa S (1984) A third rearranged and expressed gene in a clone of cytotoxic T lymphocytes. Nature 312:36—40
130. Krontiris TG, Cooper GM (1981) Transforming activity of human tumor DNA. Proc Natl Acad Sci USA 78:1181—1184
131. Murray MJ, Shilo B-Z, Sheh K. R., Cowing D, Hsu HW, Weinberg RA (1981) Three different human tumor cell lines contain different oncogenes. Cell 25:355—361
132. Perucho M, Goldfarb M, Shimiyu K, Leima C, Fogh J, Wigler M (1981) Human-tumor-derived cell lines contain common and different transforming genes. Cell 27:467—476
133. Pulciani S, Santos E, Lauver AV, Long LK, Robbins KC, Barbacid M (1982) Oncogenes in human tumor cell lines: Molecular cloning of a transforming gene from human bladder carcinoma cells. Proc Natl Acad Sci 79:2845—2849
134. Lo SC, Liotta LA (1985) Vascular tumors produced by NIH/3T3 cells transfected with human AIDS Kaposi's sarcoma DNA. Am J Pathol 118:7—13
135. Blair DG, Cooper CS, Oskarsson MK, Eader LA, Vande-Woude GF (1983) Tumorigenesis by transfected cells in nude mice: A new method of detecting cellular transforming genes. In: O'Connor TE, Rauscher FJ (eds) Oncogenes and retroviruses: evaluation of basic findings and clinical potential. Alan R. Liss, New York, pp 79—90
136. Lahita RG, Chiorazzi N, Gibofsky A, Winchester RJ, Kunkel HG (1983) Familial systemic lupus erythematosus in males. Arthritis Rheum 26:39—44
137. Lippmann SM, Arnett FC, Conley CL, Ness PM, Meyers DA, Bias WB (1982) Genetic factors predisposing to autoimmune disease: autoimmune hemolytic anemia, chronic thrombocytopenic purpura, and systemic lupus erythematosus. Am J Med 73:827—840
138. Arnett FC, Shulman LE (1976) Studies in familial systemic lupus erythematosus. Medicine 55:313
139. Block SR, Lockshin MD, Winfield JB et al (1976) Immunological observations on 9 sets of twins either concordant or discordant for SLE. Arthritis Rheum 19:454
140. Steinberg AD, Melez KA, Raveche ES et al (1979) Approach to the study of the role of sex hormones in autoimmunity. Arthritis Rheum 22:1170
141. Miller KB, Schwartz RS (1979) Familial abnormalities of suppressor-cell function in systemic lupus erythematosus. N Engl J Med 301:803
142. Morton RO, Gershwin ME, Brady C, Steinberg AD (1976) Incidence of systemic lupus erythematosus (SLE) in North American Indians. J Rheumatol 3:186
143. Reinertsen JL, Klippel JH, Johnson AH et al (1982) Family studies of B lymphocyte alloantigens in systemic lupus erythematosus. J Rheumatol 9:253
144. Lippmann SM, Arnett FC, Conley CL et al. (1982) Genetic factors predisposing to autoimmune disease. Am J Med 73:827

145. Blaese RM, Grayson J, Steinberg AD (1980) Elevated immunoglobulin secreting cells in the blood of patients with active systemic lupus erythematosus: correlation of laboratory and clinical assessment of disease activity. Am J Med 69:345
146. Budman DR, Merchant EB, Steinberg AD et al (1977) Increased spontaneous activity of antibody-forming cells in the peripheral blood of patients with active SLE. Arthritis Rheum 20:829
147. Glinski W, Gershwin ME, Budman DR, Steinberg AD (1976) Study of lymphocyte subpopulation in normal humans and patients with systemic lupus erythematosus by fractionation of peripheral blood lymphocytes on a discontinuous Ficoll gradient. Clin Exp Immunol 26:228
148. Kumagai S, Sredni B, House S et al (1981) Defective regulation of B lymphocyte colony formation in patients with systemic lupus erythematosus. J Immunol 128:258
149. Steinberg AD, Smolen JS, Sakane T et al (1983) Immune regulatory abnormalities in systemic lupus erythematosus. In: Cummings N, Michael A, Wilson C (eds) Immune mechanisms of renal disease. Plenum, New York, pp 529—548

Autoimmune Disease in New Zealand Mice

T. M. CHUSED, K. L. MCCOY, R. B. LAL, TH. R. MALEK, E. M. BROWN,
L. J. EDISON, and P. J. BAKER

Introduction

Because the pathogenic mechanisms of spontaneous autoimmune diseases in human patients have not been elucidated, researchers have studied animal models with the expectation that their experimental accessibility and defined genetic scope will facilitate understanding of the autoimmune process. These efforts have focused on several lines of inbred mice that spontaneously develop genetically conditioned autoimmune disease. Our work emphasizes the study of New Zealand mice, because their clinical disorders and genetic complexity most closely resemble human disease. Several strains of New Zealand mice were inbred, selecting for coat color, by Dr. Marianne Beilschowsky at the University of Otago in Dunedin, New Zealand during the 1950s. In the eleventh inbred generation, it was noted that the mice of the New Zealand Black (NZB) strain developed autoimmune hemolytic anemia — the first animal model of autoimmune disease [1, 2]. Subsequent crosses with other strains revealed that the F_1 hybrid of NZB with New Zealand White (NZW) mice develops lupus erythematosus in which anti-DNA and anti-gp70 autoantibodies cause immune complex glomerulonephritis [3]. Interestingly, the NZW strain is immunologically normal, at least until very late in life. As in most human autoimmune disorders, female (NZB × NZW) F_1 mice are more severely affected than males. The results of castration and sex hormone replacement experiments have shown that this is a hormonal effect [4, 5].

A number of pertinent observations on the immunologic disorder of New Zealand mice have been reported. These include the fact that B cells in NZB mice are polyclonally activated to IgM (but not IgG) production at the beginning of life [6—9]. Splenic B cells from all F_1 hybrids derived from crosses between NZB mice and other inbred strains produce one third to one half the amount of IgM produced by the NZB parent, indicating that this trait is semidominant. This abnormality is independent of T-lymphocytes, because it occurs in *nu/nu* and T cell-deprived thymectomized, irradiated, fetal liver-reconstituted NZB mice [10]. It is accompanied by increased expression of surface IgM receptors and decreased levels of surface IgD on the B cells of NZB mice [11, 12]. In addition, NZB mice are resistant to the experimental induction of immunologic tolerance prior to the onset of autoimmune disease [13—15]. Investigators using different methods and a variety of test antigens have attributed the difficulty in inducing tolerance to both T and B cell dysfunction; thus, the nature of this defect has not been clarified [16—21].

The genetic basis of autoimmune disease in New Zealand mice is extremely complex. Abnormalities such as B cell hyperactivity, tolerance resistance, and the formation of antithymocyte and antierythrocyte autoantibodies appear to be controlled by different genes or groups of genes [22—28]. It is clear, however, that NZW immune response genes within the major histocompatibility complex of the H-2^z haplotype facilitate the immunologic recognition of DNA [29]. Replacement of the H-2^z haplotype of NZW mice with the H-2^d haplotype from NZB mice (to generate the NZW strain congenic for H-2^d, named ZWD) greatly reduces the level of anti-DNA antibodies, but not of serum immunoglobulin, in the (NZB × ZWD) F$_1$ hybrid; this prolongs the survival of (NZB × ZWD) F$_1$ hybrids in comparison with the unmanipulated (NZB × NZW) F$_1$ mice [30].

An important feature of New Zealand mouse disease is that B cell hyperactivity and resistance to tolerance are fully established by 6—8 weeks of age, but overt autoimmune disease (formation of antierythrocyte and anti-DNA autoantibodies, and the development of hemolytic anemia and/or immune complex glomerulonephritis) does not appear until 6—12 months of age. We have examined NZB mice, during the interval between the development of immunologic maturity and the onset of disease, for alterations in lymphocyte cell surface antigen phenotype, abnormal lymphocyte protein synthesis, and changes in lymphocyte function. This review summarizes some of our findings and describes the results of recent studies on tolerance resistance and the analysis of NZB lymphocyte proteins by two-dimensional polyacrylamide gel electrophoresis.

Results

Changes in NZB Lymphocytes with Age

Longitudinal analysis of splenic T, B, and null cell populations in NZB mice during the first year of life by flow cytometry revealed: (a) a progressive shift in the B cell population from surface IgD bright, IgM dull to IgD dull, IgM bright; (b) progressive elevation of IgG-containing plasma cells after 6 months of age; (c) the appearance of IL-2 receptors on some B cells, but not T cells, as shown in Fig. 1; (d) a slight decrease in the ratio of Lyt-2$^+$ (suppressor, cytotoxic) to Lyt-2$^-$ (helper, inducer) T cells; (e) the sudden onset of splenomegaly caused by proliferation of null cells, beginning at about 10 months of age; and (f) an increase in cell size (determined by narrow-angle forward light scatter) of the Lyt-2$^+$ but not the Lyt-2$^-$ T cells after 10 months of age [31]. Although larger in size, two-color flow cytometry with the DNA stain Hoechst 33342 and anti-Lyt-2 showed that the Lyt-2$^+$ cells did not enter the S phase of the cell cycle. Consistent with the lack of proliferation, the total number of splenic Lyt-2$^+$ T cells did not change as NZB mice age. Alterations in the B lymphocyte population did not correlate with any other changes observed, including those in the T cell population, indicating that they follow a distinct "program."

The unusual enlargement of the Lyt-2⁺ T cells in aging NZB mice prompted us to ask whether enlargement is correlated with the onset of disease. We examined individual NZB mice for Lyt-2⁺ T cell size, antierythrocyte autoantibodies, anemia, proteinuria, and splenomegaly. Lyt-2⁺ T cell size was found to correlate with the level of anti-erythrocyte autoantibodies ($P<0.002$) and the severity of

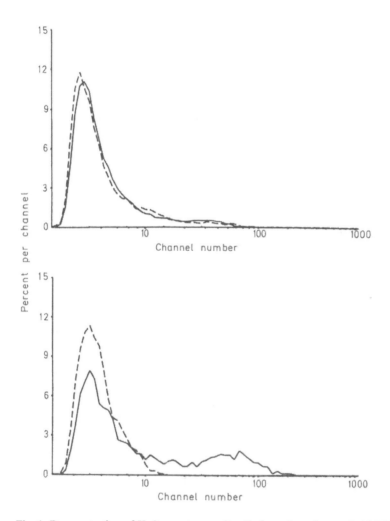

Fig. 1. Demonstration of IL-2 receptors on B cells from the spleens of old NZB mice. Spleen cells were stained for green fluorescence with directly fluoresceinated monoclonal anti-IL-2 receptor antibody and for red fluorescence with B cell-specific biotinylated monoclonal anti-B220 followed by Texas Red-conjugated avidin. The *lower panel* shows the green fluorescence staining of IL-2 receptor for B220⁺ (red positive) B cells from the spleen of a 50-week-old NZB mouse *(solid line)*. As a control for nonspecific staining, the spleen cells were first incubated with unlabeled anti-IL-2 receptor, then stained as above *(dashed line)*; this shows that the straining was specific. Approximately 22% of the B cells are brighter than the control. The *upper panel* shows the same two staining protocols for spleen cells from an 8-week-old NZB mouse, indicating that no IL-2 receptor-positive B cells were present

Autoimmune Disease in New Zealand Mice   53

hemolytic anemia ($P<0.04$), but not with proteinuria or splenomegaly [32]. NZB mice congenic for *xid,* the gene causing X-linked immunodeficiency, which inhibits B cell hyperactivity and prevents the development of autoimmune disease [33], failed to develop enlarged Lyt-2[+] T cells. Similarly, the phenomenon was not observed in (NZB × NZW) F_1 or (NZB × NFS) F_1 hybrids. Thus, the enlargement of the Lyt-2[+] T cells appears to depend on both the NZB B cell hyperactivity and recessive genetic factors.

For closer definition of the functional status of the enlarged Lyt-2[+] T cells in old NZB mice developing hemolytic anemia, their lymphocytes were exposed to concanavalin A both in vitro and in vivo. The in vitro proliferative responses to concanavalin A by both the L3T4[+] and Lyt-2[+] T cells from the old mice were reduced by approximately 75%, and induction of IL-2 receptors was decreased about 50% (Table 1). Only after in vivo treatment with concanavalin A was a significant difference between the Lyt-2[+] and L3T4[+] T cell responses observed (Table 2). IL-2 receptors were induced on the L3T4[+] T cells from old mice at 35% of the level observed in young animals; however, IL-2 receptors could not be induced on Lyt-2[+] T cells from old NZB mice. Thus, in vivo activation of Lyt-2[+], but not L3T4[+], T cells is completely blocked in old NZB mice. That this block is partially relieved upon culture of these cells suggests that in vivo it depends either on a short-lived factor or on intact lymphoid architecture.

Flow cytometric examination indicated that in old NZB and (NZB × NZW) F_1 mice splenic L3T4[+] and Lyt-2[+] T cells had similar amounts of autoantibody on

Table 1. Responses of splenic T cells from NZB mice

Age	Cells	^{3}H-TdR incorporation[a]		IL-2 receptor expression[b]	
		Con A	*Medium*	*Con A*	*Medium*
8 weeks	Unfractionated	324	9		
	Lyt-2[+] T cells	314	10	72	4
	L3T4[+] T cells	183	13	77	6
60 weeks	Unfractionated	37	2		
	Lyt-2[+] T cells	42	3	38	7
	L3T4[+] T cells	18	4	34	9

[a] cpm × 10^{-3}
[b] Percent positive

Table 2. Lack of IL-2 receptor induction in vivo on Lyt-2[+] T cells from old NZB mice

Age	Treatment	Percent expressing IL-2 receptors	
		Lyt-2[+] T cells	L3T4[+] T Cells
Young	Con A	7.2	12.9
	Saline	0.9	1.2
Old	Con A	1.3	5.5
	Saline	2.1	1.4

their cell surfaces. Since Lyt-2$^+$ T cells enlarge in NZB, but not (NZB × NZW) F$_1$, mice it is unlikely that anti-T cell autoantibodies play a role in this process.

To assess the functional capacity of enlarged Lyt-2$^+$ T cells in NZB mice, old and young animals were given concanavalin A for nonspecific activation of T suppressor cells involved in the antibody response to type III pneumococcal polysaccharide (SSS-III); the degree of suppression induced was then determined [34]. As in normal strains, the anti-SSS-III antibody response of young NZB mice was suppressed substantially by concanavalin A, whereas the response of old NZB mice with enlarged Lyt-2$^+$ T cells was paradoxically enhanced [32].

The expression of regulatory T cell activity for the antibody response to SSS-III was also used to analyze further the state of T suppressor cells in aging NZB mice. Treatment (priming) with a subimmunogenic dose of SSS-III prior to immunization induces an antigen-specific state of unresponsiveness mediated by T suppressor cells [35]. Although low-dose paralysis can be induced in nonautoimmune BALB/c mice at all ages tested, it is significantly diminished in NZB mice at 36 weeks of age, and nearly absent in NZB mice at 52 weeks of age (Table 3).

Adoptive transfer of Lyt-2$^+$ T cells from low-dose SSS-III-primed BALB/c mice to naive animals of the same strain resulted in antigen-specific suppression of the antibody response to SSS-III upon subsequent immunization of recipients. Suppression could also be transferred by primed Lyt-2$^+$ T cells from young to old animals and vice versa. By contrast, normal-sized Lyt-2$^+$ T cells from low-dose primed old NZB mice were able to transfer suppression to young NZB mice; however, enlarged Lyt-2$^+$ T cells from old NZB mice were without effect [36]. Studies in which cells were transferred from young into old NZB mice demonstrated still another immunologic defect: the antibody response of old NZB mice to SSS-III was not reduced by Lyt-2$^+$ T cells, even though the same cells were effective upon transfer to young mice. These results suggest that two defects are involved in the decline of low-dose paralysis to SSS-III in aging NZB mice: (a) enlarged Lyt-2$^+$ T cells appear to lose their ability to function as mediators of suppression; and (b) B cells become resistant to T-cell-mediated suppression. B cell resistance to suppression may be related to alteration in cell surface antigen phenotype and activation, as suggested by the expression of IL-2 receptors.

Table 3. Reduced low-dose paralysis in response to SSS-III in old NZB mice

Strain	Percent suppression by low-dose priming at age (weeks)			
	12	24	36	52
BALB/c	82	68	83	80
NZB	82	57	49	18

Tolerance Defects in New Zealand Mice

The loss of tolerance to particular self-antigens is associated with the development of autoimmune disease in NZB and (NZB × NZW) F_1 mice. Experimental induction of tolerance to foreign antigens has been studied to enhance understanding of the failure to maintain self-tolerance in autoimmune mice. Abnormalities of both B and T cells have been implicated in the resistance to tolerance induction of New Zealand mice [15—19]. To resolve this question, we developed a system that allows separate assessment of tolerance in the T and B cell compartments in vivo. Unresponsiveness was induced with monomeric bovine serum albumin (BSA). The effectiveness of tolerance induction was determined by challenging with dinitrophenyl (DNP)-conjugated BSA and measuring the serum anti-hapten and anti-carrier antibody levels of individual mice. Treatment with monomeric BSA induced tolerance in the T helper population, whereas B cells specific for DNP remained capable of responding to hapten. Obviously, a defect affecting T helper tolerance would prevent the development of tolerance to both hapten and carrier; by contrast, a defect affecting only B cells would impair tolerance only to the carrier.

Application of this system to normal NFS and NZW mice showed that doses of 10—1000 µg of monomeric BSA induced tolerance to both BSA and DNP (Table 4). In NZB mice tolerance to BSA was not induced by any dose. Unlike the anti-carrier response, the anti-DNP response of NZB mice decreased with increasing doses of BSA, so that 1000 µg BSA induced the same reduction of anti-hapten antibodies as in control mice.

The mode of inheritance of this abnormality in the induction of tolerance was determined by testing NZB F_1 hybrids. NZB, (NZB × B10.D2) F_1, and

Table 4. Resistance of NZB mice to induction of tolerance

Mouse strain	Monomeric BSA (µg)	Percent reduction of response to BSA	DNP
NFS	10	99	99
	100	99	99
	1000	99	99
NZW	10	98	99
	100	98	99
	1000	99	99
NZB	10	−28	26
	100	11	82
	1000	−45	99
NZB × B10.D2 F_1	1000	−23	79
NZB × NFS F_1	1000	33	96
NZB × NZW F_1	1000	−35	20
NZB.xid ♀	1000	99	99
NZB.xid × NZW F_1 ♀	1000	55	−56
NZB.xid × NZW F_1 ♂	1000	16	2

(NZB × NFS) F_1 mice express the same phenotype for the induction of tolerance, i.e., monomeric BSA induces tolerance to DNP but not to BSA when presented as a conjugate. Surprisingly, (NZB × NZW) F_1 mice generated an antibody response to both DNP and BSA after receiving the same treatment (Table 4). These results suggest that (NZB × NZW) F_1 mice express a major defect in T helper cell tolerance, whereas the parental NZB exhibits a less profound abnormality. The severe (NZB × NZW) F_1 defect presumably results from the combined effects of several genes.

To further characterize the lymphocyte subsets responsible for the NZB and (NZB × NZW) F_1 tolerance defects, we examined the effect of the *xid* gene on the abnormal antibody responses (Table 4). The presence of this gene, which suppresses the spontaneous polyclonal B cell activation of NZB mice [33] but does not affect T cells, causes NZB mice to become susceptible to tolerance induction. NZB.*xid* mice treated with monomeric BSA do not produce anti-BSA after challenge; this suggests that the anti-BSA response of similarly treated NZB mice may be associated with B cell hyperactivity. By contrast, male (NZB.*xid* × NZW) mice (which are phenotypically *xid*) and (NZB.*xid* × NZW) females (which are phenotypically normal) both manifest resistance to tolerance induction to BSA and DNP. The failure of the *xid* gene to correct the tolerance defect of (NZB × NZW) F_1 mice provides further evidence that this hybrid manifests substantial tolerance resistance in the T helper population.

Genetic Features of NZB Recombinant Inbred Lines

We have also initiated a study of NZB × NFS (a nonautoimmune inbred Swiss line) recombinant inbred (RI) lines and their F_1 progeny from crosses with NZW mice. Lymphocyte phenotype distribution, B cell activation, Ly1 expression by B lymphocytes, susceptibility to tolerance induction, null cell levels, leukemia virus expression, and other features were examined in young animals; older mice are now being followed for the late development of immunologic abnormalities. Although these studies are still in progress, four trends have emerged:

1. Nine of the 16 lines examined had an increase in the frequency of splenic IgM-containing plasma cells which correlated with a decrease in surface IgD expression. Only two lines had numbers of plasma cells as high as those of NZB mice. This suggests that at least two genes are involved in the B cell hyperactivity of NZB mice.
2. Elevated numbers of IgM plasma cells were significantly associated with the development of proteinuria in (RI × NZW) F_1 mice.
3. No single feature in young mice predicted the subsequent development of autoimmune disease.
4. In F_1 hybrids of the RI lines with NZW, IgM-containing plasma cell elevation early in life was associated with the later development of glomerulonephritis.

Two-Dimensional Gel Analysis of NZB Lymphocyte Proteins

To investigate the mechanism of autoimmune disease in NZB mice at the molecular level, we have analyzed radiolabeled proteins synthesized by NZB lymphocytes by two-dimensional polyacrylamide gel electrophoresis. We noted that the synthesis of two peptides (12.5 and 10.5 kd in size) decreased with age in control mice and then increased sharply in NZB mice as they developed overt autoimmune disease [37]. These nonsecreted cytoplasmic proteins were restricted to B and null cells.

An additional peptide, of 16 kd molecular weight, is restricted to the spontaneous B cell blasts found in the spleen of NZB mice. This protein was not induced by lipopolysaccharide stimulation of B cells from normal mice. Studies are currently in progress to define the role of this protein in the B cell hyperactivity of NZB mice.

Conclusions

These studies indicate that complex genetic and functional interactions unfolding over the life of the animals cause the development of autoimmune disease in New Zealand mice. Although each strain of autoimmune mice follows a unique path, our results suggest that various factors play a role in New Zealand mice:

1. Polyclonal B cell activation, which appears necessary, but not sufficient for the development of disease. Only IgM production is elevated in young animals, and this abnormality is intrinsic to B cells. The molecular basis of this phenomenon is not known but the possibility that the unique synthesis of several nonimmunoglobulin proteins, including the 16-kd peptide, by NZB B cell blasts may be related is being investigated.
2. There are age-related changes in the distribution of NZB B cell subsets. The expression of IL-2 receptors by B cells late in life when disease develops indicates a type of B cell activation distinct from that occurring in young animals. Either or both of these changes could be related to the age-dependent loss in B cell susceptibility to regulatory T cell signals.
3. New Zealand mice exhibit two types of tolerance defect. The (NZB × NZW) F_1 hybrid demonstrates a major block to the induction of tolerance in T helper cells, while the parental NZB shows partial resistance. The studies with NZB.*xid* mice suggest that NZB B cells may also manifest resistance to tolerance induction.
4. In NZB, but not (NZB × NZW) F_1 mice, Lyt-2$^+$ T suppressor cells enlarge in size become functionally impaired as antierythrocyte autoantibody and hemolytic anemia appear.
5. Finally, immune response genes permit the immunologic recognition of disease-associated self-antigens.

58 T. M. Chused et al.

Our results suggest a difference between the pathogenesis of autoimmune disease in NZB and (NZB × NZW) F_1 mice. While intrinsic B cell hyperactivity is common to both, the T cell abnormalities are distinct. The NZB stain has a much milder T helper tolerance defect than the (NZB × NZW) F_1 hybrid. It appears that the enlargement and associated loss of function of the Lyt-2$^+$ T suppressor cells in aging NZB mice coupled with the continued high expression of amplifier T cell activity (unpublished data) permits the emergence of antierythrocyte autoantibody and subsequent autoimmune hemolytic anemia. By contrast, the (NZB × NZW) F_1 mouse has a major defect in T helper tolerance. That this is present at immunologic maturity may explain the earlier onset of disease in the NZB × NZW F_1 than in the NZB mouse and the absence of Lyt-2$^+$ T cell enlargement.

Spontaneous autoimmune disease in humans, like that in New Zealand mice, is likely to have a complex genetic basis. Whether immunoregulatory defects of both T and B cells are required in humans as they appear to be in New Zealand mice is an important question for clinical research.

References

1. Bielschowsky M, Helyer BJ, Howie JB (1959) Spontaneous haemolytic anemia in mice of the NZB/BL strain. Proc Univ Otago Med Sch 37:9
2. Helyer BJ, Howie JW (1963) Spontaneous auto-immune disease in NZB/BL mice. Br J Haematol 9:119
3. Lambert PH, Dixon FJ (1968) Pathogenesis of the glomerulonephritis of NZB/W mice. J Exp Med 127:507
4. Talal N (1976) Disordered immunologic regulation and autoimmunity. Transplant Rev 31:240
5. Roubinian JR, Papoian R, Talal N (1977) Androgenic hormones modulate autoantibody responses and improve survival in murine lupus. J Clin Invest 59:1066
6. DeHeer DJ, Edginton T (1977) Evidence for a B lymphocyte defect underlying the anti-X anti-erythrocyte autoantibody response of NZB mice. J Immunol 118:1858
7. Moutsopoulos HM, Boehm-Truitt M, Kassan SS, Chused TM (1977) Demonstration of activation of B lymphocytes in New Zealand Black mice at birth by an immunoradiometric assay for murine IgM. J Immunol 119:1639
8. Izui S, McConahey PJ, Dixon FJ (1978) Increased spontaneous polyclonal activation of B lymphocytes in mice with spontaneous autoimmune disease. J Immunol 121:2213
9. Manny N, Datta SK, Schwartz RS (1979) Synthesis of IgM by cells of NZB and their crosses. J Immunol 122:1220
10. Chused TM, Moutsopoulos HM, Sharrow SO, Hansen CT (1979) Evidence of a primary B lymphocyte abnormality of NZB mice. In: Cooper M, Mosier DE, Scher I, Vitetta ES (eds) B lymphocytes in the immune response. Elsevier North Holland, New York, p 363
11. Cohen PL, Ziff M, Vitetta ES (1978) Characterization of a B cell defect in the NZB mouse manifested by an increased ratio of surface IgM to IgD. J Immunol 121:973
12. Manohar V, Brown E, Leiserson WM, Chused TM (1982) Expression of Lyt-1 by a subset of B lymphocytes. J Immunol 129:532
13. Weir DM, McBride W, Naysmith JD (1968) Immune response to a soluble protein antigen in NZB mice. Nature 219:1276
14. Staples PJ, Talal N (1969) Rapid loss of tolerance induced in weanling NZB and B/W F_1 mice. Science 163:1215
15. Staples PJ, Talal N (1969) Relative inability to induce tolerance in adult NZB and NZB/NZW F_1 mice. J Exp Med 129:123

Autoimmune Disease in New Zealand Mice   59

16. Laskin CA, Taurog JD, Smathers PA, Steinberg AD (1981) Studies of defective tolerance in murine lupus. J Immunol 127:1743
17. Taurog JD, Smathers PA, Steinberg AD (1980) Evidence for abnormalities of separate lymphocyte populations in NZB mice. J Immunol 125:485
18. Laskin CA, Smathers PA, Reeves JP, Steinberg AD (1982) Studies of defective tolerance induction in NZB mice: evidence for a marrow pre-T cell defect. J Exp Med 155:1025
19. Goldings EA, Cohen PL, McFadden SF, Ziff M, Vitetta ES (1980) Defective B cell tolerance in adult (NZB×NZW) F_1 mice. J Exp Med 152:730
20. Goldings EA (1983) Defective B cell tolerance induction in New Zealand Black mice. I. Macrophage independence and comparison with other autoimmune strains. J Immunol 131:2630
21. Laskin CA, Smathers PA, Leiberman R, Steinberg AD (1983) NZB cells actively interfere with the establishment of tolerance to BGG in radiation chimeras. J Immunol 131:1121
22. Ghaffar A, Playfair JHL (1971) The genetic basis of autoimmunity in NZB mice studied by progeny-testing. Clin Exp Immunol 8:479
23. Warner NL (1973) Genetic control of spontaneous and induced antierythrocyte autoantibody production in mice. Clin Immunol Immunopathol 1:353
24. Knight JG, Adams DD (1978) Three genes for lupus nephritis in NZB×NZW mice. J Exp Med 147:1653
25. Yoshida H, Kohno A, Ohta K, Hirose S, Maruyama N, Shirai T (1981) Genetic studies of autoimmunity in New Zealand mice. III. Associations among anti-DNA antibodies, NTA, and renal disease in (NZB×NZW) F1×NZW backcross mice. J Immunol 127:433
26. Boccieri MH, Cooke A, Smith JB, Weigert M, Riblet RJ (1982) Independent segregation of NZB immune abnormalities in NZB×C58 recombinant inbred mice. Eur J Immunol 12:349
27. Raveche ES, Novotny EA, Hansen CT, Tjio JH, Steinberg AD (1981) Genetic studies in NZB mice. V. Recombinant inbred lines demonstrate that separate genes control autoimmune phenotype. J Exp Med 153:1187
28. Maruyama N, Furukawa F, Nakai Y, Sasaki Y, Ohta K, Ozaki S, Hirose S, Shirai T (1983) Genetic studies of autoimmunity in New Zealand mice. IV. Contribution of NZB and NZW genes to the spontaneous occurrence of retroviral gp70 immune complexes in (NZB×NZW) F_1 hybrid and the correlation to renal disease. J Immunol 130:740
29. Papoian R, Talal N (1980) Ability of NZW but not NZB antigen-presenting cells to support T cell proliferative response to DNA methylated albumin. J Immunol 124:515
30. Hirose S, Nagasawa R, Sekikawa I, Hamaoki M, Ishida Y, Sato H, Shirai T (1983) Enhancing effect of H-2 linked NZW gene(s) on the autoimmune traits of (NZB×NZW) F1 mice. J Exp Med 158:228
31. Manohar V, Brown EM, Leiserson WM, Edison LJ, Chused TM (1984) Ly2$^+$ T cell enlargement and null cell proliferation occur at the onset of splenomegaly and autoantibody production in New Zealand Black mice. J Immunol 133:3020
32. McCoy KL, Baker PJ, Malek TR, Chused TM (1985) Enlargement of Lyt-2 positive T cells is associated with functional impairment and autoimmune hemolytic anemia in New Zealand Black mice. J Immunol 135:2432−2437
33. Taurog JD, Moutsopoulos HM, Rosenberg YJ, Chused TM, Steinberg AD (1979) CBA/N X-linked B-cell defect prevents NZB B-cell hyperactivity in F_1 mice. J Exp Med 150:31
34. Markham RB, Stashak PW, Prescott B, Amsbaugh DF, Baker PJ (1977) Effect of concanavalin A on lymphocyte interactions involved in the antibody response to type III pneumococcal polysaccharide. I. Comparison of the suppression induced by ConA and low dose paralysis. J Immunol 118:952
35. Baker PJ, Amsbaugh DF, Stashak PW, Caldes G, Prescott B (1982) Direct evidence for the involvement of T suppressor cells in the expression of low-dose paralysis to type III pneumococcal polysaccharide. J Immunol 128:1059
36. McCoy KL, Baker PJ, Stashak PW, Chused TM (1985) Two defects in old New Zealand Black mice are involved in the loss of low-dose paralysis to type III pneumococcal polysaccharide. J Immunol 135:2438−2442
37. Lal RB, Monos DS, Chused TM, Cooper HL (1985) Analysis of lymphocyte proteins from New Zealand Black mice by two-dimensional gel electrophoresis. J Immunol 134:2350

The NZB × SWR Model: Insights into Viral, Immunologic, and Genetic Factors*

S. K. Datta

Introduction

The primary etiologic mechanism of systemic lupus erythematosus (SLE) is unknown. SLE in humans is probably not a single entity, but a heterogeneous group of diseases with similar clinical and immunopathologic features [1]. A genetic predisposition clearly plays a role in the development of SLE, but the genetic interactions that occur in this disorder are multiple and complex, and very little is known about the mechanism of action of such genetic factors [2]. Furthermore, the etiologic role of viruses in human SLE is disputable; retroviruses have been implicated by some investigators [3—6], whereas other have not been able to reproduce such findings [7, 8]. Discrepancies are also prevalent among the vast number of studies on the immune system in SLE [1]. It is not clear whether the immunologic abnormities are the cause of the disease or its consequence. Because of this complexity, several animal models are being investigated to define the fundamentalal mechanism of the disease.

The New Zealand strains of mice, notably NZB and (NZB × NZW) F_1 hybris, have served as informative models for the study of human SLE [9]. These mice and the NZB × SWR crosses described in this paper parallel humans in the sex distribution and immunopathologic characteristics of SLE. Recently two additional strains, MRL-*lpr/lpr* and BXSB, have been vigorously investigated as models of SLE [10]. In the MRL-*lpr/lpr* strain a recessive gene, *lpr*, accelerates the development of SLE by causing massive proliferation of a population of T-lymphocytes that induces polyclonal activation of B cells [11]. No human counterpart of such a model exists. Moreover, the *lpr* gene produces full-blown SLE only in the MRL genetic background, and not in the background of other normal nonautoimmune mouse strains [12, 13]. The "normal" congenic background strain of MRL-*lpr/lpr* is the MRL-+/+ mouse. The latter strain, however, does develop nephritis and produce high levels of autoantibodies later in life [14, 15]. Thus, the extensive investigations in the MRL-*lpr/lpr* strain so far have dealt with secondary factors that can accelerate and increase the severity of SLE. The primary mechanism of autoimmunity in the MRL model lies in the "normal" MRL-+/+ background, and this strain has yet to be systematically studied. Similarly, in the BXSB model, Y chromosome-linked genes acceleralte the

---

* The studies described in this paper were supported by National Institutes of Health grant no. RO1 CA 31789.

development of SLE in male mice of a SLE-prone genetic background. Although many studies have been carried out on the secondary effects of the Y chromosome-accelerating genes, almost nothing is known about the primary underlying defects in this model.

The NZB × SWR cross, on the other hand, has unique features allowing a genetic dissection of various components that may be primarily involved in autoimmune disease. Unlike the NZB parents or crosses of NZB with other normal strains, the F_1 hybrids of NZB and the normal SWR mouse strain uniformly develop lethal glomerulonephritis. And as in human SLE, the incidence of lupus nephritis is higher in the female (NZB × SWR) F_1 hybrids [16, 17]. The only other cross of NZB that regularly develops a high incidence of lupus nephritis is the (NZB × NZW) F_1 hybrid. NZW mice, however, are not normal; they produce anti-DNA antibodies and develop nephritis later in life [18]. They also share background genes with the NZB strain, and both strains have the same virologic abnormalities, i.e., production of exceptionally high levels if retroviruses and retroviral antigen (gp70) throughout life [19]. By contrast, mice of the SWR strain do not produce any infectious retroviruses and have extremely low serum levels of gp70 [16, 20]. Moreover, they do not develop any manifestations of autoimmune disease or produce autoantibodies spontaneously [16, 17]. These features of the NZB × SWR cross have allowed us to dissect the role of various genetic, viral, and immunologic abnormalities of the NZB strain in the etiology of autoimmune disease. Furthermore, they are also helping us to identify the factors contributed by a completely normal strain in the development of lupus nephritis.

Role of Viruses

A Genetic Test of the Hypothesis in the NZB × SWR Cross

The virologic aspects of NZB and (NZB × NZW) F_1 hybrid mice have figured prominently in theories about the etiology and pathogenesis of autoimmunity. These mice express high levels of retroviruses (type-C RNA viruses) in their tissues. The genetic information coding for these retroviruses is now known to be present in the genomes of all vertebrates, including man [21]. Not all mouse strains express these viruses, although they carry latent viral genomes integrated in their chromosomes. The retroviruses that are found in virus-positive mouse strains can be classified into two broad categories. Ecotropic retroviruses can replicate in cells of the mouse. Xenotropic retroviruses, although expressed by mouse cells, can productively infect only cells of heterologous species. NZB mice express xenotropic viruses only, and not ecotropic viruses [16, 22].

Thus, NZB and NZB × NZW mice have two distinctive features: the uniform development of autoimmune disease and high level expression of retroviruses throughout life. Viral antigens (the viral envelope glycoprotein, gp70) and antiviral antibodies, together with antibodies to DNA, are detected in the renal lesions of NZB × NZW mice [19]. These observations suggested a cause-and-effect relationship between the virus and the autoimmune disease. Moreover, the proposition has also been advanced that xenotropic virus causes the disturbed immunoregulation in NZB mice, possibly by provoking an immune response against virus-producing, thymocytes [23]. Thus, the virus was thought both to initiate the disease and to provide antigens that generated nephritogenic immune complexes.

The presence of virus particles and the detection of viral antigens and antiviral antibodies in lesions do not, however, constitute proof that xenotropic viruses cause the disease of NZB mice. Transmission of autoimmunity has not been achieved with cell-free filtrates from NZB mice [24]. The reason for this is that the xenotropic retrovirus cannot infect mouse cells; it can infect only cells of heterologous species [22]. Thus, a traditional microbiological approach cannot be applied to solution of the problem. However, since copies of xenotropic viral genomes are found to be integrated in the chromosomes of mice, the relevance of the virus to autoimmunity can be ascertained by genetic techniques.

Genetic analyses became feasible with the identification of two autosomal dominant genes that govern the expression of xenotropic virus in NZB mice [25, 26]. One of these genes, *Nzv-1*, specifies high-grade expression of the virus, and the other, *Nzv-2*, specifies low-grade expression of the virus. Homozygosity for recessive alleles at both loci results in a virus-negative mouse strain, such as the SWR. Matings between NZB and virus-negative SWR mice result in three kinds of progeny in F_2 and (F_1 × SWR) backcross generations: high-virus, low virus, and virus-negative. These virologic phenotypes are stable and thus permitted us to test the hypothesis that development of autoimmunity requires the expression of xenotropic virus.

The results we obtained were clear-cut: The virological phenotype of the progeny of NZB × SWR crosses was independent of the presence of autoantibodies or glomerulonephritis. Crosses that were virologically identical with NZB mice failed to develop any signs of autoimmunization, and the progeny mice that were virus-negative were able to produce autoantibodies to erythrocytes and DNA and develop severe immune-deposit glomerulonephritis in the absence of deposits of viral gp70 antigens [16, 20]. Moreover, the other NZB traits, namely, high levels of circulating gp70 antigen and gp70 immune complexes, could also be dissociated from the development of glomerulonephritis in the NZB × SWR crosses [20]. The dissociation between virus expression and the development of autoimmune disease was not a peculiar feature of NZB × SWR crosses; similar results were found in crosses between NZB and B10.A, C57Bl/6 and AKR mice and also recombinant inbred lines derived from NZB and C58 progenitor strains [16, 27].

The genetic dissection that was feasible with the NZB × SWR cross could not be applied to the other NZB cross that regularly develops lupus nephritis, NZB × NZW. NZW mice, unlike SWR, are not normal; they themselves produce anti-DNA antibodies and develop nephritis late in life [18]. Moreover, in contrast to SWR mice, NZW mice are virologically similar to NZB in expressing high levels of xenotropic virus and circulating gp70 antigen [19]. Thus, in the

NZB × NZW cross, in addition to anti-DNA antibodies, antibodies to gp70 antibodies participate in immune complex formation and renal disease [28, 29].

Therefore, because of their contrasting virologic and immuniligic phenotypes from the NZB and NZW strains, SWR mice are valuable genetic tools that can be used to define the role of various NZB abnormalities in the etiology of autoimmune disease. Our results indicated that the xenotropic virus and gp70 antigen are *endogenous* and thus potential autoantigens in NZB mice [16, 20, 25, 26]. Like other autoantigens, such as erythrocytes and DNA, they may play secondary roles, but they are not required primarily for autoimmunization. Whether an autoimmune reaction occurs against xenotropic viral antigens or other autoantigens depends on genes ("autoimmunity genes") that are distinct from viral genes. This interpretation set the NZB model apart from examples of immune complex-mediated injury involving infection by *exogenous* viruses, in which case the infectious agent participates in both the etiology and the pathogenesis of the immunologic lesions.

The results we obtained from virologic and genetic studies with the NZB × SWR cross brought a conceptual change in the direction of research on SLE because, at that time, retroviruses were thought to be the etiologic agents of this disease [3—6, 23]. We next used the NZB × SWR cross as a genetic tool to analyze the role of various immunologic abnormalities in autoimmune disease.

Non-specific Immunologic Defects

Generalized Deficiency of Suppressor T Cells

An age-dependent deficiency of suppressor T cells was thought to be a primary defect causing a deregulation of the immune system that led to the development of autoimmune disease [30, 31]. However, these T suppressor cells are not known to be specific for any particular autoantibody. A deficiency of suppressor T cells can be caused by natural thymocytotoxic antibodies (NTA) produced in NZB mice [32]; however, NTA production can be dissociated from the production of anti-DNA and antierythrocyte antibodies in NZB crosses [33]. Moreover, other workers, including our selves, failed to find a consistent decline of T suppressor cells in old NZB mice or in the NZB × SWR crosses that develop lupus nephritis [34, 35]. Finally, genetic studies on congenic and mutant NZB mice showed that these nonspecific T cell abnormalities can be dissociated from autoimmune manifestations [36, 37]. Thus, a generalized deficiency of suppressor T cells, when present, may influence the severity of SLE, but it is not the fundamental etiologic mechanism.

Polyclonal B Cell Hyperactivity

Polyclonal hyperactivity of B-lymphocytes with increased immunoglobulin production has been observed in all the murine models and also in human SLE [1, 11, 27, 35]. This trait could be secondary to a decreased suppressor T cell or increased helper T cell function, or it could be due to a primary B cell defect. In NZB mice these generalized B cell abnormalities are complex and are influenced by unlinked sets of genes [27]. One of these B cell hyperactivity traits is manifested by spontaneous hypersecretion of IgM [38]. This abnormality is expressed from fetal life onward independently of any T cell influence, and is determined by two sets of autosomal genes [27, 35]. The NZB B cells that hypersecrete IgM have an unusual phenotype: they express Ly-l antigen, which is a surface marker of T cells, expecially those of the helper/inducer class [39, 40]. Moreover, these spontaneously hyperactive B cells belong to the same B cell subset as the one affected by an X-linked recessive gene *(xid)* in the CBA/N mutant mice [41, 42]. Introduction of the *xid* gene on the NZB background prevents the development of autoimmune disease [36]. Therefore, it has been widely postulated that intrinsic hyperactivity of a subpopulation of B cells of NZB mice results in the activation of autoreactive B cells, causing autoimmune disease [11, 35, 36]. The *xid* mutation, however, affects a relatively large subet of B cells (approx. 60% of splenic B cells), which may also encompass autoantibody producing clones of cells without a specific cause-and-effect relationship. Moreover, the Ly-l positive B cells secrete only IgM autoantibodies [43], whereas in SLE, pathogenic autoantibodies are of the IgG class [44—46]. Indeed, finer genetic segregation analysis in the NZB × SWR crosses and recombinant inbred lines showed that inheritance of the spontaneous B cell hyperactivity trait that specifies increased secretion of IgM can be dissociated from development of autoantibodies and autoimmune disease [17, 27]. Another B cell abnormality of NZB mice manifests as a precocious hyperresponse to sheep red blood cell antigens. This trait is thought to be due to a primary B cell defect in responsiveness to B cell growth and differentiation fectors [11]. This abnormality can also be genetically dissociated from autoantibody production in NZB-derived recombinant inbred lines [27].

These results suggest that a generalized polyclonal B cell abnormality is not the underlying cause of SLE and that the spontaneously activated autoantibody-producing B cells constitue a far more restricted population than was previously realized. This interpretation derives further support from genetic studies showing that the inheritance and expression of each type of antoantibody, such as anti-DNA, antierythrocyte, or anti-Sm antibody, can be independent of each other [27, 47, 48]. Thus, highly restricted abnormalities specific for the regulation of each family of autoreactive B cells have to be elucidated. We therefore focused our attention on the cells responsible specifically for anti-DNA autoantibody production.

Autoantibody-Specific Immunologic Defects

Very little is known about the specific regulation of anti-DNA antibody-producing B cells in human SLE. As a logical extension of findings in other antibody—idiotype systems [49, 50], it was proposed that idiotype—anti—idiotype network regulation may also play a role in autoimmunity [51]. However, the role of spontaneously produced anti-idiotypic antibodies against autoantibodies in autoimmune desease remains confusing because of conflicting results. Circumstantial evidence suggests that they may have a favorable effect on the disease, as they have been found during remission of SLE [52]. In other cases, however, anti-idiotypic antibodies were found to have a deleterious effect on disease [53]. In these examples the auto-antibody idiotypes were not defined. Deliberate manipulation with defined anti-idiotypic antibodies raised in the laboratory can either suppress or enhance the production of the anti-DNA idiotypes in murine models [54, 55]. An explanation of these paradoxical results may be forthcoming as we begin to understand the origin of anti-DNA antibodies and learn more about the factors that regulate the production of nephritogenic anti-DNA antibodies in SLE [56—59].

Anti-DNA Antibody Idiotypes of Lupus Mice can be Expressed by Normal Mice

The spontaneous production of anti-DNA autoantibodies is characteristic of human and murine SLE. These antibodies have been implicated in the pathogenesis of nephritis and other lesions of the disease [60]. The ability to produce these antibodies, however is not restricted to mice or humans that develop SLE. Normal individuals and also normal mice can spontaneously produce such antibodies with age or upon polyclonal stimulation of their B cells [61—63]. However, the latter situations do not usually lead to development of SLE. These observations raise several questions. Are the antibodies produced by lupus mice qualitatively different and more pathogenic than their counterparts in normal mice? Do normal and autoimmune mice possess identical clones of anti-DNA antibody-producing cells whose regulation is impaired in the lupus strains? We addressed these questions by determining whether normal mice can produce antibodies with idiotypic markers of the anti-DNA antibodies of MRL-*lpr/lpr* mice, a strain that develops a lethal form of SLE. We found that spleen and fetal liver B cells of five different normal mouse strains could synthesize idiotypes shared by anti-DNA antibodies of the genetically autoimmune strain [56]. Although the antibodies produced by normal mice had idiotypes of lupus anti-DNA antibodies, the major proportion of those antibodies did not bind DNA. We have recently found analogous results in humans [64].

These findings have implications for the origin of anti-DNA antibodies; they indicate that the autoantibody idiotypes are related to a conserved family of antibody-variable regions that are present in normal animals and they can be

66 S. K. Datta

expressed very early in ontogeny [56]. These conserved antibody V regions are not primarily directed against DNA, but like other inherited cross-reactive idiotypes, they are probably specific for common bacterial pathogens [56—58]. Spontaneously produced anti-DNA antibodies, moreover, are polyspecific [58]. They bind to a wide variety of antigens, suggesting again that DNA may not be the primary antigen for these antibodies. The binding of only a minority of antibodies in this "autoantibody" idiotype family to DNA, therefore, represents cross-reactions and not unique anti-self reactions. Our finding that the same idiotypic family encompasses both a minor DNA-binding and a major DNA non-binding population has many precedents in other idiotypic systems and can be explained by Jerne's network hypothesis [49, 56, 57]. For instance, in the case of the anti-DNA idiotypes we studied a bacterial antigen, and not DNA, may be the primary and natural target of the antibodies bearing those idiotypes (Ab1). These antibodies (Ab1) do not bind to DNA although they share idiotypes with anti-DNA antibodies. Ab2 induces the production of, and is regulated by, anti-idiotypic antibodies (Ab2). Certain members of this family of anti-idiotypic antibodies may bear the conformational determinants (internal image) of an autoantigen such as DNA. These anti-idiotypic antibodies (Ab2) in turn induce a population of antibodies (Ab3) that share idiotypes with Ab1 but are now specific for nucleic acid antigens and not the primary (bacterial) antigen. According to Jerne, Ab3 constitues a nonspecific parallel set of antibodies in the network [49]. The minor DNA-binding population in the idiotypic families we studied may belong to this parallel set of antibodies (Ab3). Although Ab1 and Ab3 have different antigenic specificities, by sharing the same idiotype they become connected as members of a regulatory idiotypic network [57, 65, 66].

In human and mouse strains that are gentically prone to develop SLE, a spontaneous shift in the idiotype family occurs, leading not only to expansion of the minor DNA-binding population but also to a qualitative change in those antibodies [59, 64]. The NZB $\times$ SWR cross system provides further clues regarding this immunoregulatory shift as described below.

Normal SWR Mice Contribute to the Production of Nephritogenic Anti-DNA Antibodies in Crosses with Autoimmune NZB Mice

Autoimmune hemolytic anemia occurs at a high frequency in NZB mice, whereas glomerulonephritis is infrequent, mild, and delayed in onset [16, 17]. By contrast, most female F_1 hybrids derived from crossing NZB mice with the normal SWR strain develop severe glomerulonephritis between 5 and 7 months, and by 1 year of age 100% of the animals die of renal lesions [16, 17]. These results suggest that the normal SWR parent makes a genetic contribution to the development of lupus nephritis in (NZB $\times$ SWR) F_1 mice. The incidence and amount of circulating anti-DNA antibodies are similar in the NZB parents and the (NZB $\times$ SWR) F_1 hybrids, but a qualitative difference in their antibodies may explain the difference in renal disease. Therefore, we analyzed a library of monoclonal anti-DNA antibodies derived from the (NZB $\times$ SWR) F_1 mice and compared them with a collection obtained from the NZB parents [57, 59]. The majority of anti-DNA antibodies derived from the (NZB × SWR) F_1 hybrids were IgG and cationic in charge. By contrast, 77% of the NZB-derived antibodies were IgM and most of them were neutral or anionic in charge. We identified a set of highly cationic IgG2b class anti-DNA antibodies from the (NZB × SWR) F_1 hybrids that had the allotype of the normal SWR parent. Isoelectric focusing of intact antibodies and their heavy and light chains showed that the highly cationic charge of these antibodies were determined by their heavy chain-variable regions. IgG anti-DNA antibodies with cationic charge are especially pathogenic in SLE [44]. Moreover, since DNA, like the glomerulus is negatively charged, the probability of its deposition and persistence in glomeruli will increase markedly it it is complexed with cationic anti-DNA antibodies [67, 68]. Therefore, those highly cationic IgG2b antibodies bearing the allotype of the normal SWR parent may account for the high incidence of severe nephritis in the F_1 hybrids. The results in the NZB × SWR corss indicate that a restricted family of pathogenic anti-DNA antibodies encoded by genes of normal, nonautoimmune mice can be become expressed when they interact with genes of an abnormal autoimmune mouse.

Conclusions

These genetic studies with the NZB × SWR cross show that certain abnormal traits present in the autoimmune NZB strain are not primarily required for the development of autoimmune disease. Production of autoantibodies to DNA or erythrocytes and development of lupus nephritis can occur in the absence of retrovirus expression or glomerular deposition of retroviral gp70 antigens. Thus, retroviruses are not the etiologic agents of SLE, as had been widely assumed prior to our studies with the NZB × SWR crosses. On the basis of these results, we initially proposed a different interpretation relating to the role of viruses in systemic autoimmunity [16, 20, 25, 69]. The retroviruses found in autoimmune NZB mice are endogenous viruses, and their gp70 antigen is a potential autoantigen. These viruses may play a secondary role in autoimmune disease by supplying autoantigens, but in the regard they seem to be no different from erythrocyte or DNA autoantigens [16, 20, 69]. Unlike the NZB × SWR cross, in other murine models of SLE such as the NZB × NZW hybrids and MRL-*lpr/lpr* mice, retroviral gp70 immune complex formation correlates with the development of nephritis [19, 28, 29]. However, the latter strains of mice and their progenitor strains all produce abnormally high levels of retroviruses and gp70 antigen, and thus have an excessive amount of these endogenous antigens, which participate secondarily in immune complex formation and deposition in the kidney.

Next, we showed that certain generalized immunologic abnormalities of the NZB strain, such as nonspecific suppressor T cell deficiency and spontaneous polyclonal B cell hyperactivity, can also be dissociated from the development of

68 S. K. Datta

SLE in the NZB × SWR crosses. These immunoligic abnormalities may modify the severity of disease when present, but they are not essential for the development of SLE. Moreover, these gross nonspecific abnormalities may be the consequence rather than the cause of the disease. If suppressor cell dysfunction is a contributing mechanism to autoimmunity in SLE, the restricted nature of SLE autoantibodies would require a selective rather that an overall loss of T suppressor cell function. Therefore, autoantibody-specific immunoregulatory defects have to be defined in this disease.

In contrast to SLE, viruses and the deficiency of nonspecific suppressor T cells do play a role in the etiology of certain organ-specific autoimmune disease. Although the latter category of autoimmune diseases has been considered to be distinct from systemic lupus in clinical, pathological, and genetic aspects, yet, in theory, the same etiologic factors have been implicated in both types of disorders. Viruses, by altering of mimicking self-antigens, can *initiate* the development of certain organ-specific autoimmune diseases, in contrast to SLE [70]. Moreover, selective depletion of nonspecific suppressor T cells can result in the development of organ-specific autoimmune diseases, but not SLE [71]. Therefore, these two categories of autoimmune diseases should also be considered to be etiologically distinct.

The investigations in the NZB × SWR model show that the development of systemic autoimmune disease is a multistep, multigene process. In the NZB × SWR hybrids, severe lupus nephritis results from the interaction of genes inherited from both the autoimmune NZB and the normal SWR parents. A similar genetic interaction occurs in the NZB × NZW hybrids [72, 73], but in this model both the parental strains are abnormal [18] and the nature of the gene products or their mechanism of action ist unknown. In the NZB × SWR model, we have been able to identify a restricted subpopulaion of nephritogenic anti-DNA antibody idiotypes that are encoded by genes of the normal SWR parents. Thus, these are one set of genes that determine the development of severe lupus nephritis in the F_1 hybrids. In addition, another set of genes allow the expansion of B cells, producing such pathogenic anti-DNA idiotypes in the F_1 hybrids since such B cell clones remain dormant in the normal SWR parents. Genes of the latter category, presumably specifying defects in immunoregulation, are probably inherited from the NZB parents or may be the result of complementation of genes inherited from both parents. Further investigations with the NZB × SWR model will help us define the immunoregulatory defects in SLE that are specific for the T and B cells involved in pathogenic autoantibody production.

Acknowledgments. I thank Drs. Robert Schwartz, David Stollar, Jerrie Gavalchin, and Jean Eastcott for stimulating collaboration in different portions of the work summarized in this paper. Thanks are also due to Gary Brenner for processing the manuscript.

References

1. Tsokos GC, Balow JE (1984) Cellular immune responses in systemic lupus erythematosus. Prog Allergy 35:93—161
2. Arnett FC, Reveille JD, Wilson RW, Provost TT, Bias WB (1984) Systemic lupus erythematosus: current state of the genetic hypothesis. Semin Arthritis Rheum 14:24—35
3. Mellors RC, Mellors JW (1976) Antigen related to mammalian type-C RNA viral p30 proteins is located in renal glomeruli in human systemic lupus erythematosus. Proc Natl Acad Sci USA 73:233—237
4. Lewis RM, Tanneberg W, Smith C, Schwartz RS (1974) C-type viruses in systemic lupus erythematosus. Nature 252:78—79
5. Strand M, August JT (1974) Type-C RNA virus gene expression in human tissue. J. Virol 14:1584—1596
6. Panem S, Ordonez NG, Kirstein WH, Katz AI, Spargi BH (1976) C-type virus espression in systemic lupus erythematosus. N Engl J Med 295:470—475
7. Philips PE (1978) Type C onco RNA virus studies in systemic lupus erythematosus. Arthritis Rheum 21 [Suppl 5]: S 76—81
8. Kimura M, Andoh T, Kai K (1980) Failure to detect type-C virus p30-related antigen in systemic lupus erythematosus: false-positive reaction due to protease activity. Arthritis Rheum 23:111—113
9. Howie JB, Helyer BJ (1968) The immunology and pathology of NZB mice. Adv Immunol 9:215—268
10. Murphy ED, Roths JB (1978) Autoimmunity and lymphoproliferation: induction by mutant gene *lpr,* and acceleration by a male-associated factor in strain B x SB mice. In: Rose NE, Bigazzi PE, Warner NL (eds) Genetic control of autoimmune disease. Elsevier/North Holland, Amsterdam, pp 207—221
11. Prud'homme GJ, Fieser TM, Dixon FJ, Theofilopoulos AN (1984) B cell-tropic interleukins in murine systemic lupus erythematosus. Immunol Rev 78:160—183
12. Izui S, Kelley VE, Kazushige M, Yoshida H, Roths JB, Murphy ED (1984) Induction of various autoantibodies by mutant gene *lpr* in several strains of mice. J Immunol 133:227—233
13. Hang L, Aguado MT, Dixon FJ, Theofilopoulos AN (1985) Indiction of severe autoimmune disease in normal mice by simultaneous action of multiple immunostimulators. J Exp Med 161:423—428
14. Pisetsky DS, Caster SA, Roths JB, Murphy ED (1982) Gene control of the anti-DNA antibody response. J Immunol 128:2322—2325
15. Giroir BP, Raps EC, Lewis RM, Borel Y (1983) Nucleoside-specific suppression in MRL/MP +/+ mice. Cell Immunol 75:337—347
16. Datta SK, Manny N, Andrzejewski C, Andre-Schwartz J, Schwartz RS (1978) Genetic studies of autoimmunity and retrovirus expression in crosses of New Zealand Black mice. I. Xenotropic virus. J Exp Med 147:854—871
17. Eastcott JW, Schwartz RS, Datta SK (1983) Genetic analysis of the inheritence of B cell hyperactivity in relation to the development if autoantibodies and glomerulonephritis in NZB x SWR crosses. J Immunol 131:2232—2239
18. Kelley VE, Winkelstein A (1980) Age-and sex-related glomerulonephritis in New Zealand White mice. Clin Immunol Immunopathol 16:142—150
19. Yoshiki T, Mellors RC, Strand M, August JT (1974) The viral envelope glycoprotein of murine leukemia virus and the pathogenesis of immune-complex glomerulonephritis of New Zealand mice. J Exp Med 140:1011—1027
20. Datta SK, McConahey PJ, Manny N, Theofilopoulos AN, Dixon FJ, Schwartz RS (1978) Genetic studies of autoimmunity and retrovirus expression in New Zealand Black mice. II. The viral envelope glycoprotein gp70. J Exp Med 147:872—881
21. Weiss R, Teich N, Varmus H, Coffin J (eds) (1982) RNA tumor viruses. Molecular biology of tumor viruses. Cold Spring Harbor, Laboratories, New York (Cold Spring Harbor Laboratories monograph no. 10C)

70   S. K. Datta

22. Levy JA, Kazan P, Varnier O, Kleinman H (1975) Murine xenotropic type-C virus. I. Distribution and further characterization of the virus in NZB mice. J Virol 16:844—853
23. Levy JA (1976) Endogenous C-type viruses: double agents in natural life processes. Biomedicine 24:84—93
24. East J (1970) Immunopathology and neoplasms in NZB and SJL/J mice. Prog. Exp Tumor Res 13:84—134
25. Datta SK, Schwartz RS (1976) Genetics of expression of xenotropic virus and autoimmunity in NZB mice. Nature 263:412—415
26. Datta SK, Schwartz RS (1977) Mendelian segregation of loci controlling xenotropic virus production in NZB crosses. Virology 83:449—452
27. Datta SK, Owen FL, Womak JE, Riblet RJ (1982) Analysis of recombinant inbred line derived from autoimmune (NZB) and high-leukemia (C58) strains: independent multigenic systems control B cell hyperactivity, retrovirus expression and autoimmunity. J Immunol 129:1539—1544
28. Izui S, McConahey PJ, Clark JP, Hang LM, Hara I, Dixon FJ (1981) Retroviral gp70 immune complexes in NZB × NZW F_2 mice with murine lupus nephritis. J Exp Med 154:517—528
29. Maruyama N, Furukawa F, Nakai Y, Yutaka S, Ohta K, Ozaki S, Hirose S, Shirai T (1983) Genetic studies of autoimmunity in New Zealand mice. IV. Contribution of NZB and NZW genes to the spontaneous occurrence of retroviral gp70 immune complexes in (NZB × NZW) F_1 hybrid and correlation to renal disease. J Immunol 130:740—746
30. Barthold DR, Kysela SJ, Steinberg AD (1974) Decline in suppressor T cell function with age in female NZB mice. J Immunol 112:9—16
31. Cantor H, McVay-Boudreau L, Hugenberger J, Naidorf K, Shen FW, Gershon RK (1978) Immunoregulatory circuits among T-cell sets. II. Physiologic role of feedback inhibition in vivo: absence in NZB mice. J Exp Med 147:1116—1125
32. Shirai T, Hayakawa K, Okumura KO, Tada T (1978) Differential cytotoxic effect of natural thymocytotoxic autoantibody of NZB mice on functional subsets of T cell. J Immunol 120:1924—1929
33. Raveche ES, Steinberg AD, Klassen LW, Tjio JH (1978) Genetic studies in NZB mice. I. Spontaneous autoantibody production. J Exp Med 147:1487—1501
34. Primi D, Hammarstrom L, Smith CIE (1978) Genetic control of lymphocyte suppression. I. Lack of suppression in aged NZB mice is due to a B cell defect. J Immunol 121:2241—2243
35. Manny N, Datta SK, Schwartz RS (1979) Synthesis of IgM by cells of NZB and SWR mice and their crosses. J Immunol 122:1220—1227
36. Taurog JD, Raveche ES, Smathers PA, Glimcher LH, Huston DP, Hansen CT, Steinberg AD (1981) T cell abnormalities in NZB mice occur independently of autoantibody production. J Exp Med 153:221—234
37. Gershwin ME, Castels JJ, Ikeda RM, Erickson K, Montero J (1979) Studies of congenitally immunologic mutant New Zealand mice. I. Autoimmune features of hereditary asplenic (Dh/+) NZB mice, reduction of naturally occurring thymocytotoxic antibody and normal suppressor function. J Immunol 122:710—717
38. Moutsopolos HM, Boehm-Truitt M, Kassan SS, Chused TM (1977) Demonstration of activation of B-lymphocytes in New Zealand Black mice at birth by an immunoradiometric assay for murine IgM. J Immunol 119:1639—1644
39. Manohor V, Brown E, Leiserson WM, Chused TM (1982) Expression of Lyt-l by a subset of B lymphocytes. J Immunol 129:532—538
40. Hayakawa K, Hardy RR, Parks DR, Herzenberg LA (1983) The "Ly-1 B" cell subpopulation in normal, immunodefective and autoimmune mice. J Exp Med 157:202—218
41. Nakajima PB, Datta SK, Schwartz RS, Huber BT (1979) Localization of spontaneously hyperactive B cells of NZB mice to a specific B subset. Proc Natl Acad Sci USA 76:4613—4616
42. Taurog JD, Montsopoulos HM, Rosenberg YJ, Chused TM, Steinberg AD (1979) CBA/N X-linked B cell defect prevents NZB B-cell hyperactivity in F_1 mice. J Exp Med 150:31—43

The NZB × SWR Model 71

43. Hayakawa K, Hardy RR, Honda M, Herzenberg LA, Steinberg AD, Herzenberg LA (1984) Ly-l B cells: functionally distinct lymphocytes that secrete IgM autoantibodies. Proc Natl Acad Sci USA 81:2494—2498

44. Ebling F, Hahn BH (1980) Restricted subpopulations of DNA antibodies in kidneys of mice with systemic lupus: comparison of antibodies in serum and renal eluates. Arthritis Rheum 23:392—403

45. Rothfield NF, Stollar BD (1967) The relation of immunoglobulin class, pattern of anti-nuclear antibody and complement-fixing antibodies to DNA in sera of patients with systemic lupus erythematosus. J Clin Invest 46:1784—1794

46. Talal N (1976) Disordered immunologic regulation and autoimmunity. Transplant Rev 31:240—263

47. Raveche ES, Novotny EA, Hansen CT, Tjio JH, Steinberg AD (1981) Genetic studies in NZB mice. V. Recombinant inbred lines demonstrate that separate genes control autoimmune phenotype. J Exp Med 153:1187—1197

48. Pisetsky DS, McCarty GA, Peters DV (1980) Mechanisms of autoantibody production in autoimmune MRL mice. J Exp Med 152:1302—1310

49. Jerne NK (1974) Towards a network theory of the immune system. Ann Immunol (Paris) 125:373—389

50. Bona CA (1981) Idiotypes and lymphocytes. Academic, New York

51. Wigzell H, Binz H, Frischknecht H, Peterson P, Sege K (1978) Possible roles of auto-anti-idiotypic immunity in autoimmune disease In: Rose NE, Bigazzi PE, Warner NL (eds) Genetic control of autoimmune disease. Elsevier/North Holland, Amsterdam, pp 327—342

52. Abdou NI, Wall H, Lindsley HB, Halsey JF, Suzuki T (1981) Network theory in autoimmunity. In vitro suppression of serum anti-DNA antibody binding to DNA by anti-idiotypic antibody in systemic lupus erythematosus. J Clin Invest 67:1297—1304

53. Wasserman NH, Penn AS, Freimuth PI, Treptow N, Wentzerl S, Cleveland WL, Erlanger BF (1982) Anti-idiotype route to antiacetylcholine receptor antibodies in experimental myasthenia gravis. Proc Natl Acad Sci USA 79:4810—4814

54. Hahn BH, Ebling FM (1983) Suppression of NZB/NZW murine mephritis by administration of a syngeneic monoclonal antibody to DNA. Possible role of anti-idiotypic antibodies. J Clin Invest 71:1728—1736.

55. Titelbaum D, Rauch J, Stoller BD, Schwartz RS (1984) In vivo effects of antibodies against a high frequency idiotype of anti-DNA antibodies in MRL mice. J Immunol 132:1282—1285

56. Datta SK, Sollar BD, Schwartz RS (1983) Normal mice espress idiotypes related to autoantibody idiotypes of lupus mice. Proc Natl Acad Sci USA 80:2723—2727

57. Datta SK (1984) Anti-DNA antibody idiotypes in normal and lupus mice. In: Sercarz E, Cantor H, Chess L (eds) Regulation of the immune system, UCLA Symposia on molecular and cellular biology, vol 18. Liss. New York, pp 877—886

58. Schwartz RS, Stoller BD (1985) Origins of anti-DNA autoantibodies. J Clin Invest 75:321—327

59. Gavalchin J, Nicklas JA, Eastcott JW, Madaio MP, Stoller BD, Schwartz RS, Datta SK (1985) Lupus-prone (SWR × NZB) F_1 mice produce potentially nephritogenic autoantibodies inherited from the normal SWR parent. J Immunol 134:885—894

60. Koffler D, Carr R, Agnello V, Thoburn R, Kunkel HG (1971) Antibodies to polynucleotides in human sera: antigenic specificity and relation to disease. J Exp Med 134:294—312

61. Rubin RL, Carr RI (1972) Anti-DNA activity of IgG F (ab')$_2$ from normal human serum. J Immunol 122:1604—1607

62. Fish F, Ziff M (1982) The in vitro and in vivo induction of anti-double-strandes DNA antibodies in normals and autoimmune mice. J Immunol 128:409—414

63. Kobayakawa T, Louis J, Izui S, Lambert PH (1979) Autoimmune responses to DNA, red blood cells and thymocyte antigens in association with polyclonal antibody synthesis during experimental African trypanisomiasis. J Immunol 122:296—301

64. Datta SK, Naparstek Y, Schwartz RS (1986) In vitro production of an anti-DNA indiotype by lymphocytes of normal subjects and patients with systemic lupus erythematosus Clin Immunol Immunopathol 38:302—318

72 S. K. Datta

65. Paul WE, Bona CA (1982) Regulatory idiotopes and immune networks: a hypothesis. Immunol Today 3:230—234
66. Hornbeck PV, Lewis GK (1983) Idiotype connectance in the immune system. I. Expression of a cross-reactive idiotype on induced anti-p-azophenylarsonate antibodies and on endogenous antibodies not specific for arsonate. J Exp Med 157:1116—1136
67. Lawrence Y, Agodoa C, Gauthier VJ, Mannik M (1985) Antibody localization in the glomerular basement membrane may precede in situ immune deposit formation in rat glomeruli. J Immunol 134:880—884
68. Barnes JL, Venkatachalam MA (1984) Enhancement of glomerular immune complex deposition by a circulating polycation. J Exp Med 160:286—293
69. Datta SK, Schwartz RS (1978) Genetic, viral and immunologic aspects of autoimmune disease in NZB mice. In: Rose NR, Bigazzi PE, Warner NL (eds) Genetic control of autoimmune disease. Elsevier/North Holland, Amsterdam, pp 193—206
70. Haspel MV, Onodera T, Prabhakar BS, McClintock PR, Essani K, Roy UR, Yagihashi S, Notkins AL (1983) Multiple organ-reactive monoclonal autoantibodies. Nature 304:73—76
71. Sakaguchi S, Fukuma K, Kuribayashi K, Mesuda T (1985) Organ specific autoimmune diseases induced in mice by elimination of T cell subset. J Exp Med 161:72—87
72. Knight JG, Adams DD (1978) Three genes for lupus nephritis in NZB × NZW mice. J Exp Med 147:1653—1660
73. Hirose S, Nagasawa R, Sakikawa I, Hamaoki M, Ishida Y, Sato H, Shirai T (1983) Enhancing effect of H-2 linked NZW gene(s) on the autoimmune traits of (NZB × NZW) F_1 mice. J Exp Med 158:228—233

Relevance of the Murine Models of Systemic Lupus Erythematosus to Human Disease

C. A. LASKIN and H. R. SMITH

Introduction

Systemic lupus erythematosus (SLE) is a complex multisystem disorder which is associated with specific genetic, environmental, hormonal, and cellular events culminating in autoantibody production and clinical disease manifestations. The precise derangements and interactions of these various factors have been the focus for considerable research in humans and also in the murine lupus models. These lupus-prone mice spontaneoulsy develop an illness which resembles the human disorder [1—3]. Although they do not necessarily reflect a perfect correlate for human SLE, they do allow insights into the pathogenetic mechanisms of SLE. Like human SLE, which is a heterogeneous disease with much variation between individual patients [4], the murine models of SLE also have a wide spectrum of presentation. Although no single mouse model completely represents the human counterpart, the mice in their entirety do demonstrate a spectrum comparable to that of patients. In this paper, we will emphasize studies in spontaneously occurring autoimmunity in mice and illustrate the general principles as they relate to human SLE. The investigations of murine SLE have demonstrated the important contribution of genetic composition, environmental influence, hormonal regulation, and cellular interaction in mediating disease [5]. It is hoped that through a better understanding of the immunopathogenesis of the murine disease, insights into the pathogenesis of the human disorder and better approaches to therapy may result.

Common Features Among the Strains

Although the murine models have certain unique charcteristics, they do share some clinical and immunologic features. All strains develop immune complex renal disease, hypergammaglobulinemia, antinuclear antibodies, decreased serum complement levels, and large amounts of circulating immune complexes of gp 70/anti-gp 70 — an oncornavirus glycoprotein of 70000 daltons (Table 1). In addition to a loss of self-tolerance associated with the development of autoimmunity, all of the mice share an inability to manifest experimentally induced tolerance [6-8]. The latter is, however, not a prerequisite for the development of

74 C. A. Laskin and H. R. Smith

Table 1. Feature common to the murine models of SLE

Clinical	Serological	Cellular
Immune complex GN	Hypergammaglobulinemia	B cell hyperactivity
Thymic atrophy	Autoantibodies	Tolerance induction defects
Lymphoid hyperplasia	Decreased serum	
Coronary artery	complement levels	
disease with	Increased circulating	
myocardial infarction	immune complex levels	
Pneumonia	gp 70 — anti-gp 70	
Decreased survival	complexes	

SLE [9]. Central to the immunopathogenesis of the disease in all strains is generalized B cell hyperactivity [10—13]. The cause of this polyclonal B cell activation and the consequential autoantibody production probably account for much of the clinical and serologic manifestations of the disease [1, 2, 10—13]. In the following pages, we will review both the clinical and the serologic aspects of murine lupus, relating these features to disease expression as seen in humans. Although we will concentrate on the more widely known strains, the final section will give brief descriptions of the lesser utilized models.

NZB Mice

Detailed analyses of New Zealand Black mice (NZB) have led to an appreciation of the complexities of the disorder both immunologically and genetically, as well as a sensitivity to the problem of differentiating early from secondary immune abnormalities. The genetic studies have suggested that there is not a single gene which leads to NZB disease [14]. In fact, at least six genes may be responsible for the disorder. One gene plays an important role in anti-ssDNA production, and an unlinked gene plays an important role in anti-T cell antibody production. The latter has associated with it a mutation which renders it insusceptible to modulation by androgens [15]. Additional genes are responsible for anti-RBC production, a high mitotic index, and hyperdiploidy. A recent additional genetic study has indicated that NZB mice which bear the single gene *xid*, fail to develop the signs of NZB disease. The congenic NZB.*xid* mice are highly inbred NZB mice that carry an X-linked gene, *xid*, which is associated with the absence of a subpopulation of B cells [16]. The failure of such NZB.*xid* mice to develop autoimmunity suggests that that B cell subset (Lyb 3^+/Lyb 5^+) ist largely responsible for autoantibody production under ordinary circumstances. Moreover, such mice maifest the T cell defects characteristic of NZB mice [16]. Therefore, the T cell regulatory defects appear to be separable from, and not dependent upon, the B cell hyperactivity so characteristic of the mice. Studies in radiation chimeras have also suggested that both T cell defects and B cell defects contribute to the development of illness [17]. Moreover, NZB features can be transferred to nonautoimmune strains of mice with bone marrow [18, 19]. These oberservations have recently been reconciled. It appears that the T cell defect of NZB mice in tolerance induction is already present in a bone marrow pre-T stem cell [20]. This prethymocyte stem cell will differentiate into an abnormal thymocyte in any thymic microenvironment, whether that be provided by an NZB or normal thymus. Therefore, the bone marrow contains the information for the ultimate production of abnormal B cells and abnormal T cells [20]. Whether or not these arise from common stem cells has yet to be determined.

The information to date suggests that NZB disease is the result of a number of separate genes. There are genes for high responses to individual self-antigens and genes for immune abnormalities. Both B cell abnormalities and T cell abnormalities contribute to the development of maximum illness. Finally, only a subset of B cells is responsible for autoantibody production. However, recent studies have shed further light upon the additional questions of age, sex, and environmental stimuli. These studies have utilized the NZB.*xid* congenic mice which ordinarily do not manifest autoimmune features. Such mice have been stimulated by repeated administration of polyclonal immune stimulants. The results have been most helpful with regard to understanding the human condition [21]. NZB.*xid* mice, which do not develop autoantibodies spontaneously, produce large amounts of autoantibodies — anti-RBC and anti-ssDNA — upon stimulation. The earlier the age of onset of stimulation, the more severe the resulting illnes. Females continue to produce such autoantibodies long after the stimulus is removed whereas males do not [21]. These results are consistent with the development of human SLE predominantly in young females. Related studies in radiation chimeras have further clarified the cellular basis for SLE in the two sexes: females need only a defect in T cells to develop SLE, whereas males need a second marrow defect in order to maifest NZB abnormalities [6]. Thus, females require a lesser genetic cellular defect to get SLE and respond to polyclonal B cell activation with more prolonged autoantibody production.

MRL/Mp-lpr/lpr Mice

The MRL mouse strains are two congenic lines, MRL-+/+ and MRL-*lpr/lpr*, which share better than 99% of the genome. They differ with respect to one autosomal recessive gene, *lpr*, which controls the expression of lymphadenopathy, autoantibody production, and premature death as seen in the MRL-*lpr/lpr* mice [22, 23]. This latter strain represents the first single-gene model for antoimmunity; lymphoproliferation as controlled by the lymphoproliferative gene, *lpr*, is the preeminent feature. Background genes however, do play an important role in the disease of MRL mice as both *lpr/lpr* and +/+ mice develop a lupus-like syndrome; the former have early onset whereas the latter develop disease much later in life [22, 23]. The *lpr* gene in the setting of other autoimmune mice (e.g., NZB-*lpr/lpr*) can quicken the onset of autoimmunity and decrease survival as compared with those NZB mice without the *lpr* gene present [24, 25]. Furthermore, *lpr* can induce the formation of autoantibodies in strains of mice which otherwise are not predisposed to autoimmune disease [24, 25]. Such mice develop lymphadenopathy, high levels of immune complexes, and premature death. These studies suggest that background genes again seem to be important in determining: (a) the types and amounts of autoantibodies produced, and (b) the extent of glomerulonephritis produced in the presence of the *lpr* gene. Thus, depending on the background genes, homozygosity for the *lpr* gene appears to be either an inducer or an accelerator of disease.

The manifestations of overt disease in MRL-*lpr/lpr* mice include decreased survival, lymphoid hyperplasia, arthritis, arteritis, thymic atrophy, coronary artery disease, and pneumonia. Whereas MRL-*lpr/lpr* females and males have early onset of disease with mean survival of 5.0 and 5.5 months, respectively, the MRL-+/+ females and males develop disease late in life and survive on average for 15 and 23 months, respectively [26, 28, 29]. Death in these mice is usually secondary to subacute proliferative glomerulonephritis and nephrotic syndrome. MRL-*lpr:lpr* mice develop massive lymphadenopathy, splenomegaly, and (initially) thymic enlargement; these organs can be 100, 7, and 2 times the weight of control +/+ organs, respectively [28, 29, 26]. Eighty-eight to 95% of an enlarged node is composed of an expanded abnormal subset of T cells bearing the phenotype of: dull Thy 1$^+$, dull Ly 1$^+$, L3T4$^-$, Lyt 2$^-$, Ig$^-$, I-A$^-$, and ThB$^-$ [7, 27, 28]. In addition, these cells express the Ly 5 family of glycoproteins that is normally expressed only on B cells and their precursors [28]. These cells are probably of T cell lineage as they do not have Ig heavy chain gene rearrangement [28]. "Normal" T cells, such as Lyt 2$^+$, and B cells are not, however, inherently lacking in the nodes of MRL-*lpr/lpr* mice as amelioration of their clinical disease and immune abnormalities with cyclophosphamide normalizes the relative composition of B and T cells in the lymph nodes and allows for the expression of Lyt 2$^+$ T cells [29]. Thus it appears that a dilutional effect occurs; the absolute number of normal cells remains unchanged.

Other clinical manifestations that are peculiar to MRL-*lpr/lpr* mice include arthritis and arteritis. Approximately 25% of these mice have swelling of the joints of the back legs which consits of destruction of articular cartilage, synovial proliferation, pannus formation and joint effusions [26]. Occasional "rheumatoid-like" nodules are seen in the periarticular tissues [26]. These mice are the only strain that develops an arthritis which, in addition, is rheumatoid factor-positive [23, 30]. Hence, this mouse also can serve as a model for the study of rheumatoid arthritis. Like other autoimmune mice, 15%—20% of MRL-*lpr/lpr* mice are found to have coronary artery disease [23, 26, 31, 32]. Furthermore, pathologically these arteries, as well as the renal arteries, are characterized by an acute necrotizing, inflammatory polyarteritis-like picture [26, 32].

Serologically, MRL-*lpr/lpr* mice display a greater number of autoantibodies and in higher titer than are seen in other murine lupus models. Blood gamma globulin (IgG and IgG$_{2a}$) levels are eight times higher than in normal nonautoimmune controls, and are the highest of the murine lupus-prone mice [23, 26]. Frequently, monoclonal gamma globulins are also seen in 43% of these mice [26]. A variety of antinuclear antibodies are seen in MRL-*lpr/lpr* mice. These consist of antibodies to both double- and single-stranded DNA and anti-Sm antibodies [33]. Among human diseases, anti-Sm antibodies are unique to SLE, whereas in murine lupus these antibodies are only seen in the MRL-*lpr/lpr* strain [33]. Also unique to this strain is the presence of an IgM or IgG rheumatoid factor on 50%

of the mice [30]. Elevated titers of immune complexes and cryoglobulins, along with depressed concentrations of complement, help contribute to the very aggressive lupus illnes seen in these mice [26].

Therefore, the MRL-*lpr/lpr* mice represent a wide spectrum of the clinical and serologic features associated with murine SLE. As a correlate for the human disease, they are unique among the mouse models in that they manifest arthritis and anti-Sm autoantibodies. However, the appropriateness of the MRL-*lpr/lpr* as a model for human SLE may be questioned as most patients do not manifest massive adenopathy or distinctive cellular abnormalities [34]. Nevertheless, the MRL-*lpr/lpr* model is still useful as it provides insights into the pathogenesis of those abnormalities in common, and immune disorders in general.

BXSB/Mp Mice

The BXSB strain is a recombinant inbred line derived from a cross between a C57Bl/6J female and an SB/Le male [22, 35, 36]. BXSB mice are unique in their presentation of SLE in that the disease in this strain is predominantly seen in males [22, 35, 36]. In contrast to the female predominance of both human SLE and other autoimmune mouse models [1, 2, 37, 38], the BXSB mals is afflicted through a Y-chromosome effect that is not hormonally mediated. Neither androgen administration to females nor castration of males has an effect upon disease [39]. The disease is, however, related to hematopoietic stem cell abnormalities and transfer of male cells to lethally irradiated BXSB mice will induce disease [40]. A Y-chromosome-linked factor is responsible for accelerated autoimmunity. This factor, Yaa, cannot by itself induce autoimmunity. Thus the F_1 from the cross of a BXSB male with a nonautoimmune female leads to offspring that manifest mild, late onset autoimmunity [35, 36]. In contrast, the male offspring of crosses between females of other autoimmune strains and BXSB males develop accelerated autoimmune features [35]. Therefore, Yaa in concert with background genes operates to accelerate autoimmunity. Yaa, however, is not without effects in "normal" mouse strains [41]. Consomic CBA/J.BXSB-Y males manifest mild coronary artery disease without autoantibodies or other significant signs of autoimmune disease [41]. In addition, the Y-chromosome of the SB/Le strain is associated with decreased survival in crosses of normal C57Bl/6 female with SB/Le males, but not in reciprocal crosses of SB/Le females with C57Bl/6 males [35]. Thus, the exact nature of the mechanism of action of the BXSB Yaa remains to be determined, but its predominant action is to accelerate, and not to induce autoimmunity. Newer approaches which may allow for characterization of the Yaa gene itself and of its gene product may answer many of the remaining questions.

The disease of these mice is characterized by shortened survival, lymphoid hyperplasia, thymic atrophy, immune complex glomerulonephritis with nephrotic syndrome, hypergammaglobulinemia, Coombs' positive hemolytic anemia, coronary artery disease with myocardial infarction, and pneumonia [22, 26, 35, 36]. An early onset of the disease is seen in males who have a mean survival of 5 months whereas the females develop disease later in life and have a mean survival of 14 months. The males develop an acute to subacute, exudative and proliferative glomerulonephritis which ultimately leads to their death [26]. The renal disease of the females is that of a chronic glomerulonephritis.

Lymph nodes in BXSB mice enlarge to 10—20 times the size of controls. Although the nodal hyperplasia is under T cell regulation, the infiltrate is predominantly B-lymphocytes [22, 26, 35]. Neonatal thymectomy of the males leads to a marked increase in the lymphadenopathy up to 5% of the total body weight of the mouse [42]. Analysis of these nodes reveals that there is a disproportionate increase of Ly 1^+, IgM$^+$, Thy 1^- B cells [42]. These Ly 1^+ B cells are almost entirely responsible for autoantibody production to DNA, erythocytes, and thymocytes in NZB mice [43]. In contrast, these enlarged nodes contain very few Ly 2^+ cells, suggesting that suppressor T cells which normally serve to regulate the B cell hyperactivity are defective.

The pathogenesis of murine lupus as seen in BXSB mice has been further elucidated by studies on the effect of the X-linked imunodeficiency gene *(xid)* on disease expression. The presence of this gene is assocated with the depletion of a subset of late maturing B cells which results in a number of immune defects, including low levels of IgM and unresponsiveness to relatively thymic independent type 2 antigens [44]. Through cross-breeding experiments, it was found that mice bearing both Yaa and the *xid* gene demonstrate marked protection against autoimmunity as manifested by prolonged survival, reduced autoantibodies, renal disease, and lymphoid hyperplasia [45]. Lymph nodes and spleens demonstrated an absence of late maturing B cells, an increase in Ly 2^+ T cells (suppressor phenotype), and a decrease in the Ly 1^+ B cells. Since the majority of Ly 1^+ B cells are found in the subset of B cells depleted by the *xid* gene, the amelioration of the disease by *xid* may be related to the absence of Ly 1^+ B cells [45].

BXSB mice may be serologically the least active of all of the lupus-prone strains. Although they do have significant hypergammaglobulinemia (IgA, IgG$_1$, IgG$_{2b}$, and IgM), high affinity autoantibodies to erythrocytes and DNA are minimally increased. In contrast to MRL-*lpr/lpr* mice, antithymocyte antibodies are found in 20% of the BXSB mice. As in the other murine lupus strains, serum complement levels are depressed, and both circulating immune complexes and cryoglobulins are elevated [22, 26]. Thus in spite of the aggressive nature and rapid onset of their disease with early death, BXSB mice fail to exhibit commensurate serologic abnormalities in keeping with the severity of the autoimmune process.

Recently, in human studies four families have been described where SLE occurred in fathers and sons [46]. Several of the female offspring of the affected fathers had autoantibodies. These kindreds resemble the disease as seen in the BXSB mouse model. That is, the disease is predominantly in the male members of the family but may become fully expressed in the serologically abnormal female members. Therefore this human correlate of the BXSB disease demonstrates that the full spectrum of human SLE can be seen within the spectrum of disease exhibited by the murine models.

Other Murine Lupus Models

A number of other murine strains and crosses develop a lupus-like illness which expands the spectrum of clinical and immune abnormalities. However, they have not been as fully characterized and studied as those discussed above. Some strains (e.g., MRL-+/+, BXSB females) and crosses such as (BXSB X MRL-*lpr/lpr*)F$_1$ and (NZW X MRL-*lpr/lpr*)F$_1$ mice develop lupus later in life [2, 22, 28]. Others, such as motheaten mice, develop disease exceptionally early and die by 8 weeks of age [47, 48]. Some autoimmune mice manifest a limited lupus syndrome, such as Hall Institute mice (antinuclear antibodies), Palmerston North (antinuclear and anti-DNA antibodies, vasculitis, and glomerulonephritis) [49, 50], SL/Ni (glomerulonephritis and arteritis) [51], Swan (antibodies to DNA and T cells) [52, 53], and certain nude strains (anti-DNA and glomerulonephritis) [53, 54]. Recently, another autosomal recessive single gene model of autoimmunity has been described which is characterized by a generalized lymphoproliferative disease *(gld)* [55, 56]. These mice have many immune abnormalities similar to *lpr* mice, but do not develop glomerulonephritis or arteritis. They do, however, have decreased survival, adenopathy, and interstitial pneumonitis [55, 56].

Collectively, these models represent a large spectrum of both clinical and immune abnormalities, the heterogeneity of which is comparable to that seen in human SLE and related disorders. It is hoped that through further analysis of these disorders, a more complete understanding of both human and murine lupus will be gained and thus allow for better therapeutic approaches.

Relevance of the Murine Models to Human SLE

None of the animal models of SLE is a perfect reflection of the human disease. Taken together, however, they provide the proper kind of information expected of an animal model. The mice provide evidence for a genetic, hormonal, environmental, and cellular basis for the illness, as has been found in humans [57].

A genetic predisposition to the development of human disease has been established by both familial studies and by analysis of major histocompatibility associations [58—62]. Similarly, detailed genetic analyses of the murine models has indicated the complexity of the genetic contribution to illness [63—66]. The background genes for autoimmunity have been studied best in the NZB strain (vida supra). Here, at least six genes are responsible for all the features of the illness [64]. Some of the genes appear to code for individual abnormalities in the mice. Thus, a single gene is responsible for the predisposition to anti-DNA production and another unlinked gene allows anti-T cell antibodies to be produced in large amounts [14]. There appears to be no linkage to H-2 or allotype in the recombinant inbred lines [66]. In the NZB mice there is no single gene that predisposes to, or causes, autoimmunity; rather a number of genes contribute [14,

64]. The studies of the single gene locus models, *lpr/lpr* and *gld/gld*, further demonstrate the complexity of the genetic requirements for disease. These models suggest that their effects vary depending upon the background genes [24, 25, 55, 56]. Homozygosity for *lpr* appears to be either an inducer or an accelerator of disease. Similarly, the Y-chromosome of the BXSB mouse is associated with an acceleration of disease upon appropriate backgrounds. Thus, the intricacies of the murine genetic contribution to illness have made the lack of a definite inheritance pattern in human disease more understandable.

Sex hormones can modify immune activity and possibly disease manifestations. The role of estrogen and androgen metabolism in SLE and its effects upon the immune system are just beginning to be understood. From a clinical viewpoint, SLE is predominantly a disease of women of child-bearing age and thus it might be expected that the sex hormones may contribute to its pathogenesis. Exacerbations of human SLE are often seen with hormonal changes, such as during or after pregnancy, at menarche, or with oral estrogen-containing contraceptive use. It has been shown that both male and female patients with SLE [67—69], SLE—Klinefelter's patients [70], and first-degree relatives of SLE patients [68] all have an increase in hydroxylation of estrogen to the potent estrogenic urinary 16 alpha metabolites. In addition, male SLE patients have elevated ratios of estradiol/testosterone [69]. Thus, some patients with SLE may have a metabolic abnormality that leads to excessive production of certain estrogenic components. The mechanisms whereby estrogens exacerbate disease have not been entirely elucidated. Nevertheless, sex hormones and their metabolism provide yet another factor that modifies disease expression in SLE.

There has been an attempt to understand the female predominance in human SLE by studying sex hormones in murine lupus. Studies of (NZB X NZW)F$_1$ mice have demonstrated that the age of the mouse is critical to disease outcome when sexual alterations are performed [38, 71, 72]. Castration of females and males at 2—3 weeks of age and treatment with the opposite sex hormone led to accelerated disease in males and retarded disease in females [71, 72]. In these studies it appeared that androgens retarded disease to a greater extent than estrogens accelerated it; however, both processes were operative. To the extent that patients were like (NZB X NZW)F$_1$ mice, a hormonal explanation for the female predominance of SLE was possible. Studies of experimental tolerance have further shown that in the presence of estrogens a single cellular defect is sufficient to transmit a defect in tolerance; in the presence of androgens, two cellular defects are necessary for a tolerance defect [6]. Therefore, females, by virtue of their estrogens, might be expected to have a predisposition to SLE with more modest cellular abnormalities and males would be protected by their androgens unless they had profound cellular abnormalities.

Not all of the murine models show hormonal effects upon disease. Sex differences are much less marked in the severity of disease in MRL-*lpr/lpr* and NZB mice than in NZB hybrids. Nevertheless, androgens tend to retard and estrogens accelerate disease in these strains, even if it is quantitatively less impressive than in the NZB hybrids. Furthermore, the disease of BXSB mice is unrelated to sex hormones [39, 40] and appears to be caused by the stem cell defect that requires the BXSB Y-chromosome [40]. Once again, the spectrum of disease and the influences exerted upon it as seen in the mouse reflect that observed in humans.

Environmental influences may determine disease manifestation. Environmental immune activators may be critical to the triggering of disease in certain patients with SLE. Photosensitivity to ultraviolet sunlight commonly exposes new cases of lupus or flares preexisting ones while a number of drugs, such as hydralazine or procainamide can unmask clinical SLE. Other chronic immune stimulators may initiate or perpetuate illness. Thus, viruses (Epstein-Barr), bacteria, or parasites which can polyclonally stimulate B cells could lead to increased immunoglobulin and autoantibody production. The search for such environmental agents has been considerable in the mouse models. Xenotropic type C RNA virus and circulating levels of the murine retroviral envelope glycoprotein, gp 70, are found in murine SLE strains [73—76]. However, features of autoimmunity have been dissociated from viral expression in F_2 and recombinant inbred lines [73]. Some viruses, such as lymphocytic choriomeningitis, can accelerate disease [77], whereas others, such as lactate dehydrogenase virus, can ameliorate disease and prolong survival [78]. Although available evidence does not support an etiologic role for viruses, it appears that antibody formation to virus and/or viral antigens causes immune complexes which can deposit in the kidney and contribute to the development of glomerulonephritis. Further studies have revealed that other potential environmental agents, such as the polyclonal B cell activators, can exacerbate autoimmunity in NZB mice [21]. Autoantibody formation can be transiently induced even in normal mice by such polyclonal B cell activators [79, 80] and persistent autoantibody production can be induced in normal mice by polyclonal B cell activators and neonatal thymectomy [81]. Thus, in the appropriate setting of immune dysregulation and/or genetic predisposition to disease, environmental agents can trigger the onset of illness. The elucidation of the precise environmental agents which may contribute to both murine and human SLE will be a great step toward our fuller understanding of its etiopathogenesis.

The cellular immune abnormalities of SLE in both the human and the mouse have been quite extensively studied for over 2 decades. Most of the cellular defects can be observed in both. These abnormalities are too numerous to be fully discussed here as they represent a wide spectrum of cellular defects attributable to lymphocytes and other hematopoietic cells [1, 3, 82]. The unifying cellular abnormality observed, however, is polyclonal B cell activation. This hyperactivity of B cells is felt to be the "final common pathway" through which autoantibody production occurs [1, 37]. Numerous dysregulated cellular events may precede the B cell activation, including loss of suppressor T cell function, heightened helper T cell function, defective cell—cell communication via abnormal macrophages and/or abnormal cytokine production, etc., but the production of autoantibodies by the B cell apprears to be common to humans and mice with SLE. This common event suggests that therapeutic approaches which are specifically directed toward such B cell activity might promise a possible means of intervention.

Summary

Other comparisons between murine lupus and the human disease can be made. However, the above comparisons illustrate that no single murine model is adequately representative of human SLE either clinically or immunologically. It is well appreciated that SLE in man is a very heterogeneous disorder with a myriad of manifestations that differ among patients and even within an individual patient over time. Collectively, the murine models of SLE do reflect the clinical heterogeneity of the human disorder. Furthermore, the variety of immune abnormalities seen in these strains emphasize the different regulatory disturbances that ultimately converge on the final common pathway of polyclonal B cell activation. Similarly, the immunopathogenesis of human SLE differs among patients. Individuals have been described who have decreased suppressor T cells both in number and function (as in NZB mice), increased phenotypic helper T cells (MRL-*lpr/lpr* mice), and normal T cell subpopulations phenotypically but still with polyclonal B cell activation [4].

Therefore, through the study of murine models of SLE we have already gained significant insights into the pathogenesis of the human disorder. Further investigation of all of these strains should in time not only help elucidate the fundamental defect(s) underlying the etiology of the human disease, but also may suggest newer avenues of therapeutic intervention.

References

1. Smith HR, Steinberg AD (1983) Autoimmunity — a perspective. Annu Rev Immunol 1:175
2. Theofilopoulos AN, Dixon FJ (1981) Etiopathogenesis of murine lupus. Immunol Rev 55:179
3. Steinberg AD, Houston DP, Taurog JD, et al (1981) The cellular and genetic basis for murine lupus. Immunol Rev 55:121
4. Smolen JS, Chused TM, Leiserson WM, Reeves JP, Alling DW (1982) Heterogeneity of immunoregulatory T cell subsets in systemic lupus erythematosus. Correlation with clinical features. Am. J. Med. 72:783
5. Steinberg AD, Raveche ES, Laskin CA, Smith HR, Santoro TJ, Miller ML, Plotz PH (1984) Systemic lupus erythematosus: Insights from animal models. Ann. Int. Med. 100:714
6. Laskin CA, Taurog JD, Smathers PA, Steinberg AD (1981) Studies of defective tolerance in murine lupus. J. Immunol. 127:1743
7. Staples PJ, Talal N (1969) Relative inability to induce tolerance in adult NZB and NZW/NZB F_1 mice. J. Exp. Med. 129:123
8. Goldings, EA, Cohen PL, McFadden SF, Ziff M, Vitetta E (1980) Defective B cell tolerance in adult (NZB X NZW)F_1 mice. J. Exp. Med. 152:730
9. Izui S, Masuda K (1984) Resistance to tolerance induction is not prerequisite to development of murine SLE. J. Immunol. 133:3010
10. Moutsopoulos HM, Boehm-Truitt M, Kassan SS, Chused TM (1977) Demonstration of activation of B lymphocytes in New Zealand Black mice at birth by an immunoradiometric assay. J. Immunol. 119:1639

Relevance of the Murine Models of Systemic Lupus Erythematosus **83**

11. Izui S, McConahey PJ, Dixon FJ (1978) Increased spontaneous polyclonal activation of B lymphocytes in mice spontaneous autoimmune disease. J. Immunol. 121:2213
12. Manny N, Datta SK, Schwartz RS (1979) Synthesis of IgM by cells of NZB and SWR mice and their crosses. J. Immunol. 122:1220
13. Theofilopoulos AN, Shawler DL, Eisenberg RA, Dixon FJ (1980) Splenic immunoglobulin-secreting cells and their regulation in autoimmune mice. J. Exp. Med. 151:446
14. Raveche, ES, Steinberg AD, Klassen LW, Tjio JH (1978) Genetic studies in NZB mice. I. Spontaneous autoantibody production. J. Exp. Med. 147:1487
15. Raveche ES, Tjio JH, Steinberg AD (1980) Genetic studies in NZB mice. IV. The effect of sex hormones on the spontaneous production of anti-T cell autoantibodies. Arth. Rheum. 23:48
16. Taurog JD, Raveche ES, Smathers PA, Glimcher LH, Huston DP, Hansen CT, Steinberg AD (1981) T cell abnormalities in NZB mice occur independently of autoantibody production. J. Exp. Med. 153:221
17. Taurog JD, Smathers PA, Steinberg AD (1980) Evidence for abnormalities in separate lymphocyte populations in NZB mice. J. Immunol. 125:485
18. Mortin JI, Siegel BW (1974) Transplantation of autoimmune potential. I. Development of antinuclear antibodies in H-2 histocompatible recipients of bone marrow from New Zealand black mice. Proc. Natl. Acad. Sci. USA 71:2162
19. DeHeer DH, Edgington TS (1977) Evidence for a B-lymphocyte defect underlying the anti-X anti-erythrocyte autoantibody response of NZB mice. J. Immunol. 118:1858
20. Laskin CA, Smathers PA, Reeves JP, Steinberg AD (1982) Studies of defective tolerance induction in NZB mice: Evidence for a marrow pre-T cell defect. J. Exp. Med. 155:1025
21. Smathers PA, Steinberg BJ, Reeves JP, Steinberg AD (1982) Efect of polyclonal immune stimulators upon NZB. *xid* congenic mice. J. Immunol. 128:1414
22. Murphy ED, Roths JB (1978) New inbred strains. Mouse News Lett 58:51
23. Murphy ED (1981) Lymphoproliferation *(lpr)*, a mutant gene in strain MRL inducing murine lupus. In: Gershwin ME, Merchant B (eds) *Immunologic defects in laboratory animals*, vol 2. Plenum, New York, pp 143—173
24. Roths JB et al. (1983) Modification of expression of *lpr* by background genome. Fed. Proc. 42:1075
25. Izui S, Kelly VE, Masuda K, Yoshida H, Roth JB, Murphy ED (1984) Induction of various autoantibodies by mutant gene *lpr* in several strains of mice. J. Immunol. 133:227
26. Andrews BB, Eisenberg RA, Theofilopoulos AN, Izui S, Wilson CB, McConahey PJ, Murphy ED, Roths JB, Dixon FJ (1978) Spontaneous murine lupus-like syndromes. Clinical and immunopathological manifestations in several strains. J. Exp. Med. 148:1198
27. Lewis DE, Giorgi JV, Warner NL (1981) Flow cytometry analysis of T cells and continuous T cell lines from autoimmune MRL/1 mice. Nature 289:298
28. Morse HC III, Davidson WF, Yetter RA, Murphy ED, Roths JB, Coffman RL (1982) Abnormalities induced by the mutant gene *lpr:* expansion of a unique lymphocyte subset. J. Immunol. 129:2612
29. Smith HR, Chused TM, Steinberg AD (1984) Cyclophosphamide-induced changes in the MRL-*lpr/lpr* mouse: effects upon cellular composition, immune function, and disease. Clin. Immunol. Immunopathol. 30:51
30. Eisenberg RA, Thor LT, Dixon FJ (1979) Serum—serum interactions in autoimmune mice. Arth. Rheum. 22:1074
31. Hang LM, Izui S, Dixon FJ (1981) (NZW X BXSB)F₁ hybrid. A model of acute lupus and coronary vascular disease with myocardial infarction. J. Exp. Med. 154:216
32. Berden JHM, Hang LM, McConahey PJ, Dixon FJ (1983) Analysis of vascular lesions in murine SLE. I. Association with serologic abnormalities. J. Immunol. 130:1699
33. Eisenberg RA, Tan EM, Dixon FJ (1978) Presence of anti-Sm reactivity in autoimmune mouse strains. J. Exp. Med. 147:582, 1978
34. Theofilopoulos AN, Prud'homme GJ, Fleser TM, Dixon FJ (1983) B-cell hyperactivity in murine lupus. II. Defects in response to and production of accessory signals in lupus-prone mice. Immunol. Today 4:317
35. Murphy ED, Roths JB (1979) A Y-chromosome associated factor in strain BXSB producing accelerated autoimmunity and lymphoproliferation. Arth. Rheum. 22:1188

36. Murphy ED, Roths JB (1978) Autoimmunity and lymphoproliferation: induction by mutant gene *lpr* and accelerated by a male-associated factor in strain BXSB mice. In: Rose NR, Bigazzi PE, Warner NL (eds) Genetic control of autoimmune disease. Elsever/North Holland, New York, p 207
37. Steinberg AD, Smith HR, Laskin CA, Steinberg BJ, Smolen JS (1982) Studies of immune abnormalities in systemic lupus erythematosus. Am. J. Kidney Dis. 2:101
38. Roubinian JR, Papoian R, Talal N (1977) Androgenic hormones moderate autoantibody responses and improve survival in murine lupus. J. Clin. Invest. 59:1066
39. Eisenberg RA, Dixon FJ (1980) Effect of castration on male-determined acceleration of autoimmune disease in BXSB mice. J. Immunol. 125:1959
40. Eisenberg RA, Izui S, McConahey PJ, Hang L, Peters CJ, Theofilopoulos AN, Dixon FJ (1980) Male determined accelerated autoimmune disease in BXSB mice: transfer by bone marrow and spleen cells. J. Immunol. 125:1032
41. Hudgins CC, Steinberg RT, Reeves JP, Steinberg AD (1985) Studies of congenic mice bearing the Y chromosome of the BXSB mouse. J. Immunol. 134:3849
42. Smith HR, Chused TM, Smathers PA, Steinberg AD (1983) Evidence for thymic regulation of autoimmunity in BXSB mice: acceleration of disease by neonatal thymectomy. J. Immunol. 130:1200
43. Hayakawa K, Hardy RR, Honda M, Herzenberg LA, Steinberg AD, Herzenberg LA (1984) Ly-1 B cells: functionally distinct lymphocytes that secrete IgM autoantibodies. proc. Natl. Acad. Sci. USA 81:2494
44. Scher I, Steinberg AD, Berning AK, Paul WE (1975) X-linked B-lymphocyte immune defect in CBA/N mice. II. Studies of mechanisms underlying the immune defect. J. Exp. Med. 142:637
45. Smith HR, Chused TM, Steinberg AD (1983) The effect of the X-linked immune deficiency gene *(xid)* upon the Y chromosome-related disease of BXSB mice. J. Immunol. 131:1257
46. Lahita RG, Chiorazzi N, Gibofsy A, Winchester RJ, Kunkel HG (1983) Familial systemic lupus erythematosus in males. Arth Rheum. 26:39
47. Shultz LD, Grren MC (1976) Motheaten, an immunodeficient mutant of the mouse. II. Depressed immune function and elevated serum innumoglobulins. J. Immunol. 116:936
48. Shultz LD, Coman DR, Bailey CL, Beamer WG, Sidman CL (1984) "Viable motheaten", a new allele at the motheaten locus. I. Pathology. Am. J. Pathol. 116:179
49. Walker SE, Gray RN, Fulton M, Wigley RD, Schnitzer B (1978) Palmerston North mice, a new animal model of systemic lupus erythematosus. J. Lab. Clin. Med. 92:932
50. Walker SE, Schnitzer B (1980) Resistance to therapy in Palmerston North mice treated with cyclophosphamide or hydrocortisone sodium succinate. Arth. Rheum. 23:539, 1980
51. Kyogoku M (1980) Pathogenesis of vasculitits in the SL/Ni mouse. In: Japan Medical Research Foundation (ed) Systemic lupus erythematosus, University of Tokyo Press, Tokyo p 281
52. Monier JC, Robert M (1974) Defective T cell functions in autoimmune Swan mice. Ann. Immunol. Inst. Pasteur (Paris) 125c:405
53. Monier JC, Sepetjian M (1975) Spontaneous antinuclear autoimmunization in Swan and nude mice: comparative study. Ann. Immunol. Inst. Pasteur (Paris) 126c:63
54. Monier JC, Costa O, Souweine G, Rigal D (1980) Lupus-like syndrome in some strains of nude mice. Thymus 1:241
55. Roths JB, Murphy ED, Eicher EM (1984) A new mutation *gld*, that produces lymphoproliferation and autoimmunity in C3H/HeJ mice. J. Exp. Med. 159:1
56. Davidson WF, Roths JB, Morse HB (1984) Single gene mutations that cause SLE-like autoimmune disease in mice. Clin. Immunol. News Let 5:17
57. Reinertsen JL, Klippel JH, Kohnson AH, Steinberg AD, Decker JL, Mann DL (1978) B-lymphocyte alloantigens associated with systemic lupus erythematosus. N. Engl. J. Med. 299:515
58. Arnett FC, Shulman LE (1976) Studies in familial systemic lupus erythematosus. Medicine 55:313
59. Block SR, Lockshin MD, Winfield JB et al. (1976) Immunological observations in 9 sets of twins either concordant or discordant for SLE. Arth. Rheum. 19:454

Relevance of the Murine Models of Systemic Lupus Erythematosus 85

60. Lippman SM, Arnett FC, Conley CL, Ness PM, Meyers DA, Bias WB (1982) Genetic factors predisposing to autoimmune disease: autoimmune hemolytic anemia, chronic thrombocytopenic purpura, and systemic lupus erythematosus. Am. J. Med. 73:827
61. Miller KB, Schwartz RS (1979) Familial abnormalities of suppressor-cell function in systemic lupus erythematosus. N. Engl. J. Med. 301:803
62. Reinertsen JL, Klippel JH, Kohnson AH, Steinberg AD, Decker JL, Mann DL (1982) Family studies of B lymphocyte alloantigens in systemic lupus erythematosus. J. Rheumatol. 9:253
63. Miller ML, Raveche ES, Laskin CA, Klinman DM, Steinberg AD (1984) Genetic studies in NZB mice. IV. Association of autoimmune traits in recombinant inbred mice. J. Immunol. 133:1325
64. Raveche ES, Novotny EA, Hansen CT, Tjio JH, Steinberg AD (1981) Genetic studies in NZB mice. V. Recombinant inbred lines demonstrate that separate genes control autoimmune phenotype. J. Exp. Med. 153:1187
65. Raveche ES, Steinberg AD, Klassen LW, Tjio JH (1978) Genetic studies in NZB mice. I. Spontaneous autoantibody production. J. Exp. Med. 147:1487
66. Bocchiere MH, Cooke A, Smith JB, Weigert M, Riblet RJ (1982) Independent segregation of NZB autoimmune abnormalities in NZB X C58 recombinant inbred mice. Eur. J. Immunol. 12:349
67. Lahita RG, Bradlow HL, Kunkel HG, Fishman J (1981) Increased 16 alpha-hydroxylation of estradiol in systemic lupus erythematosus. J. Clin. Endocrinol. Metabl. 53:174
68. Lahita RG, Bradlow HL, Fishman J, Kunkel HG (1982) Estrogen metabolism in systemic lupus erythematosus: patients and family members. Arth. Rheum. 25:843
69. Inman RD, Jovanovic L, Dawood MY, Longcope C (1979) Systemic lupus erythematosus in the male: a genetic and endocrine study. Arth. Rheum. 22:624
70. Stern R, Fishman J, Brusman H, Kunkel HG (1977) Systemic lupus erythematosus associated with Klinefelter's syndrome. Arth. Rheum. 20:18
71. Roubinian JR, Talal N, Greenspan JS, Goodman JR, Siiteri PK (1979) Delayed androgen treatment prolongs survival in murine lupus. J. Clin. Invest. 63:902
72. Steinberg AD, Melez KA, Raveche ES, Reeves JP, Boegel W (1979) Approach to the study of the role of sex hormones in autoimmunity. Arth. Rheum. 22:1170
73. Datta SK, Owen FL, Womack JE, Riblet RJ (1982) Analysis of recombinant inbred lines derived from "autoimmune" (NZB) and "high leukemia" (C58) strains: independent multigenic systems control B cell hyperactivity, retrovirus expression, and autoimmunity. J. Immunol. 129:1539
74. Izui S, McConahey PJ, Clark JP, Hang LM, Hara I, Dixon FJ (1981) Retroviral gp70 immune complexes in NZB X NZW F_2 mice with murine lupus nephritis. J. Exp. Med. 154:517
75. Datta SK, Schwartz RS (1976) Genetics of expression of xenotropic virus and autoimmunity in NZB mice. Nature 263:412
76. Izui S, McConahey PJ, Theofilopoulos AN, Dixon FJ (1979) Association of circulating retroviral gp70—anti-gp70 immune complexes with murine systemic lupus erythematosus. J. Exp. Med. 149:1099
77. Tonietti G, Oldstone MB, Dixon FJ (1970) The effect of induced chronic viral infections on the immunological diseases of New Zealand mice. J. Exp. Med. 132:89
78. Oldstone MBA, Dixon FJ (1972) Inhibition of antibodies to nuclear antigens and to DNA in New Zealand mice infected with lactate dehydrogenase virus. Science 175:784
79. Fournie GJ, Lambert PH, Miescher PA (1974) Release of DNA in circulating blood and induction of anti-DNA antibodies after injection of bacterial lipopolysaccharides. J. Exp. Med. 140:1189
80. Izui S, Lambert PH, Fournie PH, Turler H, Miescher PA (1977) Features of systemic lupus erythematosus in mice injected with bacterial lipopolysaccharides. J. Exp. Med. 145:1115
81. Smith HR, Grren DR, Raveche ES, Smathers PA, Gershon RK, Steinberg AD (1982) Studies of the induction of anti-DNA in normal mice. J. Immunol. 129:2332
82. Raveche ES, Steinberg AD (1979) Lymphocytes and lymphocyte functions in systemic lupus erythematosus. Clinics Haematol. 16:344

Part III:
Immunologic and Genetic Aspects of Human SLE

The Importance of the Study
of Monoclonal Antibodies*

D. Isenberg, Y. Shoenfeld, and R. S. Schwartz

Introduction

Systemic lupus erythematosus (SLE) is an autoimmune disease whose extensive clinical manifestations are matched by its serological abnormalities. Antibodies may be detected in the serum of SLE patients which bind to a wide variety of seemingly diverse antigenic structures. These include molecules such as nucleic acids, phospholipids, and intermediate filaments, and a variety of cells and tissues, including red and white blood cells, platelets, and synovial membranes.

In lupus, as in other autoimmune disorders, precise identification of the antigenic specificities of the autoantibodies is essential to understanding its immunopathology. However, the seemingly vast array of autoantibodies in SLE patients' sera presents a formidable barrier to the isolation and purification of individual antibodies. Occasionally, spontaneously occurring monoclonal antibodies may be found with autoantibody properties, for example, monoclonal rheumatoid factor [12] or monoclonal cold agglutinin [6]. This subject has been reviewed in detail elsewhere [49]. However, spontaneously occurring monoclonal antibodies are found too infrequently [42] to allow the properties and derivation of all autoantibodies to be studied adequately.

Monoclonal antibodies may be produced by Epstein-Barr virus (EBV) infection and subsequent immortalization of B-lymphocytes which produce autoantibodies [63]. This technique is limited because EBV-immortalized cells secrete only small quantities of immunoglobulin.

The introduction of hybridoma techniques which allow the production, purification, and isolation of monoclonal antibodies of defined specificities has opened up a new era in scientific investigations. In the last 5 years, many laboratories have employed this technique to analyze the antigenic specificities, idiotypic markers, and primary structure of lupus autoantibodies. This review will examine each of these features and the potential they provide for introducing more specific forms of therapy for SLE than currently, are available.

---

* This work was supported in part by a grant from the Bat-Sheva de Rothschild Foundation for Sciences and Humanities and by NIH Grants AM 31151 and AI 19794.

Antigenic Specificities
of Lupus Monoclonal Autoantibodies

Antipolynucleotide and Antiphospholipid Antibodies

Hybridomas from Animal Models

The potential for exploring cross-reactive and anti-DNA antibodies was not realized until the introduction of monoclonal anti-DNA autoantibodies. Andrzejewski et al. [2] were able to show that such antibodies could be derived from the MRL-*lpr/lpr* strain of lupus-prone mice without the need to preimmunize the animals. These hybridoma-derived monoclonal anti-DNA antibodies bound to a variety of nucleic acids and polynucleotides, including ssDNA, dsDNA, poly(I), poly(G), poly(C), poly(dT), and poly(dC). In a follow-up study, Lafer et al. [28], using competitive immunoassays, demonstrated that the binding of monoclonal antibodies from MRL-*lpr/lpr* mice to plates coated with ssDNA was blocked by cardiolipin, phosphatidic acid, phosphatidyl glycerol, and various polynucleotides. Furthermore, the antinuclear reaction of one of the monoclonal antibodies was specifically inhibited by cardiolipin. The same antibody prolonged the activated partial thromboplastin time, thus acting like a lupus anticoagulant. It was therefore suggested that serological diversity in SLE was restricted and could be the result of the binding of certain autoantibodies to a phosphodiester-containing epitope present in diverse molecules.

Hahn and colleagues [14] produced monoclonal anti-DNA antibodies by fusing spleen cells from NZB/NZW F_1 mice, MRL/1, or BXSB mice with mouse myeloma cells. Two of their antibodies were inhibited by both single- and double-stranded DNA, though not by single-stranded RNA or poly(I)—poly(C). Tron and his colleagues [65] also produced monoclonal anti-DNA antibodies that strongly bound both ssDNA and dsDNA. Marion and Briles [35] found that the number of hybridomas obtained from each fusion paralleled the serum anti-DNA antibody titers in NZB/NZW F_1 mice. Their monoclonals showed heterogeneous binding to ssDNA, dsDNA, and poly(I)—poly(C). Pisetsky [44] has described a monoclonal antibody from an MRL/1 fusion which reacted with various ribohomopolymers and deoxyribohomopolymers.

More recently, Morgan et al. [38] produced a large number of monoclonal anti-DNA antibodies from NZB/NZW F_1 and MRL-*lpr/lpr* fusions and subdivided them into groups according to the epitopes with which they reacted. Some monoclonals were found to be specific for ssDNA, others for dsDNA, whilst three other groups bound in varying degrees with ssDNA, dsDNA, cardiolipin, cardiolipin-cholesterol liposomes, and/or RNA.

Eliat et al. [10] obtained a monoclonal lupus antibody from an NZB/NZW F_1 fusion which bound specifically to single —, but not double —, stranded RNA. It also reacted with the random polymers poly(G, C) and poly(G, C, U). In a follow-up study, Laskov et al. [30] produced a further 12 antibodies from the NZB/NZW F_1 mouse fusions which bound to RNA.

Hybridomas from Human Fusions

The introduction of human—human hybridomas has confirmed and extended the evidence from the animal models of cross-reative anti-DNA antibodies. Shoenfeld et al. [54, 56] showed that human monoclonal anti-DNA antibodies could bind to combinations of ssDNA, ds DNA, Z-DNA, poly(I), and poly(dT). Some of these human monoclonal anti-DNA antibodies were shown to have antiplatelet activity, and 10 (48%) of 21 monoclonals tested bound to cardiolipin. Rauch et al. [51] have confirmed that human monoclonal anti-DNA antibodies from SLE patients can bind cardiolipin. Other studies have demonstrated human monoclonal anti-DNA antibodies binding to poly(dG)—poly(dC) [34].

Serum Analyses

These observations with monoclonal anti-DNA antibodies parallel experience with serum-derived anti-DNA antibodies. For example, Koike et al. [26] showed that polyspecific anti-DNA antibodies could react with ssDNA, dsDNA, and cardiolipin. Isenberg et al. [22] found that serum from 56 SLE patients often showed multiple binding to combinations of ssDNA, dsDNA, poly(dT), poly(I), RNA, and cardiolipin. Despite these observations, the question of how representative the hybridoma-derived monoclonal anti-DNA antibodies actually are, is not fully resolved. Amongst the human monoclonal anti-DNA antibodies, none which react solely with dsDNA have been described, which is perhaps surprising. Further, all the human monoclonal anti-DNA antibodies so far described are of the IgM k isotype. Since IgG anti-DNA antobodies are thought to be of importance in the immunopathology of lupus [61], these too will need to be produced in order to answer fully the question of how representative the hybridomas antibodies are.

Nucleotide Sequence

The importance of nuceotide sequence in defining antigenic specificity amongst monoclonal anti-DNA antibodies has been emphasized by Lee et al. [31]. Six hybridoma-derived anti-DNA antibodies from NZB/NZW F_1 mice were analyzed with synthetic homo- and heteropolymers of purines and pyrimidines. The reaction of each antibody was markedly influenced by the base sequence of the antigen. Similarly, Weisbart et al. [67] were able to show that a small fraction of IgG anti-DNA antibodies in SLE sera react specifically with guanosine. The autoantibody produced by Eilat and colleagues [10], which bound to single-stranded RNA, was shown to recognize an antigenic determinant containing guanine (G), cytosine (C), and uridine (U). A second monoclonal anti-RNA antibody produced by this group was shown to bind to (G, C) rich sequences of ribonucleotides.

These experiments demonstrate that monoclonal antibodies can be utilizied to demonstrate submolecular structures (epitopes) on autoantigens.

Antibodies to Other Antigenic Specificities

Hybridomas from Animal Models

Antibodies to the RNP-associated antigen Sm also are highly specific for SLE. Lerner et al. [33] have produced monoclonal antibodies from MRL-*lpr/lpr* mice that react with the Sm antigen. In an agar gel, the immunoprecipitation reaction of the mouse anti-Sm antibody with the Sm antigen was identical to the reaction of a human anti-Sm antibody. The Sm antigen was found to reside on all five of the nuclear ribonucleoproteins immunoprecipitated by both the anti-Sm serum and the monoclonal anti-Sm antibody.

Laskov et al. [30] have produced two monoclonals with specificity for histones from NZB/NZW mice. One was specific for histone H2B, both free in solution and as part of an H2A—H2B complex. The second monoclonal antibody recognized a specific conformation in the H3—H4 complex. The monoclonals did not bind RNA or DNA and may prove useful for investigations of drug-induced lupus, which is more frequently associated with antihistone antibodies than idiopathic SLE.

Hybridoma-derived monoclonal antibodies that bind to erythrocytes have been described [3]. These IgM antibodies react with an erythrocyte autoantigen revealed by bromelin treatment.

Kanai and colleagues [25] produced monoclonal antibodies that bind to poly(ADP-ribose), a biopolymer associated with chromatin and thought to participate in gene expression and DNA repair. These monoclonals, produced from MRL/*lpr/lpr* mice, also bind to single-stranded DNA and Z-DNA. Another curious cross-reaction has been observed with MRL/*lpr/lpr* monoclonal rheumatoid factors which exhibit multiple reactions with other autoantigens, including single-stranded DNA and histones [52]. This observation parallels a much earlier one [19] that rheumatoid factor isolated from serum could bind to single-stranded DNA and nitrophenyl groups. Tron et al. [66] have demonstrated that a murine monoclonal anti-DNA antibody can bind to the plasma membrane of Raji cells, an indication that the interpretation of Raji cell binding in human sera containing anti-DNA antibodies requires caution. Their observation confirmed an earlier report that antinuclear antibodies can directly interact with Raji cells [20].

Hybridomas from Human Fusions

Monoclonal anti-DNA antibodies derived from human lupus patients (and MRL-*lpr/lpr* mice) have been shown to bind to the cytoskeletal protein vimentin [1]. The cross-reactive structure in vimentin exists is unknown. A monoclonal anti-DNA antibody has also been shown to bind to erythrocytes [58]. In addition, 2 of 25 monoclonal anti-DNA autoantibodies have been found to have lymphocytotoxic activity. This activity could be inhibited by prior incubation of the antibodies with various polynucleotides, suggesting that a shared epitope might explain the apparent cross-reactivity between DNA and lymphocytic membrane [74].

Monoclonal Antibodies Derived from Normal Mice and Humans

Are anti-DNA antibodies confined to lupus-prone mice or patients with SLE? This important question has been addressed in several recent studies. Monier et al. [37] generated a hybridoma between normal spleen cells from BALB/c mice (a nonautoimmune strain) and a mouse myeloma cell line. The hybrid cells produced an IgM k anti-dsDNA antibody which bound to both ss and dsDNA and some synthetic polydeoxyribonucleotides. Rauch et al. [50] immunized BALB/c mice with cardiolipin and showed they produced cardiolipin-binding antibodies that also bound to DNA, poly(dT), and poly(I). These results suggest that the production of anti-DNA autoantibodies does not require immunization by DNA. Rauch and her colleagues [51] have also generated monoclonal anti-DNA antibodies by human—human fusion with peripheral blood lymphocytes from normal individuals and patients with rheumatoid arthritis (in addition to SLE patients, as alluded to above). The nucleic acid binding characteristics of the anti-DNA antibodies produced by the hybridomas derived from normal subjects, RA patients, and lupus patients howed similar antigen-binding characteristics.

The fusion of tonsillar lymphoid cells from a normal donor with a human myeloma cell line has been reported [4]. Supernatants from these clones also showed polyspecificity, with binding to varying combinations of ssDNA, dsDNA, RNA, poly(dG)—poly(dC), poly(dA—dT), and cardiolipin. This broad range of anti-DNA antibody specificities thus matches those found in hybridomas from lupus-prone mice and SLE patients.

This work supports the notion that normal individuals possess lymphocytes with immunoglobulin genes which code for anti-DNA autoantibodies. Further, the nucleic acid (and phospholipid) antigen-binding characteristics may not be the only factors which determine the pathogenicity of anti-DNA autoantibodies in SLE.

Possible Explanations for Cross-reactivity

There is little doubt that anti-DNA antibodies are capable of a wide variety of cross-reactions. What remains in doubt is the identity of the shared epitope. As Schwartz [57] has discussed, an obvious candidate is the phosphodiester-linked phosphate structure that occurs in polynucleotides and phospholipids. Both molecules contain phosphate groups in phosphodiester linkage, separated by three carbon atoms of adjacent sugar molecules. The individual differences in binding specificity amongst various anti-DNA antibodies might be explained by variations in the precise interphosphate distances and helical configurations.

Another possibility, discussed by Lane and Koprowski [29], is that different antigenic structures may bind partially to a "common" conformational determinant on a monoclonal antibody. The determinant is actually made up of two or more subunits; hence the monoclonal antibody would appear to be binding to many more antigens than was at first envisaged.

These may not be the only explanations, however, Faaber and colleagues [11] have shown that anti-DNA antibodies derived from lupus sera reacted with hyaluronic acid and chondroitin sulphate. They suggested that these cross-reactivations of anti-DNA antibodies may simply be binding to structures with repeating negatively charged groups.

These three explanations may not be mutually exclusive and indeed other possibilities, including a fuller consideration of antibody affinity, have yet to be evaluated.

Amino Acid Sequence Analysis of Monoclonal Anti-DNA Antibodies

N-terminal sequence analyses of four IgM human monoclonal hybridoma-derived anti-DNA monoclonal antibodies have been performed [40]. In each, the heavy chains belonged to the k-III subgroup and the light chains to the k-I subgroup. The sequences of the 40 N-terminal light chain amino acids were 95% identical, compared to 85% amongst the heavy chains. Remarkably, the heavy and light chain amino acid sequences were almost identical to those of a Waldenstrom's monoclonal IgM, known as WEA, that binds to the *Klebsiella* polysaccharide K30. Tests of antigenic specificity and idiotypic analysis have established that these monoclonal lupus and Waldenstrom's IgM are of common origin and derived from a conserved V gene. They imply that anti-DNA autoantibodies might arise from a family of anti bacterial clones that undergo polyclonal activation. The close relationship between anti bacterial and anti-DNA antibodies has also been demonstrated by Diamond and Scharff [7]. They performed amino acid sequence analyses on an antiphosphocholine antibody derived from an IgA k myeloma cell line and a mutant antibody in which a single amino acid residue, alanine, was substituted for glutamic acid at position 35 on the heavy chain V region. The mutant antibody no longer bound to phosphocholine but did bind to a variety of phosphorylated molecules, including double-stranded DNA and cardiolipin.

The likely sharing of determinants between nucleic acids and bacterial cell wall antigens is of considerable interest. Perhaps an early step in the pathogenesis of SLE is exposure to immunogenic determinants on bacteria. The antibodies thus formed may cross-react with antigenic determinants on nucleic acids. In this context, it is worth recalling that native nucleic acid is a poor immunogen [76].

94 D. Isenberg et al.

It is conceivable that pathogenic anti-"DNA" antibodies may be induced by contact with unusual fragments of DNA [53], a cross-reacting immunogen (phospholipid in a bacterial cell wall), or even by polyclonal B cell activation in the absence of any immunogen [8].

Idioytypic Analyses

General Considerations

Antigen-binding capability is one way of determining the diversity amongst autoantibodies. Another method involves the serological analysis of variable region structures (idiotypes) of immunoglobulins. Since these structures may themselves be immunogenic, it is possible to produce anti-idiotypic antibodies by immunization with monoclonal antibodies in another species. This procedure requires the removal of irrelevant antibodies by absorption.

Anti-DNA Antibody Idiotypes

Serological Studies

A number of studies of idiotypes of monoclonal anti-DNA antibodies in lupus prone mice have reported concordant results. Marion and colleagues [35] utilized a rabbit antiserum against an idiotype of a monoclonal anti-DNA antibody of NZB/NZW F_1 origin. They showed that a common idiotype was shared by 8 out of 13 monoclonal antibodies with similar ligand-binding specificities. This common idotype, known as DNA-3, was found in the serum of all tested NZB/NZW F_1 mice over the age of 6 months. Tron et al. [65] developed monoclonal anti-idiotypic antibody by immunizing A/J mice with a monoclonal NZB/NZW F_1 anti-DNA autoantibody designated F-227. It detected the F-227 idiotype in each of the 24 NZB/NZW F_1 sera tested. Finally, Rauch and colleagues [48], prepared an anti-idiotype by immunizing rabbits with an MRL-*lpr/lpr* monoclonal DNA antibody known as H-130. This reagent reacted with 8 of 12 other MRL-derived monoclonal autoantibodies. It also detected the idiotype in the serum of all 40 MRL-*lpr/lpr* sera tested. The proportion of serum anti-DNA antibodies with the H-130 idiotype ranged from 22% to 50%, indicating that H-130 is a predominant idiotypic family within the population of MRL-*lpr/lpr* anti-DNA antibodies.

A monoclonal antibody to an idiotype present on IgG anti-DNA antibodies from NZB/NZW F_1 mice detected similar determinants found on polyclonal and monoclonal IgG anti-DNA antibodies from the unrelated MRL-*lpr/lpr* and BXSB strains [17]. This public idiotype was found to be close to the antigen-binding regions on anti-DNA antibodies carrying a cationic charge (pI > 7). The relation to cationic charge is of interest because IgG2a anti-DNA antibodies eluted from the glomeruli of NZB/NZW and MRL-*lpr/lpr* mice constitute a restricted subpopulation with cationic charge [9].

More recent studies have extended these observations in mice to human anti-DNA antibodies. Three anti-idiotypic reagents were prepared by immunization of rabbits or a mouse with human monoclonal anti-DNA autoantibodies derived from two SLE patients [55]. Each anti-idiotypic antibody appeared to detect a different idiotypic determinant. Of 60 human monoclonal anti-DNA autoantibodies tested with the three anti-idiotypic antibodies, 40 reacted in one or more competitive immunoassay, and 15 reacted with all three reagents. These three reagents were then used to screen the serum from 98 SLE patients. Serum levels of one idiotype, designated 16/6/R, were elevated in 40 of 74 (54%) patients with active SLE, compared with 6 of 24 (25%) patients with inactive lupus [24]. Further, in 8 of 12 patients followed serially, some concordance was found between the idiotype levels and clinical activity.

In a recent prospective study [75], the 16/6 idiotype was also found to reflect clinical activity in four of seven patients judged severely ill during the year of the investigation (see Fig. 1 for an example). In another study, Solomon et al. [60] prepared a mouse monoclonal antibody against an idiotypic determinant on anti-dsDNA antibodies purified from the serum of a lupus patient. This reagent (3I) detected cross-reacting idiotypes in sera from eight of nine lupus patients. Further studies using the 3I anti-idiotype indicated that it was able to detect anti-DNA antibodies in sera of some SLE patients that lacked anti-DNA antibodies by ordinary assays [18]. The authors suggested that these antibodies might be inhibited from binding double-stranded DNA by either excess antigen or autologous anti-idiotype.

The two anti-idiotypic antibodies described above, anti 16/6/R and mouse monoclonal anti 32/15, were used to study the presence of idiotypes (16/6 and 32/15) in the healthy first-degree relatives of 48 SLE patients [71]. In this study, 40% of SLE patients and 24% of 147 healthy first-degree relatives had increased levels of 16/6 idiotype. With anti 32/15, 24% of patients and 7% of their relatives had raised levels.

In a study of the origins of DNA antibody idiotype 16/6, Datta and colleagues [5a] reported the in vitro production of the idiotype following pokeweed mitogen stimulation of peripheral blood lymphocytes from normal subjects and lupus patients. Using biosynthetic labelling, immunoprecipitation and SDS polyacrylamide gel electrophoresis their findings indicate that the 16/6 idiotype exists on two distinct populations of antibodies. The first population is of uncertain antigenic specificity, though it is tempting to speculate that they are directed against common environmental pathogens, and it dominates the 16/6 idiotype set that appears after pokeweed mitogen stimulation of lymphocytes from normal individuals and lupus patients in relapse. In contrast, the second population is found on antibodies binding to nucleic acids and becomes prominent during a clinical relapse of SLE. The mechanism behind this 'switch' and its significance in relation to the immunopathology of SLE remain to be determined.

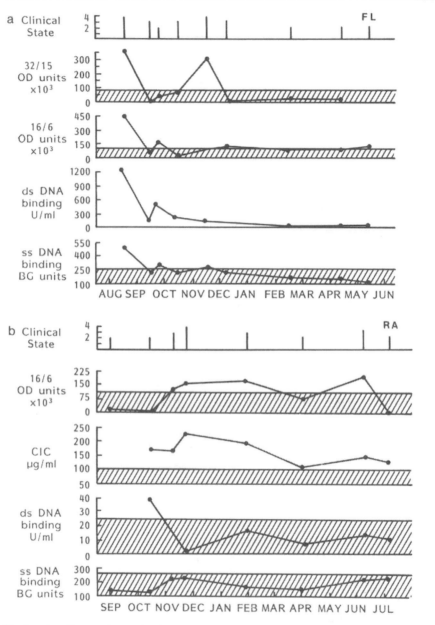

Fig. 1. a, b. a Prospective study of an SLE patient (FL) comparing the clinical state (*1*, inactive; *2*, mildly active; *3*, moderately active; *4*, severely active) with DNA antibody idiotypes 16/6-R and 32/15-M, dsDNA binding (Amersham kit), and ssDNA binding (arbitary units, from an ELISA assay). Normal ranges are represented by the *hatched areas* (16/6-R normal = 115 OD units x 10^3. There is good correlation between all four measurements during the initial disease flare, but only 32/15-M is elevated during the second flare. **b** Prospective study of an SLE patient (RA) comparing clinical state with DNA antibody idiotype 16/6-R, circulating immune complexes (CIC), dsDNA (Amersham kit), and ssDNA (measured as described). Normal ranges are represented by the *hatched areas*. The 16/6 idiotype and CIC levels reflect disease activity in contrast to the ssDNA and dsDNA levels

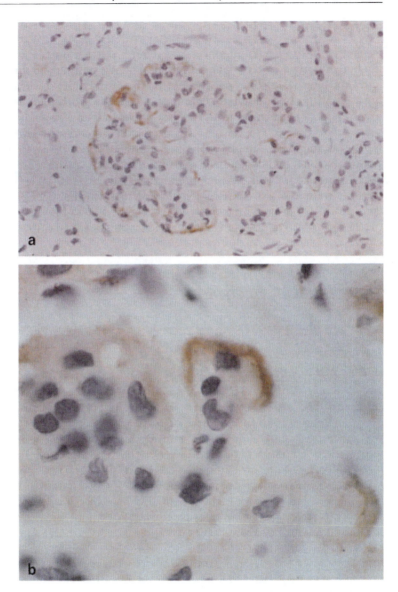

Fig. 2. a, b. a 16/6-R deposition in the glomerular basement membrane of a lupus patient. A horseradish peroxidase second-step antibody was used to identify the sites to which anti-16/6-R had bound (*brown* = positive). *Note:* No binding to 2/4 disease controls with anti-16/6-R has been found. b High-power view of the 16/6-R deposition in the glomerular basement membrane.

Tissue Studies

Studies have also been undertaken to examine whether cross-reactive anti-DNA antibody idiotypes can be found on tissue-bound immunoglobulins from kidney and skin biopsies of SLE patients. In the first study [72], 11 of 26 (42%) renal bipsies had the 16/6 idiotype demonstrable in the glomerular basement membrane (Fig. 2), in the focal tuft proliferation, or in the mesangium. In 5 of the 26 bipsies (19%), the 32/15 idiotype was detectable. In contrast, neither of the idiotypes was found on immunoglobulins deposited in 24 disease control bipsies. Four polyclonal and two monoclonal anti-idiotypic reagents were used to screen skin bipsies from 24 SLE patients. Immunoglobulins at the dermal—epidermal junction were found to share idiotypes in almost half the specimens. In comparison, 30% of 23 discoid lupus biopsies also shared these idiotypes, unlike any of the 15 IgM-positive disease controls, which were negative [73].

Other Antibody Idiotypes

Sharing of idiotypes by lupus autoantibodies is not confined to anti-DNA antibodies. Pisetsky et al. [43a] showed that two monoclonal anti-Sm antibodies of MRL-*lpr/lpr* origin, designated Y2 an Y12, shared an idiotype. They also showed that this idiotype could be detedted in the sera of both anti-Sm positive and anti-Sm negative MRL mice, though not in the sera of BALB/c mice of the same allotype. With a different anti-Y2 anti-idiotype, they showed that the Y2 determinant was found in the sera of MRL-*lpr/lpr* and MRL—+/+ mice, as well as in the sera of some normal mouse strains [46]. Overall, however, the Y2 idiotype defined only a minor component of the anti-Sm autoantibody response; most antibodies with this determinant express other antigenic specificities. In a study of an MRL-*lpr/lpr* derived monoclonal anti-RNP antibody (4LI), a commonly expressed idiotypic determinant was identified in the pooled serum of MRL-*lpr/lpr* mice [45]. Some cross-reactivity of this idiotype with those found on the anti-Sm monoclonal antibodies Y2 and Y12 was also demonstrated. Finally, cross-reactive idiotypes on two anti-Ro/SSA mouse monoclonal antibodies have also been described [47]. One of these idiotypes was also found in the serum of several SLE patients and in the serum from C2-deficient families.

The extensive idiotypic cross-reactions found in the lupus mouse models are understandable, given the inbred nature of the strains. That these observations extend to heterogeneous human lupus patients seems unusual. However, such results have been reported with other idiotypic systems. For example, cross-reactive idiotypes have been found on rheumatoid factors [27], IgM cold agglutinins [68], anti-acetylcholine receptor antibodies [32], anti thyroglobulin antibodies [36], and autoantibodies to factor VIII [62]. These observations, taken together, support the concept that autoantibodies originate from germ line genes that are dispersed throughout the human population. Furthermore, idiotypic markers of autoantibodies are not confined to autoimmune mice or to patients with autoimmune diseases; normal mice and normal individuals have been shown to possess these cross-reactive idiotypes [5, 43a, 45]. The production of autoantibodies is thus likely to be related to the abnormal expression of particular immunoglobulin genes, perhaps because of defects in immunoregulation.

Idiotypic and Anti-Idiotypic Antibodies
— Therapeutic Considerations

The treatment of SLE remains unsatisfactory in many cases. A variety of compounds, including gold, vitamin B_{12}, vitamin E, and testosterone were tried before the introduction of the anti malarial drugs and corticosteroids [39]. These latter drugs, plus other forms of immunosuppressive reagents, and plasma exchange, form the backbone of therapy for patients with moderate or severe disease. However, corticosteroids and the other major immunosuppressives (azathioprine, cyclophosphamide, and methotrexate) are no panacea. Their effects on the immune system are wide ranging and they may induce many side-effects, including susceptibility to infection, bone marrow suppression, hair loss, and neoplasia.

We thus require far more specific therapeutic modalities which will act directly on autoantibody-producing cells or possibly the T-lymphocytes that control them. Initial attempts to achieve more specific control with monoclonal antibodies have been made in lupus mouse models. It is worth remembering that, following Jerne's hypothesis [24], one might anticipate that anti-idiotypic antibodies could be detected in healthy individuals. Just this phenomenon has been reported [69]. In one case, Zouali and Eyquem [70], showed that anti-DNA antibody anti-idiotypes became detectable in the serum as the patient went into remission, but were not present during active disease. This sort of reciprocal arrangement of DNA antibody idiotype and auto anti-idiotypic antibodies has recently been described among 16 patients with severe SLE [59].

Hahn and Ebling [15] reasoned that immunizing lupus-prone mice with a syngeneic monoclonal anti-DNA antibody that bears a high frequency idiotype would induce the production of an immunoregulatory anti-idiotype antibody. They gave repeated (every 2 weeks) injections of an IgG2a monoclonal anti-DNA antibody to NZB/NZW F_1 female mice. The treatment resulted in temporary suppression of circulating anti-dsDNA antibodies, a reduction in proteinuria, and fewer deaths from nephritis. Jacob and Tron [23] showed that monthly injections of a syngeneic anti-DNA antibody bearing a commonly found idiotype (designated PME77) to 3-month-old NZB/NZW F_1 mice induced the production of auto anti-idiotypic antibodies and suppressed PME77 production. However, suppression of the PME77 idiotype did not change the total DNA binding capacity measured on the sera of the immunized mice. More recently Zouali and colleagues [70] have shown that administering a syngeneic anti-DNA IgG together with a synthetic immunoadjuvant, muramyl dipeptide, a major reduction in both idiotype expression and total DNA antibody levels could be achieved.

Hahn and Ebling [16] were also able to show temporary suppression of antibodies to DNA, and significantly prolonged survival, due to a delay in the onset of nephritis, by innoculation of NZB/NZW F_1 mice with a monoclonal anti-idiotypic antibody. These benefits, however, were abrogated by an apparent change in the dominant idiotype on pathogenic DNA antibodies. In contrast, anti-idiotypic therapy in MRL-*lpr/lpr* mice, which was directed against the high frequency idiotype H-130, failed to suppress either the idiotype or total anti-DNA antibodies [64]. In fact, an augmentation of H-130 idiotype and anti-DNA antibody levels were observed in normal BALB/c and young MRL/++ mice. Whether this undesirable effect can be overcome by administration of a combination of anti-idiotypic reagents is unknown. In other systems, an ongoing antibody response is particularly resistant to anti-idiotypic modulation [41, 43]. More encouragingly Saski et al. [53a] were able, in *in vitro* experiments, to selectively eliminate anti-DNA antibody producing cells by conjugating an anti-idiotypic antibody with the cytotoxic agent neocarzinostatin.

Conclusions

Monoclonal antibodies derived by hybridoma techniques are now well established tools for immunological investigtion. In the context of SLE and its murine counterparts, they have been invaluable in demonstrating the broad antigenic specificities of a single kind of autoantibody. This in turn has highlighted the basic question of what provides the immunizing stimulus in SLE. It has become increasingly clear that DNA itself may not be required for the production of anti-DNA antibodies; it is, in fact, an unlikely candidate. The possibility of an infectious agent as an initiator of the autoimmune reaction must be seriously considered. Idiotypic analysis of monoclonal autoantibodies has helped re-examine the genetic background of the disease. It has also become obvious that normal individuals possess B-lymphocytes capable of producing auto reactive immunoglobulins.

Caution remains necessary, especially in the field of human—human hybridoma technology. The low rate of successful fusions with the currently available myeloma partners and a paucity of monoclonal IgG autoantibodies are problems that have not been surmounted. With these caveats in mind, there can be little doubt that monoclonal antibodies are valuable probes. They should ultimately help to provide us with a clearer understanding of the immunopathology of SLE and, in turn, more rational and specific therapy.

References

1 André-Schwartz J, Datta SK, Shoenfeld Y, Isenberg DA, Stollar BD, Schwartz RJ (1984) Binding of cytoskeletal proteins by monoclonal anti-DNA lupus autoantibodies. Clin Immunol Immunopathol 31:261—271

2 Andrzejewski C Jr, Stollar BD, Lalor TN, Schwartz RS (1980) Hybridoma autoantibodies to DNA. J Immunol 124:1499—1502

3 Bussard AE, Pages J (1978) Establishment of a permanent hybridoma producing a mouse autoantibody. Prog Clin Biol Res 26:167—169

4 Cairns E, Block J, Bell DA (1984) Anti-DNA autoantibody producing hybridomas of normal human lymphoid cell origin. J Clin Invest 74:880—887

5 Datta SK, Stollar BD, Schwartz RS (1983) Normal mice express idiotypes related to autoantibody idiotypes of lupus mice. Proc Natl Acad Sci USA 80:2723—2727

5a Datta SK, Naparstek Y, Schwartz RS (1986) In vitro production of anti-DNA idiotype by lymphocytes of normal subjects and patients with systemic lupus erythematosis. Clin Immunol Immunopathol 38:302—318

6 Dellagi K, Brouet JC, Schenmetzher C (1981) Chronic haemolytic anaemia due to a monoclonal IgG cold agglutinis with anti-Pr specificity. Blood 57:189—191

7 Diamond B, Scharff MD (1984) Somatic mutation of the T15 heavy chain gives rise to an antibody with autoantibody specificity. Proc Natl Acad Sci USA 81:5841—5844

8 Eastcott JW, Schwartz RS, Datta SK (1983) Genetic analysis of the inheritance of B cell hyperactivity in relation to the development of autoantibodies and glomerulonephritis in NZB x SWR crosses. J Immunol 131:2232—2239.

9 Ebling FM, Hahn B (1980) Restricted subpopulations of DNA antibodies in kidneys of mice with systemic lupus. Comparison of antibodies in serum and renal eluates. Arthritis Rheum 23:392—403

10 Eilat D, Asofsky R, Laskov R (1980) A hybridoma from an autoimmune NZB/NZW mouse producing monoclonal antibody to ribosomal RNA. J Immunol 124:766—768

11 Faaber P, Capel PJA, Rijke GPM, Vierwinden G, Van de Putte IBA, Koene RAP (1984) Cross reactivity of anti-DNA antibodies with proteoglycans. Clin Exp Immunol 55:502—508

12 Grey HM, Kohler PE, Terry WD, Franklin GC (1968) Human monoclonal G cryoglobulins with anti-α-globulin activity. J Clin Invest 47:1875—1884

13 Guanieri M, Eisner D (1974) A DNA that reacts with antisera to cardiolipin. Biochem Biophys Res Commun 58:347—353

14 Hahn BH, Ebling F, Freeman S, Clevinger B, Davie J (1980) Production of monoclonal murine antibodies to DNA by somatic cell hybrids. Arthritis Rheum 23:942—945

15 Hahn BH, Ebling FM (1983) Suppression of NZB/NZW murine nephritis by administration of a syngeneic monoclonal antibody to DNA. J Clin Invest 71:1728—1736

16 Hahn BH, Ebling FM (1984) Suppression of murine lupus nephritis by administration of an anti-idiotypic antibody to anti-DNA. J Immunol 132:187—190

17 Hahn B, Ebling FM (1984) A public idiotypic determinant is present on spontaneous cationic IgG antibodies to DNA from mice of unrelated lupus-prone strains. J Immunol 133:3015—3019

18 Halpern R, Schiffenbauer J, Solomon G, Diamond B (1984) Detection of masked anti-DNA antibodies in lupus sera by a monoclonal anti-idiotype. J Immunol 133:1852—1856

19 Hannestad K (1969) α M rheumatoid factors reacting with nitrophenyl groups and denatured deoxyribonucleic acid. Ann NY Acad Sci 168:63—75

20 Horsfall AC, Venables PJW, Mumford PA, Maini RN (1981) Interpretation of the Raji call assay in sera containing anti-nuclear antibodies and immune complexes. Clin Exp Immunol 44:405—415

21 Isenberg DA, Shoenfeld Y, Madaio MP, Rauch J, Reichlin M, Stollar BD, Schwartz RS (1984) Anti-DNA antibody idiotypes in systemic lupus erythematosus. Lancet 2:417—422

22 Isenberg DA, Shoenfeld Y, Schwartz RS (1984) Multiple serologic reactions and their relationship to clinical activity in systemic lupus erythematosus. Arthritis Rheum 27:132—138

23 Jacob L, Tron F (1984) Induction of anti-DNA autoanti-idiotypic antibodies in (NZB × NZW)F$_1$ mice: possible role for specific immune suppression. Clin Exp Immunol 58:293—299

24 Jerne NK (1974) Towards a network theory of the immune system. Ann Immunol 125C:373—389

25 Kanai Y, Akatsuka T, Kubota T, Goto S, Stollar BD (1985) MRL/Mp-lpr/lpr mouse derived monoclonal antibodies that recognize determinants shared by poly (ADP-ribose) single-stranded DNA and left handed Z-DNA. Clin Exp Immunol 59:139—145

26 Koike T, Tomioka H, Kumagi A (1982) Antibodies cross reactive with DNA and cardiolipin in patients with systemic lupus erythematosus. Clin Exp Immunol 50:298—302

27 Kunkel HG, Agnello V, Joslin FG, Winchester J, Capra JD (1973) Cross idiotypic specificity among monoclonal IgM proteins with anti-α-globulin activity. J Exp Med 137:331—342

28 Lafer EM, Rauch J, Andrzejewski C Jr, Mudd D, Furie B, Furie B, Schwartz RS, Stollar BD (1981) Polyspecific monoclonal lupus autoantibodies reactive with both polynucleotides and phospholipids. J Exp Med 153:897—909

29 Lane D, Koprowski H (1982) Molecular recognition and the future of monoclonal antibodies. Nature 296:200—202

30 Laskov R, Muller S, Hochberg M, Giloh H, Van Regenmortel MHV, Eilat D (1984) Monoclonal autoantibodies to histones from autoimmune NZB/NZW F$_1$ mice. Eur J Immunol 14:74—81

31 Lee JS, Lewis JR, Morgan AR, Mosmann TR, Singh B (1981) Monoclonal antibodies showing sequence specificity in their interaction with single stranded DNAs. Nucleic Acid Res 9:1707—1721

32 Lefvert AK (1981) Anti-idiotypic antibodies against the receptor antibodies in myasthenic gravis. Eur J Immnuol 13:493—497

33 Lerner EA, Lerner MR, Janeway CA Jr, Steitz JA (1981) Monoclonal antibodies to nucleic acid containing cellular constituents: probes for molecular biology and autoimmune disease. Proc Natl Acad Sci USA 78:2737—2741

34 Littman BH, Muchmore AV, Steinberg AD, Greene WC (1983) Monoclonal lupus autoantibody secretion by human-human hybridomas. J Clin Invest 72:1987—1994

35 Marion TN, Lawton AR III, Kearney JR, Briles DE (1982) Anti-DNA autoantibodies in (NZB × NZW) F$_1$ mice are clonally heterogeneous, but the majority share a common idiotype. J Immunol 128:668—674

36 Matsuyama T, Fukumori J, Tanaka H (1983) Evidence of unique idiotypic determinants are similar idiotypic determinants on human anti-thyroglobulin antibodies. Clin Exp Immunol 51:381—386

37 Monier JC, Brochier J, Moreira, Sault C, Roux B (1984) Generation of hybridoma antibodies to double stranded DNA from non autoimmune Balb/c strain mice: studies on anti-idiotype. Immunol Lett 8:61—68

38 Morgan A, Buchanan RRC, Lew AM, Olsen I, Staines NA (1985) Five groups of antigenic determinants on DNA identified by monoclonal antibodies from (NZB × NZW) F$_1$ and MRL/Mp-*lpr/lpr* mice. Immunology 55:75—83.

39 Morrow WJW, Youniou P, Isenberg DA, Snaith ML (1983) Systemic lupus erythematosus: 25 years of treatment related to immunopathology. Lancet 2:206—211

40 Naparstek Y, Duggan D, Schattner A, Madaio M, Goni F, Frangione B, Stollar BD, Kabat EA, Schwartz RS. (1985) Immunochemical similarities between monoclonal anti-bacterial Waldenstrom's macroglobulins are monoclonal anti-DNA lupus auto antibodies J Exp Med 161:1525—1538

41 Owen FL, Nisonoff A (1978) Effect of idiotype specific suppressor T cells on primary and secondary responses. J Exp Med 148:182—194

42 Pick AI, Shoenfeld Y, Frolichman R, Weiss H, Vana D, Schreibman S (1979) Plasma cell dyscrasia, analysis of 423 patients. JAMA 241:275—278

43 Pierce SK, Klinman NR (1977) Antibody-specific immunoregulation. J Exp Med 146:509—519

43a Pisetsky DS, Lerner EA (1982) Idiotypic analysis of a monoclonal anti-Sm antibody. J Immunol 129:1489—1492

The Importance of the Study of Monoclonal Antibodies 103

44 Pisetsky DS (1983) Specificity and idiotypic analysis of a monoclonal anti-DNA antibody. Clin Immunol Immunopathol 27:348—356

45 Pisetsky DS, Salistad DM, Chambers JC (1984) Characterization and idiotypic analysis of an anti-RNP monoclonal antibody. Clin Exp Immunol 56:593—600

46 Pisetsky DS, Semper KF, Eisenberg RA (1984) Idiotypic analysis of a monoclonal anti-Sm antibody. J Immunol 133:2085—2089

47 Qian G, Fu SM, Reichlin M (1984) Cross reactive idiotype of anti Ro/SSA antibodies: identification of a V region marker preferentially expressed in SLE. Arthritis Rheum (abst) 27:516

48 Rauch J, Murphy E, Roth JB, Stollar BD, Schwartz RS (1982) A high frequency idiotype marker of anti-DNA autoantibodies in MRL-lpr/lpr mice. J Immunol 129:236—241

49 Rauch J, Schwartz RS, Stollar BD (1982) Applications of hybridoma technology to autoimmunity. In Katz D (ed) Monoclonal antibodies and T cell products, CRC, Boca Raton, FL, pp 91—111

50 Rauch J, Tannenbaum H, Stollar BD, Schwartz R (1984) Monoclonal anti-cardiolipin antibodies bind to DNA. Eur J Immunol 14:529—534

51 Rauch J, Massicotte H, Tannenbaum H (1985) Hybridoma anti-DNA autoantibodies from patients with rheumatoid arthritis and systemic lupus erythemtosus demonstrate similar nucleic acid binding characteristics. J Immunol 136:180—186

52 Rubin RL, Balderas RJ, Tan EM, Dixon FJ, Theofilopoulos AN (1984) Multiple autoantigen binding capabilities of mouse monoclonal antibodies selected for rheumatoid factor activity. J Exp Med 159:1429—1440

53 Sano H, Morimoto C (1982) DNA isolated from DNA/anti-DNA antibody immune complexes in systemic lupus erythematosus is rich in guanine-cytosine content. J Immunol 128:1341—1345

53a Saski T, Muryoi T, Takai O, Tamate E, Ono Y, Koide Y, Ishida N, Yoshinaga K (1986) Selective elimination of anti-DNA antibody-producing cells by anti-idiotypic antibody conjugated with neocarzinostatin. J Clin Invest 77:1382—1386

54 Shoenfeld Y, Hsu-Lin C, Gabriels J, Silberstein LF, Furie BC, Furie B, Stollar BD, Schwartz RS (1982) Production of autoantibodies by human-human hybridomas. J Clin Invest 70:205—208

55 Shoenfeld Y, Isenberg DA, Rauch J, Madaio MP, Stollar BD, Schwartz RS (1983) Idiotypic cross-reactions of monoclonal human lupus autoantibodies. J Exp Med 158:718—730

56 Shoenfeld Y, Rauch J, Massicotte H, Datta SK, Andre-Schwartz J, Stollar BD, Schwartz RS (1983) Polyspecificity of monoclonal lupus autoantibodies produced by human-human hybridomas. N Engl J Med 308:414—420

57 Schwartz RS (1983) Monoclonal lupus autoantibodies. Immunol Today 4:68—69

58 Silberstein LE, Shoenfeld Y, Schwartz RS, Berkman EM (1985) Chronic cold agglutinin disease of mixed IgG/IgM type: immunologic studies and the response to splenectomy. Vox Sang 48:105—109

59 Silvestris F, Bankhurst AD, Searles RP, Williams RC Jr (1984) Studies of anti-F(ab)$_2$ antibodies and possible immunologic control mechanisms in systemic lupus erythematosus. Arthritis Rheum 27:1387—1396

60 Solomon F, Schiffenbauer J, Keiser HD, Diamond B (1983) The use of monoclonal antibodies to identify stored idiotypes on human antibodies to native DNA from patients with systemic lupus erythematosus. Proc Natl Acad Sci USA 80:850—854

61 Sontheimer RD, Gilliam JN (1978) DNA antibodies class, subclass and complement fixation in systemic lupus erythematosus with and without nephritis. Clin Immunol Immunopathol 10:459—467

62 Sultan Y, Kazatchkine MD, Maisonneuve P, Nydegger UE (1984) Anti-idiotypic suppression of autoantibodies in factor VIII (antihaemophilic factor) by high dose intravenous gammaglobulin. Lancet 2:765—768

63 Steinitz M, Klein G, Koskimies S, Makel A (1977) EB virus induced B lymphocyte cell lines producing specific antibody. Nature 269:420—422

64 Teitelbaum D, Rauch J, Stollar BD, Schwartz RS (1984) In vivo effects of antibodies against a high frequency idiotype of anti-DNA antibodies in MRL mice. J Immunol 132:1282—1285

65 Tron F, Le Guern C, Cazenave PA, Bach JF (1982) Intrastrain recurrent idiotypes among anti-DNA antibodies of (NZB × NZW) F_1 hybrid mice. Eur J Immunol 12:761—766

66 Tron F, Jacob L, Bach JF (1984) Binding of a murine monoclonal anti-DNA antibody to Raji cells. Implications for the interpretation of the Raji cell assay for immune complexes. Eur J Immunol 14:283—286

67 Weisbart RH, Chan G, Kacena A, Saxton RE (1984) Characterization of mouse and human monoclonal antibodies cross reactive with SLE serum antibodies to guanosine. J Immunol 132:2909—2912

68 Williams RC Jr, Kunkel HG, Capra JD (1968) Antigenic specificities related to the cold agglutinin activity of gamma M globulins. Science 161:379—381

69 Zouali M, Eyquem A (1983) Expression of anti-idiotypic clones against auto anti-DNA antibodies in normal individuals. Cell Immunol 176:137—147

70 Zouali M, Eyquem A (1983) Idiotypic anti-idiotypic interactions in SLE.Ann Immunol 134C:377—397

70a Zovali M, Jolivet M, Le Clerc C, Ravisse P, Audibert F, Eyquem A, Chedio L (1985) Suppression of murine lupus autoantibodies to DNA by administration of muramyl dipeptide and syngeneic anti DNA IgG. J Immunol 135:1091—1096

71 Isenberg DA, Shoenfeld Y, Walport M, Mackworth-Young C, Dudeney C, Todd-Pokropek A, Brill A, Weinberger A, Pinkas J (1985) Detection of cross reactive anti-DNA antibody idiotypes in the serum of lupus patients and their relatives. Arthritis Rheum 24:256—262

72 Isenberg DA, Collins C (1985) Detection of cross reacting anti-DNA antibody idiotypes on renal tissue bound immunoglobulins from lupus patients. J Clin Invest 76:287—294

73 Isenberg DA, Dudency C, Wojnaruska F, Boghal BS, Rauch J, Schattner A, Naparstek Y, Duggan D (1985) Detection of cross reactive anti-DNA antibody idiotypes on tissue bound immunoglobulins from skin biopsies of lupus patients. J Immunol 135:261—264

74 Shoenfeld Y, Zamir R, Joshua H, Pinkhas H (1985) Human monoclonal anti-DNA antibodies react as lymphocytotoxic antibodies. Eur J Immunol 15:1024—1027.

75 Isenberg DA, Colaco CB, Dudeney C, Todd-Pokropek A, Snaith ML (1986) A study of the relationship between anti-DNA antibody idiotypes and anti-cardiolipin antibodies with disease activity in systemic lupus erythematosus. Medicine (Baltimore) 66:46—55

76 Stollar BD (1981) Anti-DNA antibodies. Clin Rheum Dis 1:243—260.

ANA Subsets in Systemic Lupus Erythematosus

M. REICHLIN and J. B. HARLEY

Introduction

Antinuclear antibody (ANA) is a hallmark of systemic lupus erythematosus (SLE), being almost invariably detected in the sera of active untreated SLE patients. The recent history of research in the serology of SLE is marked by the resolution of the heterogeneous group of antigen-antibody reactions characteristic of these patients into individual antigen-antibody systems. This has involved purification and biochemical characterization of the reactive antigens of several of the frequently occuring nuclear targets of autoimmune attack in these patients. The detection and analysis of unfractionated ANA as well as antibodies to the two forms of DNA [native or double-stranded (ds) and denatured or single-stranded (ss)] will not be discussed in this chapter as they have been adequately described in other publications [1, 2].

This chapter will describe the biochemical and antigenic analysis of three groups of autoantigens as well as their clinical associations. These include:

1. The RNA protein antigens, nRNP, Sm, Ro/SSA, and La/SSB/Ha
2. Histones
3. Cardiolipin

An extraordinary effort has been expended in the last 6 years which has resulted in an impressive collection of molecular information about these antigens, the localization of reactive epitopes within these molecules, and numerous relationships of clinical phenomena to the presence and/or the titer of autoantibodies to these antigens.

Antibodies to Sm and nRNP

Antibodies to the Sm and nRNP antigens frequently occur together in SLE sera and knowledge of their molecular structure is so intertwined that it is prudent to discuss them together. Several techniques have been used to detect antibodies to Sm and nRNP. Historically, the first method used was passive hemagglutination of sheep erythrocytes coated with a partially purified nuclear extract of calf thymus tissue. This has been called ENA (for extractable nuclear antigen), and the weakness of the method results from the uncertainties generated by the presence of antigens other than Sm and nRNP in the preparations. This method has been largely replaced by the double diffusion method of Ouchterlony in which sera were diffused against concentrated saline extracts of thymus or spleen tissue with the formation of strong precipitin lines. The nature of the lines was established by line fusion with monospecific serum. Cellular localization of the antigens was determined by cell fractionation studies and some biochemical properties of the antigens established. Thus, sera of anti-Sm and anti-nRNP specificities were characterized and have provided the reference reagents underlying further analysis of the nature of the antigens. The future analysis of the significance of these antibodies lies in more sensitive and quantitative approaches such as the ELISA method, although little has been published at the present time utilizing this technique.

The Sm and nRNP antigens are nuclear in origin, and recent work has elucidated their structure. Early characterization of the Sm antigen showed it to be periodate sensitive, but trypsin [3], RNAase, and DNAase did not affect its antigenicity in prcipitin reactions. The ability of the nRNP antigen to precipitate [4] or coat cells for a hemagglutination reaction [5, 6] was ablated by either RNAase or trypsin. The frequent simultaneous occurrence of antibodies to Sm and nRNP was noted [7], and their molecular association demonstrated by immunochemical methods [8]. These early studies [8] and later more elegant immunoaffinity studies have shown that Sm and nRNP antigenic determinants exist in a molecular complex and that there exists a molecular form of Sm free of nRNP [9—11].

Two major advances have enhanced the understanding of the antigenic structure of these antigens. One is the work of Lerner and Steitz, who characterized the RNA components of RNA-protein particles that carry the Sm and nRNP epitopes [12]. The second development was the application of the Western blot technique as well as other quantitative analytical methods (elution from SDS polyacrylamide gels) to a study of the antigenicity of the protein components of the Sm and nRNP particles [9—11, 13].

The particle bound by anti-nRNP is composed of an RNA component designated U_1 complexed to at least seven proteins varying in molecular weight from 12 to 68 # kd; the Sm particle is composed of the same seven proteins as well as U_2, U_1, U_4, U_5, and U_6, RNAs containing 196, 171, 145, 120, and 95 nucleotides, respectively. As already mentioned, there is a smaller antigenic version of the Sm particle apparently lacking RNA but having several small protein bands and a total molecular weight of 70 # kd. Precipitation reactions of nRNP with its antibody require the whole particle, both RNA and protein. Protein alone is sufficient for the precipitation of Sm with anti-Sm. Takano and colleagues [10] have shown direct binding of protein components of molecular weight 68 and 30 kd with anti-nRNP and direct binding of protein components of 30 and 13 kd to anti-Sm. Douvas found nRNP antigenicity associated with a 30-kd protein and Sm antigenicity related to a 13-kd protein by the immunoblot technique [11]. Differences in elution conditions (3 M KSCN vs. 0.01 M HCl) may account for some of the differences in antigenicity noted by these two groups. There is no evidence for the direct binding of RNA to either antibody. The antigenic epitopes for both Sm and nRNP may be represented only on protein molecules, but more work is necessary to settle this issue. Moreover, it is quite possible that individual patients may have antibodies that bind to different epitopes on the same protein or even different protein subunits within the same particle. Recently, a hybridoma producing anti-Sm was formed by fusion of spleen cells from an autoimmune MRL/1 mouse with an appropriate myeloma cell line [13]. This mouse monoclonal antibody precipitates the same RNA-protein particle as does the human antibody, and the immunoblot technique indicates that the monoclonal antibody binds a 26-kd protein. The monoclonal antibodies of human-human hybridomas with activity against the Sm and nRNP antigens should provide powerful tools for the definitive analysis of these autoantigens.

A schematic representation of the general structure and several specific members of this RNA protein family are represented in Fig. 1. As illustrated, a single RNA molecule is associated with six to eight protein molecules. Each particle has a unique RNA molecule, five shared protein molecules, and one to three distinctive proteins. It is easy to understand why antibodies to Sm bind all the particles since the epitopes for Sm antigenicity are carried on one or more of the protein molecules shared by all the particles. Although there is still some controversy about which proteins carry Sm antigenicity, there are data supporting the antigenicity of the shared 28–30-, 18-, and 13-kd proteins. Contrariwise, antibodies specific for the U_1 particle (anti-nRNP) react only with the unique polypeptides which are constituents of that particle: the 68-, 33-, and 22-kd proteins.

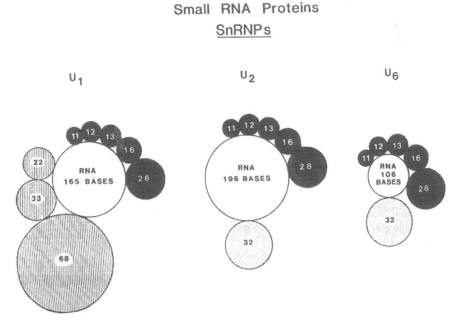

Fig. 1. Schematic representation of small RNA protein particles. The *central circles* are RNA molecules while the *outer circles* are proteins. *Blackened circles* are proteins shared by all particles, while *stippled* or *lined circle* proteins are unique to each particle

The clinical significance of antibodies to nRNP and Sm has been carefully studied and is briefly summarized here. There is agreement among most workers in this area that antibodies to the Sm antigen are highly specific for SLE patients [14].

A careful clinical analysis of a large group of patients in a referral center [15] reveals that not all patients with anti-Sm satisfy preliminary criteria for the diagnosis of SLE as set forth by the ARA [16]. This may mean that patients with rheumatic diseases other than SLE have anti-Sm in their sera or that the antibodies to Sm appear early in the course of lupus and prolonged follow-up will reveal that eventually all anti-Sm patients will satisfy clinical criteria for the diagnosis of SLE. Only extensive longitudinal study of such patients will answer this question.

No characteristic clinical features are apparent for this group of patients, although there are reports that the nephritis of such patients is mild and follows a benign course [17, 18]. It has also been reported that antibodies to Sm are associated with central nervous system involvement when it occurs as an isolated clinical manifestation of the disease [19]. A recent report provides evidence for fluctuation of anti-Sm levels with disease activity, suggesting participation in immune complex disease and use as a possible indicator of clinical activity in some patients [20].

Patients who have antibodies only to nRNP have a low frequency of antibodies to DNA and a low frequency of clinically apparent renal disease [5, 6, 21]. SLE patients with anti-nRNP in their sera develop nephritis only when antibodies of other specificities are present, notably anti-DNA [22, 23]. Nephritis also occurs when anti-nRNP is associated with antibodies to Sm or Ro/SSA.

Much attention has centered on a group of patients with overlapping features of SLE, scleroderma, and polymyositis, who have been designated as having mixed connective tissue disease (MCTD) by Sharp and his associates [5, 6]. These patients all possess antibodies to nRNP in their sera and, like other patients with anti-nRNP who lack overlapping features, have a low frequency of antibodies to DNA and a low frequency of nephritis.

Two reports of immune complex nephropathy in patients with MCTD and anti-nRNP have appeared [24, 25] but in neither report were antibodies to Ro/SSA [26] or ssDNA [27] sought in the sera of the nephritic patients. Both of these systems have been shown to participate in immune complex nephritis and to occur in 10%—15% of patients with anti-nRNP. Special tests are required for their detection, and unless specifically sought, they are easily overlooked.

MCTD patients present with very heterogeneous clinical features, a point noted in the initial description and re-emphasized in the follow-up of the original 25 patients [28]. The only uniform finding in these patients is, by definition, the presence of antibodies to nRNP. No immunologic, clinical, genetic, or biochemical charcteristic has yet been described that gives this syndrome definition. The finding(s) that will distinguish MCTD from its component connective tissue diseases (SLE, myositis, and PSS) awaits recognition.

Antibodies to the U_1 particle are not a specific marker for MCTD since they also occur in 40% of SLE patients [4, 7, 14, 22, 29]. Two papers have appeared which describe a second antibody in anti-nRNP (U_1) sera which has as a target a

70-kd protein that is part of the matrix [30] or that binds a component of the matrix that is thought to be heterogeneous nuclear ribonucleoprotein associated with the nuclear matrix [31]. In the former case [30], matrix proteins were isolated after a prior extraction and removal of saline soluble proteins and were run out in SDS gels in preparation for western blotting. A 70-kd protein was demonstrated in every MCTD sera that contained antibodies to U_1 RNP [30]. In the second instance, the antimatrix antibodies were recognized as giving a distinctive large speckled pattern of immunofluorescence after extraction of HEp-2 nuclei with 0.1 N HCl. The reactive antigen was further characterized as heterogeneous nuclear ribonucleoprotein [30]. In both instances, the evidence was good that this antimatrix antibody is distinct from anti-U_1, nRNP. Whether such antimatrix antibodies occur exclusively in the sera of MCTD patients or are invariably linked with the presence of anti-U_1 nRNP awaits further study, although it is suggested by Fritzler, Ali, and Tan (1984) that such antibodies to the matrix are also found in SLE patients with anti-U_1 nRNP, albeit in lower titer than in MCTD patients. Clearly, this is an area for further study.

An intersting issue involves the clinical features of patients who have both anti-nRNP and anti-Sm precipitins in their sera. As pointed out in 1973 (8), such sera are more common than those with only an anti-Sm precipitin. Recent elegant work by Reeves and colleagues [32] shows that sera with only anti-Sm precipitins have substantial amounts of anti-nRNP antibodies as deduced from the binding of intrinsically radiolabeled 68-kd protein, which is a specific component of the U_1 particle by specific antibody. They also confirmed this, showing substantial quantities of anti-nRNP by using nRNP coated plates in an ELISA which cannot be blocked by isolated Sm particles free of nRNP determinants. Confirmatory data have been obtained in our laboratory (unpublished observations). These sera, apparently monospecific for anti-Sm by precipitation, have substantial quantities of anti-nRNP. Previous studies of precipitation seemed to indicate three types of sera: (a) anti-nRNP alone; (b) anti-nRNP and anti-Sm; and (c) anti-Sm alone. The above biochemical and immunochemical studies suggest a simpler picture. Sera either contain anti-nRNP alone or both anti-nRNP and anti-Sm. This conforms with our clinical experience that patients with anti-Sm alone are indistinguishable from those with both anti-Sm and anti-nRNP precipitins, having similar frequencies of all clinical features, including nephritis [23]. Only the patients with anti-nRNP alone have a favorable clinical course and prognosis.

Autoantibodies against these antigens have been shown to be present at high concentration in some sera, accounting for more than 20% of the total immunoglobulin [33, 34].

Antibodies to Ro/SSA and La/SSB

Precipitating antibodies against Ro/SSA were probably first appreciated by B. R. Jones [35] who found that rare sera from Sjögren's syndrome patients formed a precipitin against salivary gland tissue in double diffusion assay. Anderson and colleagues [36] demonstrated the presence of two common precipitin activities in systemic lupus erythematosus as well as in Sjögren's syndrome [37].

These precipitin reactions were rediscovered in two laboratories and have been extensively studied [38—40]. They have become identified as Ro or SSA and La or SSB [41]. In the past few years, it has become clear that particular disease manifestations and clinical findings are related to these precipitating antibodies. Not only are they found in a major fraction of patients with Sjögren's syndrome and systemic lupus erythematosus; they are also found in subacute cutaneous lupus and both clinical expressions of the neonatal lupus syndrome: cutaneous lupus and complete congenital heart block [42, 43].

Relationships of Anti-Ro/SSA and Anti-La/SSB to Clinical Manifestations

Whether the anti-Ro/SSA and anti-La/SSB autoantibodies are intimately related to the course and expression of SLE or whether they are interesting epiphenomena unrelated to the immunopathogenesis of the disease is a subject of much current investigation. The presence of large quantities of these autoantibodies is suggestive of an immunopathogenetic role but their presence in asymptomatic normal individuals at the least indicates that the autoantibody by itself is not sufficient for disease expression. On the other hand, there are data implicating a relationship of these autoantibodies in some SLE patients with nephritis, with cutaneous disease, and with systemic disease in patients who lack many of the other autoantibodies associated with SLE or in those who have complement component C2 deficiency and develop SLE.

A study of 55 SLE patients with Ro/SSA and/or La/SSB precipitins found that patients with anti-Ro/SSA alone had much more serious renal disease than the patients who had both anti-Ro/SSA and anti-La/SSB [44]. Most of the patients with anti-Ro/SSA alone (77%) had anti-DNA antibodies, while fewer (33%) with both anti-Ro/SSA and anti-La/SSB had anti-DNA. The possibility that anti-Ro/SSA is related to nephritis is enhanced by the relative enrichment of anti-Ro/SSA in renal eluates from SLE patients with nephritis and anti-Ro/SSA [45].

There are SLE patients with a restricted collection of autoantibodies. They have no antinuclear antibody when epithelial tissues such as mouse kidney or rat liver are used as substrates to detect antinuclear antibody. Indeed, a subset of these sera do not bind antigens on proliferating cell substrates (HEp-2, KB cells) prepared by the standard technique. These individuals have been referred to as

ANA Subsets in Systemic Lupus Erythematosus   111

having "ANA-negative SLE" and most of them have anti-Ro/SSA precipitins [46]. Systemic disease in these patients has been related to the presence of anti-Ro/SSA and/or anti-La/SSB [47].

The basis for the relationship between complement component deficiency and systemic lupus erythematosus is not known. Recently, it has been shown that patients with C2 deficiency who also manifest findings of SLE have a very high frequency of Ro/SSA precipitins [48]. Unexpectedly, none of these patients had La/SSB precipitins.

Cutaneous disease of any type in SLE and especially the subset of patients now diagnosed as having subacute cutaneous lupus erythematosus are related to the coexistence of anti-Ro/SSA [42]. These patients have widespread cutaneous lesions whicn are usually photosensitive. Annular and papulosquamous lesions are the major morphologic types and are usually easily distinguished from discoid lupus lesions. Ro/SSA often accompanied by La/SSB precipitins are present in over 60% of these patients and this is the most common serologic finding. These patients appear to be at lower risk for nephritis and neuropsychiatric disease than do patients with SLE but without these skin lesions.

The cutaneous disease of neonatal lupus bears certain similarities to subacute cutaneous lupus erythematosus. Photosensitive cutaneous lesions (annular, macular, or discoid) are characteristic. Over 90% of infants of mothers have anti-Ro/SSA and over 50% have anti-La/SSB. The lesions usually appear after the first few weeks of life and resolve within 6 months in parallel with the clearing of the maternal autoantibodies from the infant's circulation [49—52]. Recently, an animal model of neonatal cutaneous lupus has been developed by transplanting human skin to nude mice [53]. When anti-Ro/SSA containing sera are infused, immunoglobulin deposits develop on the basal keratinocytes only in the human tissue. Exposure to ultraviolet light increases the deposition of immunoglobulin.

The other major manifestation of the neonatal lupus syndrome is complete congenital heart block, which may occur in the presence or absence of cutaneous findings. Congenital complete heart block occurs in one of 20000 births [54]. Over 80% of the isolated cases appear to be related to the presence of Ro/SSA precipitins in the maternal circulation [55]. Immunofluorescent evaluation of a recent case has shown immunoglobulin deposition in cardiac tissue [56]. Finally, quantitative analysis of the anti-Ro/SSA antibody in a family with twins discordant for complete congenital heart block revealed an unexpected relative decrease of the anti-Ro/SSA level in the affected infant [57]. The Ro/SSA antigen has been demonstrated in cardiac tissue by two independent methods, thereby allowing models of pathogenesis which require participation of the Ro/SSA antigen [57, 58]. Collectively, these data constitute the strongest evidence for the direct involvement of autoantibodies in the expression of clinical lupus.

Almost equally powerful data implicate anti-Ro/SSA in the systemic manifestations of Sjögren's syndrome. In one series of patients, Ro/SSA precipitins were more often found in patients with many clinical and laboratory features of extraglandular disease including vasculitis, salivary gland enlargement, lympadenopathy, purpura, anemia, leukopenia, and thrombocytopenia. Other serologic abnormalities were also more frequent in Ro/SSA precipitin positive patients, including hyperglobulinemia, rheumatoid factor, antinuclear antibody, cryoglobulinemia, and hypocomplementemia [59]. Analysis of a second series of patients using a quantitative assay has confirmed some of these observations [60].

None of these data, however, directly implicates anti-Ro/SSA in the clinical expression of Sjögren's syndrome. Data from a carefully evaluated patient with Sjögren's syndrome in association with primary biliary cirrhosis have shown that the anti-Ro/SSA titer decreased as immune complex titers rose and that anti-Ro/SSA was deposited in the parotid gland [61].

Serology of the Ro/SSA and La/SSB Autoantigens

Until recently, the anti-Ro/SSA and anti-La/SSB autoantibodies were only detected by precipitation in agar, either by Ouchterlony double diffusion or counterimmunoelectrophoresis. These techniques have shown that anti-Ro/SSA and anti-La/SSB are closely associated. Indeed, nearly all, if not all, sera containing anti-La/SSB precipitins also contain anti-Ro/SSA in parallel fashion to anti-nRNP being present in all anti-Sm sera as described above. There is, however, no apparent predilection for Ro/SSA or La/SSB precipitins to occur with nRNP precipitins.

Other relationships with the Ro/SSA and La/SSB precipitins are known. Ro/SSA precipitin is coincident with rheumatoid factor in over half of the patients, whether the underlying diagnosis is SLE or Sjögren's syndrome [59, 60, 62]. The mechanism for this relationship is not known, but it has been suggested that Ro/SSA and immunoglobulin cross-react [63].

Sera with La/SSB precipitins almost always stain the nucleus with a speckled pattern. That at least this pattern represents anti-La/SSB activity has been confirmed by inhibition of the nuclear speckled pattern by purified antigen and by the demonstration that a mouse monoclonal anti-La/SSB heteroantibody binds in the same pattern on cells from the appropriate species [64].

The Ro/SSA precipitin containing sera were originally described as binding a cytoplasmic antigen which was also appreciated by studies using RNA gels to detect antibody [38, 76]. Other workers, however, have noted a speckled nuclear pattern [66, 67]. In addition, many sera with anti-Ro/SSA do not produce any antinuclear fluorescent pattern [68]. The determination of exactly what the range and location of possible anti-Ro/SSA reactive determinants are must await the applklication of purified reagents (Ro/SSA antigen, anti-Ro/SSA antibody, and monoclonal antibodies) to this problem.

A variety of alternative technologies has been applied to the detection of anti-Ro/SSA and anti-La/SSB autoantibodies. A modified radioimmunoassay was used to detect anti-La/SSB but did not substantially improve sensitivity over double diffusion [69, 70]. RNA gels have been used to detect these autoantibodies since the seminal studies of Lerner et al. (1979, 1981). A number of groups have adapted the solid phase assay technology to the detection of anti-La/SSB [60, 64, 70]. These assays require purified antigen and, therefore, are probably restricted to the research laboratory, but recent application of a monoclonal anti-La/SSB antibody to trap La/SSB antigen was over 1000-fold more sensitive than

ANA Subsets in Systemic Lupus Erythematosus   113

double diffusion in agar gel [64] and could be broadly applied. These studies have also shown that patients with anti-Ro/SSA precipitins almost uniformly have some La/SSB binding activity [64].

Solid phase assays to detect anti-Ro/SSA have been hindered by the difficulties in purifying Ro/SSA; nevertheless, two groups have established these assays [71, 72]. In addition to the known associations of La/SSB to Ro/SSA and Sm to nRNP precipitins, this approach has shown that anti-Ro/SSA is associated with anti-Sm [72].

With the availability of more sensitive solid phase techniques for antibody detection and the knowledge that some individuals have Ro/SSA and/or La/SSB precipitins, it is not surprising that low levels of anti-Ro/SSA and anti-La/SSB have been detected in the normal population [73, 74].

Questions of sensitivity and specificity using the solid phase assays are only now being answered. From the limited data available, the fidelity between solid phase assay and precipitation is very good for assessment of anti-La/SSB, while anti-Ro/SSA appears to be much more complicated [75]. The serum binding levels of anti-Ro/SSA were not completely reliable predictors of precipitin formation. Amongst sera with equivalent binding levels of anti-Ro/SSA, those with higher rheumatoid factor and antinuclear antibody titers tended to form precipitins, which is consistent with the possibility that these other autoantibodies participate in Ro/SSA precipitin formation [75].

Molecular Properties of Ro/SSA and La/SSB

The present understanding of the molecular properties of the Ro/SSA and La/SSB antigens has been constructed from their initial descriptions [36, 38—40], from the marriage of molecular biology with the serology of these autoantigens [12, 76], and from the recent conclusions reached using purified autoantigen preparations [70, 71, 73, 77]. Both Ro/SSA and La/SSB are composed of RNA and protein components. The antigenic activity of both are resistant to RNAse treatment and, since the protein components react with autoimmune antisera under conditions which separate the RNA and protein, it is thought that the RNA is not required for antigenic reactivity. The undenatured Ro/SSA antigen is resistant to trypsin while the La/SSB antigen is rapidly degraded. Indeed, the La/SSB antigenic activity is rapidly lost in extracts maintained at room temperature while Ro/SSA is much more stable.

Gel filtration has shown that the Ro/SSA particle has a Stokes radius which predicts a molecular weight of approximately 100 kd and that the La/SSB is approximately 60 kd. The protein portion of Ro/SSA and La/SSB are composed of single polypeptides of 55—60 and 42—45 kd respectively. The Ro/SSA peptide has the unusual property of incomplete denaturation in sodium dodecylsulfate and, when denaturation does not proceed to completion, a second Ro/SSA band is appreciated at an apparent 40 kd which upon complete denaturation has an apparent molecular weight of 60 kd [71]. The La/SSB protein is degraded to a 29-kd peptide after which it loses antigenity [113]. Recently, an antigenic epitope of La/SSB has been localized to a restricted region of the peptide [114].

The RNA component of Ro/SSA is known as hY RNA for human (h) cytoplasmic (Y) RNA. It is uridine rich and in man is composed of at least four unique RNA species between 83 and 112 bases, of which three of the RNA species have been sequenced [79—81]. Helical regions near the 3' and 5' ends are protected from RNAse digestion when the hY RNA is complexed with the Ro/SSA protein [82]. The genes for hY1 and hY3 RNAs are adjacent on the human genome [81].

The function of Ro/SSA in the cell is unknown. Estimates of the number of molecules of hY RNA have been in the range of 10^5 per cell, which means that the hY RNAs are a minor RNA species accounting for less than 1% of the ribosomal RNA and explains why the hY RNAs were not known before their description using the autoimmune sera [79]. The hY RNAs are transcripts of RNA polymerase III [81].

The La RNAs are more complicated. In many cells, there are RNA species termed 4.5S RNA which bind the La/SSB protein. Though 4.5S RNA appears to be the major RNA in mice [79] and 5.0S in man [83], 4.5S RNA is partially homologous to the Alu family DNA, which are highly repetitive interspersed sequences found in mammalian genomes [84]. The 5.0S RNA has been shown to be a precursor form of ribosomal RNA [83]. There are, however, many other RNAs also immunoprecipitated by anti-La/SSB largely between 80 and 120 nucleotides [76]. Some of these have been shown to be precursor RNA molecules, leading to the hypothesis that all RNA polymerase III transcripts are at least initially associated with the La/SSB protein. The common structural feature of the RNA which binds it to the La/SSB protein is an oligouridylate stretch found at the 3' end of the polymerase III transcripts [65].

Viral encoded RNAs have also been shown to complex with the La/SSB protein. In particular, two adenovirus RNAs and two Epstein-Barr virus RNAs containing 160 to 173 nucleotides bind the La/SSB protein [76—78]. These observations form a foundation upon which a possible relationship of viral infection to SLE pathogenesis can be elucidated.

Antibodies to Histone

Antibodies to histones have long been recognized as occurring in patients with SLE, both the idiopathic disease [85, 86] and that induced by drugs, principally procainamide and hydralazine. Several technical problems have complicated studies concerning antibodies to histone. The major one is the relative contribution of DNA and histone in the antigenicity of DNA-histone. This has been a problem because isolated individual histones, total histones, and the histone-DNA complex all have different structures. It is now known that five of the histones, H_1, H_2A, H_2B, H_3, and H_4 have a highly organized structure in chromatin in which an octamer of H_2A, H_2B, H_3, and H_4 (2 moles of each) is internal to double helical DNA which is wound about the histone complex. The overall structure resembles beads on a string (called nucleosomes) in which each bead is a histone octamer with its DNA coat while a single mole of H_1 is bound to the internucleosomal DNA [87]. Only certain COOH and NH_2 terminal ends of the various histone polypeptides are exposed in intact chromatin.

It is known that antibodies reactive with histones occur in both drug-induced and idiopathic SLE. The questions to be addressed are: (a) What is known of the reactive epitopes in histones and are they the same or different in the two forms of LE? (b) In what proportion of the two forms of LE do antihistones appear and is there anything about their quantity or specificity that helps distinguish the two forms of LE? Complete answers to these questions are still not known but much has been learned in the past 7 years and a description of the knowledge follows.

Fritzler and Tan [88] developed a method of studying antihistone antibodies which involved indirect immunofluorescence of acid-extracted nuclei in tissue sections and reconstitution of such tissue sections with purified histones. In drug-induced SLE, 23 of 23 patients showed complete loss of immunofluorescence with acid extraction and 22 showed virtually complete reconstitution of the titer with isolated histones. The H_2A-H_2B mixture was most effective in restoring reactivity. In idiopathic SLE, only 12 of 20 sera showed complete loss of immunofluorescence with acid extraction while of the remaining eight, four showed a decrease in ANA titer and four showed no change. Of the 12 that showed complete loss of fluorescence, only four regained the original titer and the other eight continued to be negative despite the histone reconstitution. Thus, drug-induced LE sera uniformly reacted with a histone-dependent antigen in ANA tests which accounted for most of the antibody. The idiopathic LE sera clearly reacted with several antigens, only one of which depended on histone for its antigenic integrity. This study did not distinguish between a determinant of pure histone and histone-DNA complex.

Subsequent studies in several laboratories have utilized isolated histones as antigen and are less ambiguous about whether the antigen is a histone-DNA complex or pure histone. On the other hand, it is less easy to judge how much of the total reactivity to histone-dependent antigen is dependent on antibodies to histone alone, since only histone is utilized as antigen.

Indeed, the next relevant study utilized isolated histones and/or histone fractions for assay in an ELISA and revealed several interesting correlations [89]. Firstly, antihistones were not present in the other rheumatic diseases, including rheumatoid arthritis (RA), progressive systemic sclerosis (PSS), and overlap syndromes. Secondly, antihistone antibodies correlated with activity, being present in 87% of active untreated patients and only 18% of inactive patients. Moreover, in individual patients studied longitudinally, antihistone titers fell as disease activity waned. Finally and most surprisingly, antibodies to histones were not present in 9 of 9 cases of drug-induced LE. The authors suggested that the earlier study of Fritzler and Tan [88] measured antibodies to a histone DNA complex and not to isolated histones to reconcile the discordant results of the two studies. Finally, in this study antibody activity was greatest against the H_1 and H_2B fraction, a finding which has been reproduced by some but not other laboratories.

Rubin, Joslin, and Tan [90] developed a solid phase radioimmunoassay and showed that IgM antihistones against total histone was present in most patients with drug-induced and idiopathic LE but was also present in smaller numbers of RA and PSS patients. In these patients and with this method, a complex of H_2A and H_2B was the major antigen and largely accounted for the reaction of unfractionated histones. Krippner [91] performed a similar study and similarly found that IgM antihistone was not specific for SLE patients, while IgG antibodies were highly specific for SLE but occurred in only 21% of patients and no correlation was apparent with disease activity. Moreover, no difference was seen between total histones and any of the isolated fractions. The authors did not use mixtures of histones known to complex in vivo (e.g., H_2A and H_2B or H_3 and H_4). The reasons for these discrepancies are unresolved but data on which a consensus has been reached are summarized at the end of this section.

Three recent reports have studied isolated histones and subfragments produced chemically or proteolytically as antigens. They suggest that only the portions of the histone molecule exposed in the nucelosomal unit of chromatin are antigenic. Hardin and Thomas [92] utilized immunoblotting of isolated histone fractions as antigens with SLE sera and showed that (a) histones H_1 and H_2B were major antigens and (b) the exposed COOH terminal of the H_1 molecule and NH_2 terminal of the H_2B molecules were the major determinants reactive with antibodies in SLE sera. Further studies with these techniques applied to drug-induced LE sera yielded similar results, with more reactivity also apparent against the exposed NH_2 and COOH termini of the H_3 molecule in addition to the COOH terminus of H_1 and the NH_2 terminus of H_2B. Such data suggested a very similar specificity pattern for the antihistones of drug-induced and spontaneous LE [93]. Finally, a similar study with ELISA methodology rather than immunoblotting with isolated histones and their peptide fragments suggested the major activity was in exposed NH_2 and COOH termini. In this latter study [94], histones H_2A, H_2B, H_3, and H_4 had similar activities quantitatively (H_1 was not studied) and a further caveat similar to the previous study [93] was that sera from drug-induced and SLE patients behaved identically.

A final recent clinical study of antibodies to histones in idiopathic SLE found that the predominant antigenic moieties were H_1, H_2B, and H_3 and that the highest levels of antihistones were found in patients with photosensitivity [95]. This raised the interesting possibility that immune responses to histones might result from nuclear damage mediated by solar radiation and that antibodies are a marker of this photodamage.

In summary, these studies suggest little difference in the fine specificity of antibodies to histones between drug-induced and idiopathic LE. The exposed COOH and NH_2 termini of histones H_1, H_2B, and H_3 may be major antigens. It is likely that such antibodies are the major immune response in drug-induced LE and one of numerous immune responses in idiopathic LE. The diagnostic specificity, correlations with activity and clinical subsets, and relationships of antibodies to histones all require further study.

Anticardiolipin Antibodies

Antibodies now known to be reactive with lipid have long been appreciated in patients with SLE. Classically, these sera contain activities which prolong the partial thromboplastin time or render a biological false-positive VDRL. Both activities in SLE patients are due to the involvement of lipid in the assay. Indeed, it has been possible to distinguish the positive VDRL reactions of patients with syphilis from those with a biological false-positive reaction [96, 97].

Though thrombotic episodes, thrombocytopenia, pulmonary hypertension, and recurrent spontaneous abortion had previously been associated with the lupus anticoagulant (98—103), the development of a sensitive assay for anticardiolipin antibodies which is more than 100-fold more sensitive has allowed these observations to be confirmed and extended [104]. Both arterial and venous thrombosis as well as thrombocytopenia and fetal wastage have been related to anticardiolipin levels. Included in this group are numerous patients with cerebral infarction without an alternative predisposing cause and who may not satisfy criteria for the diagnosis of SLE [104—106]. In a study of 121 patients, Harris et al. were able to show that the risk for thrombosis, fetal loss, and thrombocytopenia correlated with the anticardiolipin autoantibody level [107]. The observation that anticardiolipin antibody levels prospectively predict risk of fetal loss reinforces their importance [108]. Elevated levels of anticardiolipin antibody have been found in idiopathic thrombocytopenic purpura as well as in SLE [109].

The mechanism of vascular occlusion is not clear. Carreras et al. (1982) have shown that patient serum with anticoagulant activity inhibits prostacyclin production which could predispose to thrombosis [110]. Inhibition of prekallikrein activity and fibrinolysis are also suggested mechanisms of thrombogenesis [111].

Available data suggest that therapy may change the risk of thrombosis and fetal loss. Discontinuing anticoagulant therapy led to thrombotic episodes in six patients within 2 months [112]. In addition, Lubbe et al. have shown that fetal survival was associated with the reduction in lupus anticoagulant activity in patients treated with prednisolone and aspirin [102].

Summary

It is increasingly apparent that specific antibodies are of aid in defining clinical subsets in SLE patients. While the correlations of specific antibodies with clinical manifestations are strong, the development of quantitative, sensitive techniques for the measurement of autoantibodies should make such associations even more useful in the future.

References

1 Reichlin M (1985) Antinuclear antibodies. In: Kelley (ed) Textbook of rheumatology. Saunders, Philadelphia, pp 690—706

2 Reichlin M (1981) Current perspectives on serological reactions in SLE patients. Clin Exp Immunol 44:1—10

3 Tan EM, Kunkel HG (1966) Characteristics of a soluble nuclear antigen precipitating with the sera of patients with systemic lupus erythematosus. J Immunol 96:464—471

4 Mattioli M, Reichlin M (1971) Characterization of a soluble nuclear ribonucleoprotein antigen reactive with LE sera. J Immunol 197:1281—1290

5 Sharp GC, Irvin WS, LAroque O, Velez C, Daly V, Kaiser AD, Holman HR (1971) Association of autoantibodies to different nuclear antigens with clinical patterns of rheumatic disease and responsiveness to therapy. J Clin Invest 50:350—359

6 Sharp GC, Irvin WS, Tan EM, Gould RG, Holman HR (1972) Mixed connective tissue disease — an apparently distinct rheumatic disease syndrome associated with a specific antibody to an extractable nuclear antigen (ENA). Am J Med 52:148—159

7 Reichlin M, Mattioli M (1974) Antigens and antibodies characteristic of systemic lupus erythematosus. Bull Rheum Dis 24:756—760

8 Mattioli M, Reichlin M (1973) Physical association of two nuclear antigens and mutual occurrence of their antibodies: the relationship of the Sm and RNA protein (Mo) systems in SLE sera. J Immunol 110:1318—1324

9 Takano M, Agris PF, Sharp GC (1980) Purification and biochemical characterization of nuclear ribonucleoprotein antigen using purified antibody from serum of a patient with mixed connective tissue disease. J Clin Invest 65:1449—1456

10 Takano M, Golden SS, Sharp GC, Agris PF (1981) Molecular relationship between two nuclear antigens, ribonucleoprotein and Sm: purification of active antigens and their biochemical characterization. Biochemistry 21:5929—5935

11 Douvas AS (1982) Autoantibodies occurring in two different rheumatic diseases react with the same ribonucleoprotein particle. Proc Natl Acad Sci USA 79:5401—5405

12 Lerner MR, Steitz JA (1979) Antibodies to small nuclear RNAs complexed with proteins are produced by patients with systemic lupus erythematosus. Proc Natl Acad Sci USA 76:5495—5499

13 Lerner EA, Lerner MR, Janeway Jr CA, Steitz JA (1981) Monoclonal antibodies to nucleic acid-containing cellular constituents: probes for molecular biology and autoimmune disease. Proc Natl Acad Sci USA 78:2737—2741

14 Notman DD, Kurata N, Tan EM (1975) Profiles of antinuclear antibodies in systemic diseases. Ann Intern Med 83:464—469

15 Munves EF, Schur PH (1983) Antibodies to Sm and nRNP: prognosticators of disease involvement. Arthritis Rheum 26:848—853

16 Cohen AS, Reynolds WE, Franklin EC, Kulka PJ, Ropes MW, Shulman LE, Wallace SE (1971) Preliminary criteria for the classification of systemic lupus erythematosus. Bull Rheum Dis 21:643—648

17 Powers R, Akizuki M, Boehm-Truitt MJ, Daly V, Holman HR (1977) Substantial purification of the Sm antigen and association of high titer antibody to Sm with a clinical subset of systemic lupus erythematosus. Arthritis Rheum 20:131 (abstract)

18 Winn DM, Wolfe JR, Lindberg DA, Fristoe FA, Kingsland L, Sharp GC (1979) Identification of a clinical subset of systemic lupus erythematosus by antibodies to the Sm antigen. Arthritis Rheum 22:1334—1337

19 Winfield JB, Brunner CM, Koffler D (1978) Serologic studies in patients with systemic lupus erythematosus and central nervous system dysfunction. Arthritis Rheum. 21:289—294

20 Barada FA Jr, Andrews BS, Davis JS, Taylor RP (1981) Antibodies to Sm in patients with systemic lupus erythematosus. Arthritis Rheum 24:1236—1244

ANA Subsets in Systemic Lupus Erythematosus 119

21 Reichlin M, Mattioli M (1972) Correlations of a precipitin reaction to an RNA protein antigen and a low prevalence of nephritis in patients with systemic lupus erythematosus. N Engl J Med 286:908—911

22 Parker MD (1972) Ribonucleoprotein antibodies: frequency and clinical significance in systemic lupus erythematosus, scleroderma, and mixed connective tissue disease. J Lab Clin Med 82:769—775

23 Maddison PG, Mogavero H, Reichlin M (1978) Patterns of clinical disease associated with antibodies to nuclear ribonucleoprotein. J Rheumatol 5:407—411

24 Fuller TJ, Richman AV, Auerbach D, Alexander RW, Lottenberg R, Longley S (1977) Immune complex glomerulonephritis in a patient with mixed connective tissue disease. Am J Med 62:761—764

25 Bennett RM, Spargo BH (1977) Immune complex nephropathy in mixed connective disease. Am J Med 63:534—541

26 Maddison PG, Reichlin M (1979) Deposition of antibodies to a soluble cytoplasmic antigen in the kidneys of patients with systemic lupus erythematosus. Arthritis Rheum 22:858—863

27 Koffler D, Agnello V, Kunkel HG (1974) Polynucleotide immune complexes in serum and glomeruli of patients with systemic lupus erythematosus. Am J Pathol 74:109—124

28 Nimelstein SH, Brody S, McShane D, Holman HR (1980) Mixed connective tissue disease: a subsequent evaluation of the original 25 patients. Medicine (Baltimore) 59:239—248

29 Hardin JA, Rahn D, Shen C, Lerner MR, Wolin SL, Rosa MD, Steitz JA (1982) Antibodies from patients with connective tissue diseases bind specific subsets of cellular RNA-protein particles. J Clin Invest 70:141—147

30 Solden MHL, Van Eekelan CAG, Habets WJA, Vierwinden G, Van de Putte LBA, Van Venrooy WJ (1982) Antinuclear matrix antibodies in mixed connective tissue disease. Eur J Immunol 12:783—786

31 Fritzler MG, Ali R, Tan EM (1984) Antibodies from patients with mixed connective tissue disease react with heterogeneous nuclear ribonucleoprotein or ribonucleic acid (hnRNP/RNA) of the nuclear matrix. J Immunol 132:1216—1222

32 Reeves WH, Fisher DE, LAhita RG, Kunkel HG (1985) Autoimmune sera reactive with Sm antigen contain high levels of RNP-like antibodies. J Clin Invest 75:580—587

33 Maddison PJ, Reichlin MR (1977) Quantitation of precipitating antibodies to certain soluble nuclear antigens in SLE. Their contribution to hypergammaglobulinemia. Arthritis Rheum 20:819—824

34 Gaither KK, Harley JB (1985) Affinity purification and immunoassay of anti-Ro/SSA. Protides Biol Fluids Colloq 33:413—416

35 Jones BR (1958) Lacrimal and salivary precipitating antibodies in Sjögren's syndrome. Lancet 2:773—776

36 Anderson JR, Gray KG, Beck JS, Kinnear WI (1961) Precipitating autoantibodies in Sjögren's disease. Lancet 2:456—460

37 Anderson JR, Gray KG, Beck JS, Buchanan WW, McElhinney AJ (1962) Precipitating autoantibodies in the connective tissue diseases. Ann Rheum Dis 21:360—369

38 Clark G, Reichlin M, Tomasi TB (1969) Characterization of a soluble cytoplasmic antigen reactive with sera from patients with systemic lupus erythematosus. J Immunol 102:117—122

39 Mattioli M, Reichlin M (1974) Heterogeneity of RNA protein antigens reactive with sera of patients with systemic lupus erythematosus: description of a cytoplasmic non-ribosomal antigen. Arthritis Rheum 17:421

40 Alspaugh MA, Tan EM (1975) Antibodies to cellular antigens in Sjögren's syndrome. J Clin Invest 55:1067—1073

41 Alspaugh MA, Maddison P (1979) Resolution of the identity of certain antigen-antibody systems in systemic lupus erythematosus and Sjögren's syndrome: an interlaboratory collaboration. Arthritis Rheum 22:796—798

42 Sontheimer RD, Maddison PJ, Reichlin M, Jordan RE, Stastny P, Gilliam JN (1982) Serologic and HLA associations of a distinct clinical subset of lupus erythematosus: subacute cutaneous lupus erythematosus. Ann Intern Med 97:664—671

43 Lee LA, Bias WB, Arnett FC, Huff JC, Norris DA, Harmon C, Provost TT, Weston WL (1983) Immunogenetics of the neonatal lupus syndrome. Ann Intern Med 99:592—596

44 Wasicek CA, Reichlin M (1982) Clinical and serological differences between systemic lupus erythematosus patients with antibodies to Ro versus patients with antibodies to Ro and La. J Clin Invest 69:835—843

45 Maddison PJ, Reichlin M (1979) Deposition of antibodies to a soluble cytoplasmic antigen in the kidneys of patients with systemic lupus erythematosus. Arthritis Rheum 22:858—863

46 Maddison PJ, Provost TT, Reichlin M (1981) Serological findings in patients with "ANA-negative" systemic lupus erythematosus. Medicine 60:87—94

47 Provost TT, Ahmed R, Maddison PJ, Reichlin M (1977) Antibodies to cytoplasmic antigens in lupus erythematosus. Serological marker for systemic disease. Arthritis Rheum 20:1457—1463

48 Provost TT, Arnett FC, Reichlin M (1983) Homozygous C2 deficiency, lupus erythematosus, and anti-Ro/SSA antibodies. Arthritis Rheum 26:1279—1282

49 Kephart D, Hood A, Provost TT (1981) Neonatal lupus: serologic findings. J Invest Derm 77:331—333

50 Miyagawa S, Kitamura W, Yoshioka J, Sakamoto K (1981) Placental transfer of anticytoplasmic antibodies in annular erythema of newborns. Arch Dermatol 117:569—572

51 Provost TT (1983) Neonatal lupus. Arch Dermatol 119:619—622

52 Lumpkin LR, Hall J, Hogan JD, Tucker SB, Jordan RE (1985) Neonatal lupus erythematosus: a report of three cases associated with anti-Ro/SSA antibodies. Arch Dermatol 121:377—381

53 Lee LA, Weston WL, Stevens JO, Kreuger GG, Emam M, Norris DA (1985) Differential in vivo binding of specific lupus sera in human skin. Arthritis Rheum 27:S35

54 Michaëlsson M, Engle MA (1972) Complete congenital heart block: an international study of the natural history. Cardiovasc Clin 4:87—101

55 Scott JS, Maddison PJ, Taylor PV, Esscher E, Scott O, Skinner RP (1982) Connective-tissue disease, antibodies to ribonucleoprotein and congenital heart block. N Engl J Med 309:209—212

56 Litsky SE, Noonan JA, O'Connor WN, Cottrill CM, Mitchell B (1985) Maternal connective tissue disease and congenital heart block. Demonstration of immunoglobulin in cardiac tissue. N Engl J Med 312:98—100

57 Harley JB, Kaine JL, Fox OF, Reichlin M, Gruber B (1985) Ro/SSA antibody and antigen in congenital complete heart block. Arthritis Rheum 28:1321—1325

58 Wolin SL, Steitz JA (1984) The Ro small cytoplasmic ribonuclear particles: structures and clues to the pathogenesis of congenital heart block. Clin Res 32:470A

59 Alexander E, Arnett FC, Provost TT, Stevens MB (1983) Sjögren's syndrome: association of anti-Ro (SSA) antibodies with vasculitis, hematologic abnormalities and serologic hyperreactivity. Ann Intern Med 98:155—159

60 Harley JB, Alexander E, Arnett F, Fox O, Reichlin M, Yamagata H (1984) Sjögren's syndrome (SS): quantitative anti-Ro/SSA, -La/SSB, and -nRNP(Sm). Clin Res 32:538A

61 Penner E, Reichlin M (1982) Primary biliary cirrhosis associated with Sjögren's syndrome: evidence for circulating and tissue-deposited Ro/anti-Ro immune complexes. Arthritis Rheum 25:1250—1253

62 Maddison PJ, Mogavero H, Provost TT, Reichlin M (1979) The clinical significance of autoantibodies to a soluble cytoplasmic antigen in systemic lupus erythematosus and other connective tissue diseases. J Rheumatol 6:189—195

63 Mamula MJ, Fox OF, Harley JB (1985) Cross-reactivity of Ro/SSA and immunoglobulin G. Arthritis Rheum 28:S37

64 Harley JB, Rosario MO, Yamagata H, Fox OF, Koren E (1985) Immunologic and structural studies of the lupus/Sjögren's syndrome autoantigen, La/SSB, with a monoclonal antibody. J Clin Invest 76:801—806

65 Stefano JE (1984) Purified lupus antigen La recognizes an oligouridylate stretch common to the 3' termini of RNA polymerase III transcripts. Cell 36:145—154

66 Harmon CE, Deng JS, Peebles CL, Tan EM (1984) The importance of tissue substrate in the SS-A/Ro antigen-antibody system. Arthritis Rheum 27:166—172

ANA Subsets in Systemic Lupus Erythematosus 121

67 Wermuth DJ, Geoghegan WD, Jordan RE (1985) Anti-Ro/SSA antibodies: association with a particulate (large speckled like thread) immunofluorescent nuclear staining pattern. Arch Dematol 121:335—338

68 Scopelitis E, Biundo JJ (1984) Inconsistent staining of HEp-2 cells with anti-SS-A antibody. Arthritis Rheum 27:1318—1320

69 Akizuki M, Boehm-Truitt MJ, Kassan SS, et al. (1977) Purification of an acidic nuclear protein and demonstration of its antibodies in subsets of patients with sicca syndrome. J Immunol 119:932—938

70 Venables PJW, Charles PW, Buchanan RRC, Yi P, Mumford PA, Schrieber L, Room GRW, Maini RN (1983) Quantitation and detection of isotypes of anti-SS-B antibodies by ELISA and Farr assays using affinity purified antigens. Arthritis Rheum 26:146—155

71 Yamagata H, Harley JB, Reichlin M (1984) Molecular properties of the Ro/SSA antigen and ELISA for quantitation of antibody. J Clin Invest 74:625—633

72 Maddison PJ, Skinner RP, Vlachoyiannopoulos P, Brennand DM, Hough D (1985) Antibodies to nRNP, Sm, Ro(SSA), and La(SSB) detected by ELISA: their specificity and interrelations in connective tissue disease sera. Clin Exp Immunol 62:337—345

73 Harley JB, Yamagata H, Reichlin M (1984) Anti-La/SSB antibody is present in some normal sera and is coincident with anti-Ro/SSA precipitins in systemic lupus erythematosus. J Rheumatol 11:309—314

74 Gaither KK, Fox OF, Reichlin M, Harley JB (1985) An hypothesis for differences in the occurrence of autoantibodies against extractable antigens. Arthritis Rheum 28:S68

75 Harley JB (1985) Autoantibodies in Sjögren's syndrome: comparison of autoantibody determination methods shows that antinuclear antibody and rheumatoid factor are associated with Ro/SSA precipitin formation. Protides Biol Fluid Proc Colloq 33:343—346

76 Lerner MR, Boyle JA, Hardin JA, Steitz JA (1981a) Two novel classes of small ribonucleoproteins detected by antibodies associated with lupus erythematosus Science 211:400—402

77 Lerner MR, Andrews NC, Miller G, Steitz JA (1981b) Two small RNAs encoded by Epstein-Barr virus and complexed with protein are precipitated by antibodies from patients with systemic lupus erythematosus. Proc Natl Acad Sci USA 78:805—809

78 Rosa MD, Gottlieb E, Lerner MR, Steitz JA (1981) Striking similarities are exhibited by two small Epstein-Barr virus-encoded ribonucleic acids and the adenovirus-associated ribonucleic acids VAI and VAII. Mol Cell Biol 1:785—796

79 Hendrick JP, Wolin S, Rinke J, Lerner MR, Steitz JA (1981) Ro small cytoplasmic ribonucleoproteins are a subclass of La ribonucleoproteins: Further characterization of the Ro and La small ribonucleoproteins from uninfected mammalian cells. Mol Cell Biol 1:1138—1149

80 Kato N, Hoshino H, Harada F (1982) Nucleotide sequence of 4.5S RNA (C8 or hY5) from HeLa cells. Biochem Biophys Res Commun 108:363—370

81 Wolin SL, Steitz JA (1983) Genes for two small cytoplasmic Ro RNAs are adjacent and appear to be single copy in the human genome. Cell 32:735—744

82 Wolin SL, Steitz JA (1984) The Ro small cytoplasmic ribonucleo proteins: identification of the antigenic protein and its binding on the Ro RNAs. Proc Natl Acad Sci USA 81:1996—2000

83 Rinke J, Steitz JA (1982) Precursor molecules of both human 5S ribosomal RNA and transfer RNAs are bound by a cellular protein reactive with anti-La lupus antibodies. Cell 29:149—159

84 Jelinek WR, Toomey TP, Leinwand L, Duncan CH, Biro PA, Chondary PV, Weissman SM, Rubin CM, Houck CM, Deininger PL, Schmidt CW (1980) Ubiquitous, interspersed repeated sequences in mannalian genomes. Proc Natl Acad Sci USA 77:1398—1402

85 Kunkel HG, Holman HR, Deicher HRG (1960) Multiple autoantibodies to cell constituents in systemic lupus erythematosus. Ciba Found Symp 8:429—437

86 Stollar BD (1971) Reactions of systemic lupus erythematosus sera with histone fractions and histone-DNA complexes. Arthritis Rheum 14:485—492

87 Kornberg RD, Klug A (1981) The nucleosome. Sci Am 244:52—64

88 Fritzler MJ, Tan EM (1978) Antibodies to histones in drug induced and idiopathic lupus. J Clin Invest 62:560—567

89 Gioud M, Ait Kaci M, Monier JC (1982) Histone antibodies in systemic lupus erythematosus. Arthritis Rheum 25:407—413

90 Rubin RL, Joslin FG, Tan EM (1982) Specificity of anti-histone antibodies in systemic lupus erythematosus. Arthritis Rheum 25:779—782

91 Krippner H, Springer B, Merle S, Pirlet K (1984) Antibodies to histones of the IgG and IgM class in systemic lupus erythematosus. Clin Exp Immunol 58:49—56

92 Hardin JA, Thomas JO (1983) Antibodies to histones in systemic lupus erythematosus: localization of prominent autoantigens on histone H_1 and H_2B. Proc Natl Acad Sci USA 80:7410—7414

93 Craft JE, Bernstein RM, Hardin JA (1985) Autoimmunity to histones in drug induced lupus provides a model for antihistone responses to spontaneous lupus. Clin Res 33:505A.

94 Gohill J, Fritzler MJ, Crane-Robinson C (1985) Histone epitopes binding antibodies from drug induced and idiopathic lupus erythematosus. Arthritis Rheum 28:117S

95 Bernstein RM, Hobbs RN, Lea DJ, Ward DJ, Hughes GRV (1985) Patterns of antihistone antibody specificity in rheumatic disease. Arthritis Rheum 28:285—293

96 Johansson EA, Lassus A (1974) The occurrence of circulating anticoagulants in patients with syphilitic and biologically false positive antilipoidal antibodies. Ann Clin Res 6:105—108

97 Labro MT, Andrieu M, Weber M, Homberg JC (1978) A new pattern of non-organ and non-species-specific anti-organelle antibody detected by immunofluorescence: the mitochondrial antibody number 5, Clin Exp Immunol 31:357—366

98 Bowie EJW, Thompson JH Jr, Pascuzzi CA, Owen CA Jr (1963) Thrombosis in systemic lupus erythematosus despite circulating anti-coagulants. J Lab Clin Med 62:412—430

99 Mueh JR, Herbst KD, Rapapurt SI (1980) Thrombosis in patients with the lupus anticoagulant. Ann Intern Med 92:156—159

100 Firkin BG, Howard MA, Radford N (1980) Possible relationship between lupus inhibitor and recurrent abortion in young women. Lancet 2:366

101 Boey ML, Colaco CB, Gharavi AE, Elkon KB, Loizou S, Hughes GRV (1983) Thrombosis in SLE: Striking association with the presence of circulating "lupus anticoagulant". Br Med J 287:1021—1023

102 Palmer SJ, Butler WS, Laggins GC (1983) Fetal survival after prednisolone suppression of maternal lupus anticoagulant. Lancet 1:1361—1363

103 Asherson RA, Mackworth-Young CG, Boey ML, Hull RG, Saunders A, Gharavi AE, Hughes GRV (1983) Pulmonary hypertension in systemic lupus erythematosus. Br Med J 287:1024—1025

104 Harris EN, Gharavi AE, Boey ML, Pattel BM, Mackworth-Young CG, Loizou S, Hughes GRV (1983) antibodies: detection by radioimmunoassay and association with thrombosis in systemic lupus erythematosus. Lancet 2:1211—1214

105 Harris EN, Asherson RA, Gharavi AE, Morgan SH, Derue G, Hughes GRV (1985) Thrombocytopenia in SLE and related autoimmune disorders: association with anti-cardiolipin antibodies. Br J Haematol 59:227—230

106 Lockshin M, Goei S, Qamar T, Jovanovic L, Druzin M, Magid M (1985) Anti-cardiolipin antibody, placental insufficiency and fetal death in SLE pregnancies. Arthritis Rheum 28:S39

107 Harris EN, Chan JKH, Asherson RA, Gharavi AE, Hughes GRV (1985) IgG anticardiolipin antibody: possible predictor for thrombosis, thrombocytopenia, and recurrent abortion (abstract). Arthritis Rheum 48:S39

108 Lockshin MD, Druzin M, Qamar T, Magid MS, Jovanovic L, Ferenc M (1985) Antibody to cardiolipin as a predictor of fetal distress in death in patients with systemic lupus erythematosus. N Engl J Med 313:152—156

109 Harris EN, Gharavi AE, Hegde U, Derue G, Morgan SH, Englert H, Chan JKH, Asherson RA, Hughes GRV (1985) Anticardiolipin antibodies in autoimmune thrombocytopenic purpura. Br J Haematol 59:231—234

110 Carreras LO, Vermylen JG (1982) "Lupus" anticoagulant and thrombosis — possible role of inhibition of prostacyclin formation. Thromb Haemostas (Stuttgart) 48:28—40

111 Sanfelippo MJ, Drayna CJ (1982) Prekallikrein inhibition associated with the lupus anticoagulant. Am J Clin Pathol 77:275—279
112 Asherson RA, Chan JKH, Harris EN, Gharavi AE, Hughes GRV (1985) Anticardiolipin antibodies: recurrent thrombosis after cessation of anticoagulant therapy. Ann Rheum Dis 44:823—825
113 Venables PJW, Smith PR, Maini RN (1983) Purification and characterization of the Sjögren's syndrome A and B antigens. Clin Exp Immunol 54:731—738
114 Chambers JC, Keene JD. Isolation and analysis of cDNA clones expressing human lupus La antigen. Proc Natl Acad Sci USA 82:2115—2119

Complement and Complement Deficiencies

G. Tappeiner

Introduction

A decrease in complement (C) activity is frequently found in patients with active systemic lupus erythematosus and is mainly due to C consumption by immune complexes. On the other hand, in some individuals there is a lack of C function due to the absence of a particular component of the system. This is not due to consumption but rather to a hereditary deficiency in the synthesis of the component.

The first hereditary deficiency, a C2 deficiency, was found in a healthy individual upon routine testing of C levels in normal controls [1]. Subsequently, the genetically transmitted lack of $C\bar{1}$-inh was found in patients with hereditary angioedema and identified as the cause of this condition [2, 3].

As determinations of total C function and of individual C components became increasingly available for patients with various inflammatory diseases, more persons and families with hereditary deficiency states were identified and a pattern of associated diseases has begun to emerge [4]. To date, complete deficiencies of all the components of the classical pathway of activation, of C3 and C3b inactivator, and of the terminal sequence have been identified. In addition, there is the well-known deficiency of $C\bar{1}$-inh, which is never homozygous and thus never complete but is invariably associated with its typical manifestation, hereditary angioedema [3]. So far, no complete deficiency of any of the components of the alternative pathway of C activation has been found; in the rare instances of heterozygous deficiency of an alternative pathway component there was no associated disease.

The Complement System

Complement is an effector system consisting of a number of proteins, the majority of which possess enzymatic properties. Most are normally present in an inactive proenzyme form and are activated in a cascade of specific biochemical interactions. The reaction is controlled by several specific inactivator proteins.

The C system may be activated through two distinct pathways, the classical and the alternative (Fig. 1). Components of the classical pathway are C1 with its subunits C1q, C1r, and C1s, C4, and C2. The alternative pathway is composed of the factors B (C3b proactivator), $\overline{\text{D}}$ (C3b proactivator convertase), and P (properdin). The components of the common terminal sequence have been assigned the symbols C5, C6, C7, C8 and C9 according to the order in which they enter the activation reaction. Sometimes, fragments from two or more components come together to form an active entity; this is symbolized by the numbers of the components set together (e.g., C5b67). Activation of either pathway results in activation of C3. Activated complement components are symbolized by a bar over the symbol of the component or assembly of components (e.g., $\overline{\text{D}}$, $\overline{\text{C42}}$). If a more specific indication of the biochemical state is to be given, (a) denotes the smaller fragment of a cleaved proenzyme and (b) the larger one (e.g., C3a, C3b). Further small letters denote further degradation products. Inhibitors of complement proteins have as yet no systematic nomenclature; they include C1 esterase inhibitor ($\overline{\text{C1}}$ inh), C3b inactivator (C3b ina), and inhibitors of C3 in its function in the alternative pathway, called factor H and factor I.

Complement receptors are simply named after their ligand (e.g., C1q-receptor) with the exception of the receptors for C3 and its fragments, which are termed CR1, CR2, and CR3.

Pathways of Activation

As mentioned above, C may be activated via one of two routes, the "classical" and the "alternative pathway" (Fig. 1) [5]. Activation through the classical pathway is initiated by the binding of the C1q subunit of C1 to antigen-bound or otherwise aggregated antibodies of the IgG or the IgM class. This produces a steric rearrangement in C1 that gives it a serine esterase activity. $\overline{\text{C1}}$ cleaves C4 and C2 and the cleavage products of both come together to form the classical C3 convertase, $\overline{\text{C4b2a}}$. $\overline{\text{C1}}$ is controlled by $\overline{\text{C1}}$-inh; a lack of this inhibitor protein leads to excessive activation and thus, consumption of the natural substrates for $\overline{\text{C1}}$, namely C4 and C2.

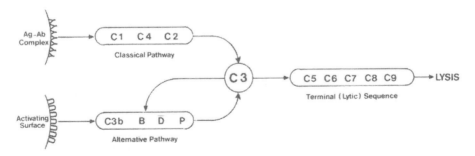

Fig. 1. The complement system, schematic representation of the pathways of activation. Inhibitors are not included. For details, see text

126 G. Tappeiner

Activation of C via the alternative pathway occurs on surfaces with certain molecular structures, including polysaccharides, lipopolysaccharides, and certain immunoglobulins as well as walls of parasites, fungi, bacteria, viruses, and certain animal tumor cells. The ability to activate the alternative pathway resides in the carbohydrate moiety of these structures, but not much is known as yet about the molecular determinants involved.

Alternative pathway activation depends upon the availability of the active fragment of C3, C3b. This is provided by continuous hydrolytic degradation of native C3. C3b together with Bb, released from factor B through the action of factor $\overline{\text{D}}$, forms the alternative C3 convertase, $\overline{\text{C3bBb}}$, which is then stabilized by binding factor P.

The reaction is controlled by a number of inhibitors; activation via the alternative pathway is initiated by the escape of C3b from inactivation on appropriate surface structures. In this context, it should be mentioned that in certain pathologic conditions such as membranoproliferative glomerulonephritis or partial lipodystrophy, an autoantibody called C3 nephritic factor (C3 NeF) appears. This autoantibody protects the alternative C3 convertase from degradation by factor H and thus increases the efficiency of C3 activation [6].

Both classical and alternative pathway activation lead to the production of a C3 activating enzyme (C3 convertase). Thus, C3 activation is the pivotal event in C activation (Fig. 1): it is achieved by either pathway, and it provides further C3b to increase the efficiency of alternative pathway activation, creating a positive feedback amplification loop, and to recruit the components of the terminal sequence C5—C9. Under normal circumstances, this amplification mechanism is controlled by C3b ina, which reduces the available C3b, and factor H, which degrades alternantive C3 convertase. A lack of C3b ina results in unchecked consumption and consequently a lack of C3.

The terminal events in C activation are the cleavage of C5 and the assembly of the membrane attack complex C5b—9 without further enzyme activation [7].

Finally, it should be mentioned that complement may also be activated by a number of enzymes: this includes plasmin (acting on C1), but also various proteases (e.g., trypsin).

Biologic Activities

As discussed above, activation of C results in the production of a number of active proteins, either through assembly or through release from their precursors, that are responsible for the biologic effects of this mediator system. It is of relevance to our present understanding of hereditary C deficiencies and their disease associations that specific functions can be ascribed to individual C components.

Cytolysis requires the activation of the terminal components through C8; the presence of C9 is not an absolute requirement for the lytic activity of C, although it greatly accelerates the reaction [7]. Lysis is caused by the penetration and perforation of the cell membrane by C5b—8 [7]. The cytolytic activity of C is responsible for host defense against certain microorganisms; furthermore, it is the underlying principle of C-mediated hemolysis, the classical tool in the study of the complement system and in many serologic and microbiologic tests.

Immune adherence of immune complexes to nonsensitized cells (e.g., erythrocytes) is mediated by C4b or C3b. This mechanism is thought to be important in the clearance of immune complexes [8]. On the other hand, insoluble immune complexes can be solubilized by activation of C3 through the alternative pathway [9] in the presence of an intact classical pathway [10]. The biologic importance of this is not yet clear, but can be assumed to be related to the processing of immune complexes. C3b also enhances phagocytosis and pinocytosis by cells carrying a surface C3b-receptor (monocytes, macrophages, neutrophils) [11]. Furthermore, C3b stimulates the release of leukocytes from the bone marrow, the release of lysosomal enzymes, and superoxide production by leukocytes [12]. C5a and C567 are directly leukocytotactic [13, 14].

A small fragment of C2 has kinin-like activity and may be responsible for edema formation in C1 inh D (hereditary angioedema) [15]. C5a and, to a lesser extent, C3a are anaphylatoxins and induce mediator release from mast cells and basophils, smooth muscle contraction, and an increase in vascular permeability. Furthermore, factor H and fragments of C3 and C5 stimulate the generation and release of arachidonic acid metabolites [16].

Neutralization of viruses or of virus-infected cells is another function of C. It may proceed via antibody-mediated C activation or be directly mediated by the components of the classical pathway and C3 [17].

Data obtained *in vitro* indicate that activated C components, in particular C4, C3, and C5, exert a regulatory influence on interacting antigen-specific lymphocytes and their accessory cells; this mechanism may be important in the regulation of the immune response but has not yet been clearly defined [18].

Finally, most C components (exceptions being the late ones) are produced by monocytes and macrophages. *In vitro* data indicate that intricate control mechanisms, exerted in part by the C proteins themselves, are operative in the regulation of C production [18].

Genetics of the Complement System

The discovery of hereditary C deficiencies and, later, of genetically determined polymorphisms of C components have permitted the investigation of complement genetics. Such polymorphisms have so far been found in humans in C4, C2, Bf, C3, C6, and C7. While there are two alleles of C4, C4A and C4B [19, 20], C2 [21] and Bf [22] are encoded by one structural gene on each chromosome. "Silent" or "null" genes are frequent in C4 [19] and C2 [23] and have in rare instances been found in C6 [24] and Bf [25].

It is well established that C4 [26], C2, and Bf [27] are encoded within the HLA region (on the short arm of chromosome 6) between the HLA B and D regions;

indeed, these C components are also referred to as HLA class III antigens. Accordingly, certain disease associations with certain C allotypes have already been identified.

Besides the existence of silent alleles, there is some genetic polymorphism in C2 and a remarkable degree of it in C4 and Bf. It is also worth noting that the red cell antigens, Chido and Rodgers, are derived from C4A and C4B molecules [28]. The locus of the C3 gene is on chromosome 19 [29]; nothing definite is known about the gene loci of the other components. The original assumption that C6 and C8 also have their gene loci within the HLA complex, based on one observation each, has since been disproved.

Complement Deficiencies — General Considerations

Complement deficiency (CD), defined as a decrease in C function (e.g., of total hemolytic complement or of opsonization), may be acquired or inborn and may be due to a variety of causes. The most widely encountered form of CD is consumption hypocomplementemia, which results from acitvation (= consumption) of C by substances such as bacterial endotoxins or immune complexes. Thus, this type of hypocomplementemia is found in certain types of vasculitis or in autoimmune diseases like SLE or rheumatoid arthritis in which the presence of immune complexes is a regular feature. According to its pathogenesis, the levels of nearly all components of C are decreased to a certain extent, but it rarely leads to complete absence of any individual component. This type of hypocomplementemia may be a valuable tool in assessing the amount of ongoing inflammation, and it is reversible upon successful treatment of the underlying condition. The peculiar "'SLE-related syndrome with early C component depression" [30], in which an SLE-like disease is associated with low classical pathway but normal or high terminal sequence component levels, also belongs here.

Another group of CDs comprises functional defects of a particular component; such a condition may be acquired or hereditary and has so far been described for $C\bar{1}$ inh, C1q, C5, and C8.

Finally, CD may be due to a genetically determined partial or complete lack of a particular component. In the case of inhibitor deficiencies, the missing control and thus the hypercatabolism of C is responsible for the hypocomplementemic state. The general assumption that these deficiencies are due to "empty" or "null" alleles of the genes coding for the deficient compoment has been proven in several, but not all instances.

Diagnosis of Complement Deficiencies

Although the clinical presentation and history of a patient may suggest the presence of a hereditary CD, the diagnosis of this status must be confirmed in the laboratory.

In most hereditary CDs, total hemolytic complement (CH50) levels are at or near zero. Exceptions include $C\overline{1}$ inh D, C9 D, C5 dysfunction, and possibly C3b ina D. However, CH50 levels may also be extremely low in acquired C deficiencies. In order to establish the cause of zero CH50, a determinantion of individual C components, either immunochemically or functionally, must be done. In acquired CD, serum concentrations of all components will be decreased in varying degrees. In hereditary CD only one component will be absent, while the others are present at more or less normal levels. The exceptions to this rule are:

1. $C\overline{1}$ inh D, in which $C\overline{1}$ inh is below 30% or, if the inhibitor is present but functionally defect, above 250% of normal and in which C4 is and C2 may be low; rarely, $C\overline{1}$ inh D may be caused by a functionally defect $C\overline{1}$ inh at an immunochemically normal level.
2. C1r D, in which C1s is also low.
3. C3b ina D, which leads to markedly reduced C3 levels.

In C5 dysfunction, which affects opsonization but not hemolytic activity or immunochemical levels of C5, the appropriate tests must be done.

C9 D leads to a decreased but not absent CH50 in the absence of detectable C9, in accordance with the function of C9 in the hemolytic pathway.

The hemolytic activity of sera from patients with hereditary CD can be reconstituted stoichiometrically by the addition of the missing component in purified form.

Deficiencies of Classical Pathway Components

C1q Deficiency

A genetic lack of C1q function may be due to the complete absence of this subcomponent but usually if not always is represented by a functionally abnormal protein which may be identified by its reaction of partial identitiy with normal C1q upon immunodiffusion against antiserum to C1q. So far, seven patients from six families have been found to suffer from C1q D and SLE. The first was a 4-year-old girl with functionally deficient C1q, the genetic basis of which was not established. She suffered from a butterfly rash, vasculitis-like lesions on her palms and soles, photosensitivity, recurrent infections and had ANA [31].

Another is a boy, born from first-degree cousins, who developed typical SLE with antinuclear, anti-Sm, and anti-native DNA antibodies, rheumatoid factor, and kidney involvement; however, no skin pathology was mentioned. Treatment with prednisone resulted in a remission of the disease [32]. This patient and his healthy sister also had nonfunctional C1q; hemolytic activity of their sera could be reconsituted by the addition of normal C1q.

130 G. Tappeiner

A 37-year-old man with C1q D developed typical SLE with discoid lesions of the face, a maculopapular eruption on his trunk and extremities, oral ulceration, photosensitivity and arthralgias, and antinuclear and anti-Sm antibodies [33]. His brother had died from renal failure secondary to SLE at the age of 10 years.

A 17-year-old girl had classical SLE with skin rash, oral ulceration, hair loss, fever, arthralgias, and seizures [34]. There were ANA but no anti-DNA antibodies; C3 and C4 levels were normal, while total hemolytic activity and C1q were absent. In addition, she suffered from recurrent infections.

In one large family, two sisters and their brother had a functionally deficient C1q [35]. The boy had had glomerulonephritis in childhood and suffered from membranous glomerulopathy. The two girls developed an SLE-like syndrome in their third decades, of which one of them died. This defect C1q was of abnormally low molecular weight and could be shown to bind to aggregated IgG but not to C1r/C1s. A further young girl with C1q D and SLE has been briefly described [36].

Besides the association with SLE, several facts are striking in C1q D: first, healthy individuals with C1q D seem to occur but are rare; second, some cases of C1q D have been reported in which there was no SLE but glomerulonephritis [37, 38]; and third, recurrent pyogenic infections have been a significant problem in some C1q D individuals with SLE or glomerulonephritis.

C1r Deficiency

A complete absence of C1r has been reported in eight individuals from four families. Of these, five suffered from SLE, or SLE-like syndromes, one had chronic glomerulonephritis, and two were clinically healthy.

In one large Puerto Rican family, one boy developed widespread CDLE of his head and the upper portion of his trunk at the age of 13 that went on to lupus panniculitis and facial ulceration [39—41]. Although there was no clinical evidence of renal disease, a kidney biopsy revealed subacute focal membranous glomerulonephritis. He had a brother who had not been studied but was said to have died of a similar disease at the age of 12. Two other siblings had died in infancy from unspecified causes. His 24-year-old sister also had facial ulceration and a history of arthritis and of skin rashes. A history of recurrent pyogenic infections was obtained from all of them. Both patients had no ANA and were negative for lupus band tests and LE cell preparations; however, the kidney biopsy showed immunoglobulin and C deposition. Both siblings had depressed CH50, undetectable C1r, and depressed C1s; C1q, C4 and C3 were normal or elevated. Addition of C1 restored CH50. An autosomal recessive mode of inheritance of the C1r D was established [41].

In another Puerto Rican family, one boy had had arthralgias since early childhood and presented with diffuse mesangioproliferative glomerulonephritis with focal IgG and C3 deposits at the age of 14 [42]. Laboratory data included high-titered ANA, anti-Sm antibodies, but not anti-DNA antibodies. Rheumatoid factors and circulating immune complexes were positive. Again, CH50 and C1r were absent and C1s was depressed while the other components studied were normal or elevated; CH50 was reconstituted by the addition of C1r. Again, an autosomal recessive pattern of inheritance was suggested by family studies in which heterozygosity for C1r D could be assigned on the basis of C1r, C1s, and CH50 levels.

In the third family, four individuals had C1r D, though two of them were clinically healthy [43]. One boy and one girl had discoid skin lesions, oral ulcerations, arthritis, and photosensitivity. In addition, the girl had hypertension and had suffered three episodes of meningitis; she was ANA negative. Besides the skin lesions, the boy showed Raynaud's phenomenon and had a history of episodes of glomerulonephritis and of pneumonia and cellulitis. Again, in all C1r D individuals, C1s was below 50% of normal values. The relationship between C1r D and low C1s levels is not yet understood, but a regulatory influence of C1r on C1s metabolism or a direct genetic linkage seems possible. One Causasian girl with advanced chronic glomerulonephritis and C1r D was also reported, but the familial nature of the defect was not demonstrated in an incomplete study of the family [44].

C1s Deficiency

Two families in which complete C1s D occurs have been noted. In one family, a 6-year-old girl seems to have suffered from SLE, but only laboratory data such as positive ANA, positive lupus band test, and negative CH50 that could be restored by the addition of C1s to her serum, have been reported [45].

In the second family, four individuals were C1s D, two of them without clinical signs of disease [46]. The other two had polyarthritis, Raynaud's phenomenon, discoid skin lesions and ANA, but no signs of internal organ involvement. Remarkably, another sibling also had SLE but no evidence of complement abnormalities.

C̄1 inh Deficiency

The deficiency of C̄1 inh and its associated disease, hereditary angioedema, is well investigated and is probably the most frequently diagnosed and best-known complement deficiency [3].

Besides this classical disease association, 17 individuals with C̄1 inh D have been reported who have developed LE [47—54]. In six of them there was discoid LE with cutaneous lesions, alopecia, and solar sensitivity; splenomegaly occured in two of them, all had ANA. The remainder (eleven patients) had typical SLE with typical clinical and immunologic features; however, four of the patients had only renal lesions typical of LE with no cutaneous or immunologic signs and symptoms. Three of the patients were male, two of them identical twins suffering from DLE.

All patients for whom data are available have suffered from hereditary angioedema as well as LE; it is felt that about 2% of patients with heredirary angioedema also develop SLE [48], a proportion that is clearly very much higher than the 0.4—1.6 cases per year per 100000 seen in the general population [55]. Recurrent infections do not seem to have been a problem in this group. Treatment with danazol, the therapy of choice for hereditary angioedema, has been found to be of benefit for those with LE in C$\bar{1}$ inh D as well [56].

According to the nature of the C$\bar{1}$ inh D, C4 and CH50 are and C2 and C3 may be low in these patients. Acquired C$\bar{1}$ inh D has been found in a few patients associated with malignant, usually lymphoproliferative disease [57]. Though they may suffer from angioedema, no such case with SLE has so far been described.

C4 Deficiency

So far, a hereditary lack of C4 has been documented in 15 individuals from 12 families [59—67]. Of these, two were clinically healthy, one had Schönlein-Henoch's purpura [62] that has gone on to renal failure, and one had glomerulonephritis but has fully recovered. The remaining 11 patients suffer from SLE. From the observations made so far, it appears that there is a peculiar type of SLE associated with C4 D.

Age of onset of SLE in C4 D persons is usually within the first few years of life but has occurred as late as in the third decade. Both sexes are affected, but there may be a somewhat higher incidence of females as the four individuals who do not have SLE are male. On the other hand, the prognosis seems to be far worse in males, all of whom have died, than in females, most of whom survive. Overall, the propensity to develop SLE seems to be higher in C4 D than in all other hereditary CDs.

Clinically there is marked sensitivity to sunlight and to cold, the latter resulting in severe Raynaud's phenomenon, often with atrophy and even mutilations of the distal phalanges (Fig. 2).

Skin lesions include all those seen in acute and in subacute LE, but lesions characteristic for LE in C4 D (and, perhaps, in C1q D) have been observed. The involvement of hands and feet is usually remarkable. Besides the atrophy of the distal phalanges as mentioned above (Fig. 2), there are often red, infiltrated plaques with pronounced hyperkeratosis on palms and soles (Fig. 3) that heal with atrophic scars. Infiltrated plaques on sun-exposed areas such as the face and the backs of the hands tend to be raised, infiltrated, and covered by smooth, atrophic, whitish-opaque epidermis (Figs. 4, 5). Later, scarring and hyperkeratosis become prominent and tend to involve the lips (Fig. 6). Internal organ involvement is variable but usually mild; evidence has been obtained in the patient with Schönlein-Henoch's purpura (but not yet in an SLE patient) that nephritis did develop in the presence of C3NeF [62].

Antinuclear antibodies are low titered or absent in these patients. Remarkably, anti-Ro (SS-A) antibodies are found twice as frequently in this group as in unselected SLE patients [68]; rheumatoid factor may also be positive. One patient had high-titered anti-DNA and kidney disease. Deposits of immunoglobulin and complement may or may not be found in skin biopsies.

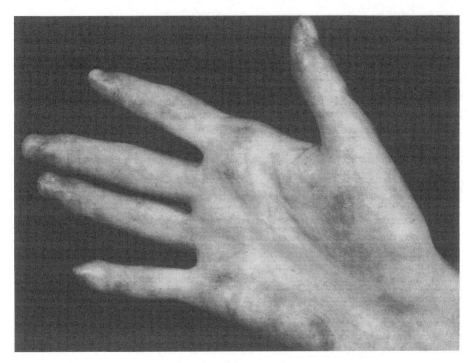

Fig. 2. SLE in C4 D. Palmar erythema and epidermal atrophy; pronounced atrophy of distal phalanges with sclerotic and hyperkeratotic skin lesions

Immune functions such as lymphocyte response to mitogens or mixed lymphocyte cultures and opsonizing activity have been found to be diminished in individual patients [69]. However, no clear immunologic defect has yet been identified, although there is a possible role of classical pathway components [16] and in particular of C4 [70] in the immune response. The gene loci for the two alleles of C4, C4A and C4B, are closely linked with each other and are situated between the HLA B and D loci. Null genes seem to occur relatively frequently on either allele, and some preliminary observations indicate that the presence of such null genes, leading to incomplete C4 D, does not increase the risk of developing LE [71]. The completely C4 D genotype has been found with several HLA types, usually in one family only and, in one family, a C4 D gene that was not HLA-associated has been identified [72].

Only two of these HLA types are found more frequently. The main association of C4 D seems to be with HLA A30, B18 (DR7) and with A2, B40 [4]. Heterozygotes for C4 D cannot always be identified on the basis of C4 levels. The development of anti-C4-antibodies has been observed in two of these patients following pregnancy or blood transfusions [67].

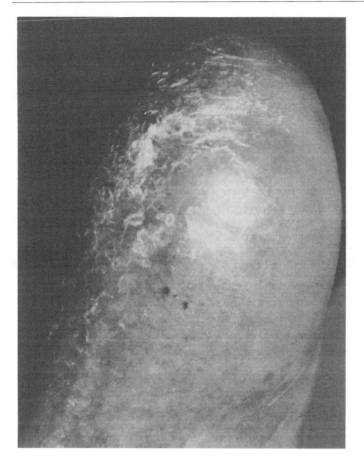

Fig. 3. SLE in C4 D. Distal phalangeal lesion, detail. Note the pronounced sclerosis and atrophy of the skin, with loss of dermatoglyphics and marked hyperkeratosis

C2 Deficiency

The hereditary lack of C2 was the first CD to be identified [1]. It is probably also the most common one, with an estimated frequency of the C2 D gene of 1% in the general population [73]; thus, about one in 10000 individuals should have a complete genetic C2 D [74]. These figures alone indicate that C2 D is not necessarily associated with clinical disease. Indeed, many individuals with C2 D remain in good health [4, 75].

Many different diseases have been found in association with C2 D: chronic discoid LE with atrophoderma, dermatomyositis, glomerulonepthritis, Schönlein-Henoch's purpura and chronic vasculitis, cold urticaria, common variable immunodeficiency, inflammatory bowel disease, and Hodgkin's lymphoma [4, 75]; however, these were sporadic case reports. Two conditions only are frequently associated with C2 D: LE, usually SLE, and recurrent infections. Of the

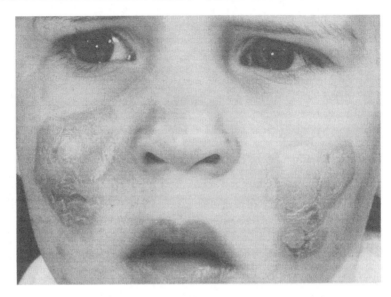

Fig. 4. SLE in C4 D. Infiltrated plaques covered with smooth, opaque, atrophic epidermis on both cheeks and small erythematous lesions on cheeks and nose

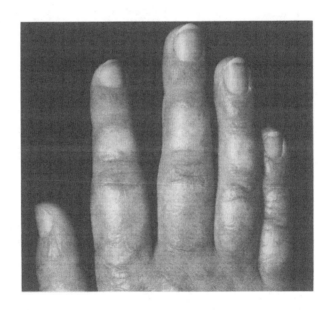

Fig. 5. SLE in C4 D. Infiltrated plaques covered with smooth, opaque, atrophic epidermis on the back of the hand (not shown) and fingers. Though there is epidermal involvement of the distal phalanges, there are no atrophic changes

reported infections, roughly two-thirds have been caused by pneumonococci; streptococci, meningococci, salmonellae, and *Hemophilus* have also been implicated [74].

The most frequent disease association of C2 D is with SLE. These patients share certain characteristics and are quite similar to those with SLE in C4 D.

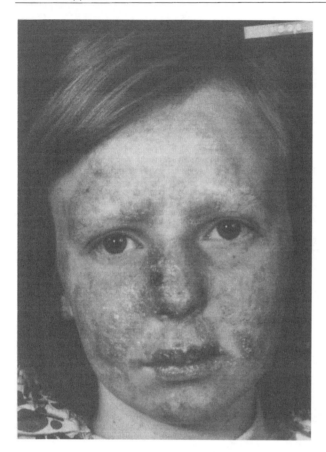

Fig. 6. SLE in C4 D. Infiltrated, scarred lesions covered with atrophic epidermis with pronounced scaling and erosion. Note the extensive involvement of the lips

Onset of SLE is early in life; there is marked photosensitivity and Raynaud's phenomenon. Skin involvement is pronounced, usually in the form of the papulosquamous lesions of subacute LE, though the whole gamut of LE skin pathology from malar erythema to chronic discoid lesions may be seen. Internal organ involvement, if present, tends to be mild, but cases of fulminant nephritis have occurred [4, 75].

The term "lupus-like disease in C2 D" has been used to describe some of these patients, but its use does not seem justified anymore since most if not all of them certainly fulfill the criteria necessary for a diagnosis of SLE.

Antinuclear antibodies tend to be low-titered or absent, but as in C4 D LE patients, anti-Ro antibodies have been found in about 50% of these patients [68, 76]. A lower incidence of immunoglobulin and complement deposits at the dermo-epidermal junction zone in discoid skin lesions in C2 D patients has also been noted [73, 77]. There is good evidence for a silent allele at the C2 gene locus as the cause for C2 D [23]. A strong linkage disequilibrium exists between C2 D and HLA A10, B18, DR2, BfS, C4A*4, C4B*2 [78, 79]. Heterozygous C2 D leads to about half-normal values of serum C2 levels [80], and a statistically significant higher incidence of SLE and juvenile rheumatoid arthritis has been found in heterogzygous C2 D individuals [81]. However, the C2 D gene per se has not been associated with the presence of ANA or rheumatoid arthritis nuclear antigen in one large family [82].

Deficiencies of C3, C3b ina, and CR1

The genetically determined absence of C3 and, functionally similar, of C3b ina, has serious consequences for host defense against pyogenic infections. All individuals so affected have suffered from severe recurrent infections, mainly with encapsulated bacteria such as pneumococci, *Hemophilus influenzae, Streptococcus pyogenes* and *Klebsiella aerogenes* and, to a lesser extent, with *Neisseria meningitidis* [4, 74]. Two sisters with homozygous C3 D, with a lupus-like syndrome that includes malar rash, arthralgias, and photosensitivity but no antinuclear antibodies, have been observed [83]. The disease seems to follow a mild course; both patients are not particularly susceptible to infections.

Remarkably, many of the C3 D patients are reported to suffer from erythematous lesions on the face and trunk during episodes of infections, but these lesions do not seem to represent LE [75].

C3 ina D has not so far been found in association with autoimmune disease.

A deficiency in CR1, the C receptor binding C4b and C3b, has been found on erythrocyte surfaces of patients with SLE and with rheumatoid arthritis [84]. This deficiency, manifest as a decrease in the number of functional receptors, improved but did not disappear upon successful treatment of the associated condidtion. It is not yet clear whether this CR1 deficiency is genetically determined or acquired and whether it represents a consequence of or a predisposing factor to the associated disease.

Late and Alternative Pathway Component Deficiencies

Hereditary deficiencies of the late C components, i.e., C5—C9, seem to occur most frequently in blacks; they are usually not associated with autoimmune or chronic immune complex diseases [4, 75]. C5 D has so far been found in three kindreds. One of the C5 D individuals had classical SLE; however, her kidney function was not severely impaired despite an active glomerulonephritis [86].

All C5 D individuals did tend to develop recurrent infections with staphylococci, streptococci, *Proteus, Pseudomonas, Enterobacter, Candida,* and, most frequently, disseminated gonococcal infections [4, 75].

138 G. Tappeiner

A peculiar dysfunctional state of C5 that only impairs its opsonizing but not its hemolytic activity has been identified in healthy individuals in association with Leiner's disease (generalized seborrheic dermatitis or erythroderma, profuse diarrhea, and malabsorption) but not with LE [75].

Deficiencies of C6, C7, and C8 cause an increased susceptibility to invasive infections with gram-negative diplococci and pneumococci. One patient with SLE has been reported each for C6 D and for C7 D [87, 88] and two for C8 D [89, 90]. Their diseases had no remarkable features except for ANA negativity in one C8 D individual. In addition, one patient with C7 D and the CRST syndrome has been found [91].

C9 deficiency is found in 56 per 100 000 Japanese and sporadically elsewhere. There is no associated disease.

Complete and incomplete deficiencies of properdin have been identified in a total of 12 individuals so far; except occasional meningococcal meningitis, there was no associated pathology (for ref., see [92]). Incomplete deficiency of factor B has been noted in isolated cases, but again was not found with immune complex disease.

Treatment

With the notable exception of $\overline{C1}$ inh D, treatment of hereditary CD and their associated diseases is problematic and often unsuccessful. The biochemical and clinical abnormalities in $\overline{C1}$ inh D can be reversed quickly but only for a short time by the administration of $\overline{C1}$ inh in purified form and perhaps also in the form of fresh-frozen plasma; this therapy is of use in the treatment of an attack of angioedema or its prevention. The endogenous production of $\overline{C1}$ inh as well as the production of a functionally active $\overline{C1}$ inh in functional $\overline{C1}$ inh D can be increased by the administration of androgens, usually the attenuated androgens danazol or stanazolol [3]. This results in a dose-dependent increase of $\overline{C1}$ inh serum levels and thus a suppression of angioedema attacks. Interestingly, this type of treatment also reverses the SLE present in some of these patients, indicating that it is not the genetic defect but rather the actual lack of $\overline{C1}$ inh that predisposes to its development.

Treatment of the autoimmune diseases in deficiencies of classical pathway components has so far only been tried by conventional corticosteroid and immunosuppressive therapy and generally did not seem to alter the course of the illness, even though isolated favorable reports have appeared [32]. In our experience with C4 D paptients, corticosteroids and immunosuppression were of limited usefulness, but physical measures such as complete protection from exposure to sunlight and cold and prevention or early treatment of infections were important in their management [63, 66]. In one C2 D patient with a lupus-like syndrome, persistent immunoglobulin deficiency developed after therapy with prednisolone and phenytoin [93].

Complement and Complement Deficiencies **139**

Treatment of infectious disease in deficiencies of C3 through C8 does not seem to pose special problems, but recurrence of infection is to be expected.

Conclusions

All genetic C component deficiencies have been associated with SLE. It is difficult to assess at present whether this reflects an increased risk of SLE development for every CD individual or whether it only reflects a bias in the detection of CD, since LE patients are certainly the most likely group to have their complement status determined.

We have proposed previously [4] that several groups of CD may be distinguished according to their associated pathologies, and these groups can be correlated with the biological function of the missing component:

1. C$\overline{1}$ inh D always results in hereditary angioedema.
2. Deficiencies of the classical pathway components C1, C4, and C2 and, to a much lesser degree, of C$\overline{1}$ inh are not invariably associated with disease but they greatly increase the risk of acquiring autoimmune or immune complex disease. By far the most frequent of these is SLE, followed by glomerulonephritis and various types of vasculitis. There may also be a somewhat higher risk of infectious disease in this group. It is remarkable that these LE patients have certain peculiar features in common regardless of which component is deficient.
3. Deficiencies of C3 and, functionally similar, of C3b ina, lead to a high risk of recurrent severe pyogenic infections.
4. C5 dysfunction leads to Leiner's disease.
5. Deficiencies of the components of the lytic pathway, C5 to C8, predispose to recurrent disseminated infections with pneumococci and gram-negative diplococci.
6. There is no particular associated pathology in C9 deficiency.

While the few reported cases of SLE in deficiencies other than classical pathway components appear to represent fortuitous associations, it seems surprising at first sight that conditions in whose pathology immune complexes are thought to play an important role are frequently found in association with a blocked C cascade. Obviously, other effector mechanisms compensate for the missing C function; furthermore, internal organ involvement, especially kidney disease, is usually remarkably mild in CD SLE patients; and finally, alternative pathway activation may play a role. One case of nepthritis in C4 D in which alternative pathway activation was mediated by C3NeF has been documented [62].

Several explanations are possible for the close association between SLE and deficiencies of classical pathway components. A fascinating hypothesis arises from research into the modification of immune complexes by the incorporation of C3b. This requires an intact classical pathway, prevents the formation of large lattices and causes the immune complexes to bind to the complement receptor CRl promoting their clearance by the fixed macrophage system and preventing their interaction with other structures (eg., vascular endothelia, glomeruli) (for ref., see [92]).

Another is derived from the assumption that C-type and perhaps other viruses provide the antigen in SLE. Since the classical pathway is an important mechanism in virus defence, its blockage would facilitate the establishment of a virus infection. This possibility may be supported by the observation of the Cls D family in which both deficient and "normal" individuals had SLE [45], and possibly by the therapeutic influence of danazol treatment of $C\overline{1}$ inh D on LE. It is also possible that CDs do not by themselves predispose to the development of SLE but that they rather are genetic markers for an underlying immunogenetic defect. This would be reasonable as far as C4 and C2 are concerned and is corroborated by the observation of LE in heterozygous C4D individuals, but it does not take $C\overline{1}$ inh D and C1 subcomponent D into account.

From a clinical point of view, patients with C2 D seem to do better that those with C4 D. However, several reports would suggest that viral infection may be an important and often unrecognized problem in patients with classical pathway component deficiency and SLE [63, 91].

At present, the validity of either hypothesis cannot be assessed; obviously, all three mechanisms may contribute in the development of SLE in CD, and other so far unrecognized factors may be of importance.

References

1 Klemperer MR, Woodworth HC, Rosen FS, Austen KF (1966) Hereditary deficiency of the second component of complement (C'2) in man. J Clin Invest 45:880—890
2 Donaldson VH, Evans RR (1963) A biochemical abnormality in hereditary angioneurotic edema. Absence of serum inhibitor of C'l-esterase. Am J Med 35:37—44
3 Frank MM, Gelfand JA, Atkinson JP (1979) Hereditary angioedema: the clinical syndrome and its magnagement. Ann Intern Med 84:580—593
4 Tappeiner G. (1982) Disease states in genetic complement deficiencies. Int. J. Dermatol. 21:175—191
5 Lachmann PJ, Hughes-Jones NC (1985) Initiation of complement activation. In: Müller-Eberhard HJ, Miescher PA (eds) Complement. Springer, Berlin Heidelberg New York Tokyo, pp 147—166
6 Pangburn MK, Müller-Eberhard HJ (1985) The alternative pathway of complement. In: Müller-Eberhard, Miescher PA (eds) Complement. Springer, Berlin Heidelberg New York Tokyo, pp 185—214
7 Müller-Eberhard HJ (1985) The membrane attack complex. In: Müller-Eberhard HJ, Miescher PA (eds) Complement. Springer, Berlin Heidelberg New York Tokyo, pp 227—279
8 Cooper NR (1969) Immune adherence by the fourth component of complement. Science 165:396—398
9 Takahashi M, Czop J, Ferreira A, et al. (1976) Mechanism of solubilization of immune aggregates by complement. Transplant Rev. 32:121

10 Takahashi, M, Takahashi S, Brade V, et al. (1978) Requirements for the solubilization of immune aggregates by complement. The role of the classical pathway. J Clin Invest. 62:349

11 Mantovani B, Rabinovitch M, Nussenzweig V (1972) Phagocytosis of immune complexes by macrophages. Different roles of the macrophage receptor sites for complement (C3) and for immunoglobulin (IgG). J Exp Med 135:780

12 Goldstein IM, Roos D, Kaplan HB, Weissman G (1975) Complement and immunoglobulin stimulate superoxide production by human leukocytes independently of phagocytosis. J Clin Invest 56:1155—1163

13 Mayer MM (1968) Chemotactic and anaphylatoxic fragment cleaved from the fifth component of guinea pig complement. Science 162:361

14 Zvaifler J (1973) The immunopathology of joint inflammation in rheumatoid arthritis. Adv. Immunol 16:265

15 Donaldson VH, Rosen FS, Bing DH (1977) Role of the second component of complement (C2) and plasmin in kinin release in hereditary angioneurotic edema (H.A.N.E.) plasma Trans Am Assoc Phys 90:174

16 Weigle WO, Goodman MG, Morgan EL, Hugh TE (1985) Regulation of immune response by components of the complement cascade and their activated fragments. In: Müller-Eberhard HJ, Miescher PA (eds) Complement. Springer, Berlin Heidelberg New York Tokyo, pp 323—344

17 Cooper NR, Nemerow GR (1985) Complement, viruses and virus-infected cells. In: Müller-Eberhard HJ, Miescher PA (eds) Complement. Springer, Berlin Heidelberg New York Tokyo, pp 345—366

18 Hartung HP, Hadding U (1985) Synthesis of complement by macrophages and modulation of their functions through complement activation. In: Müller-Eberhard HJ, Miescher PA (eds) Complement. Springer, Berlin Heidelberg New York Tokyo, pp 279—472

19 O'Neill GH, Yang SY, Dupont B (1978) Two HLA-linked loci controlling the fourth component of human complement. Proc Natl Acad Sci. USA 75:5165—5169

20 Roos MH, Mollenhauer E, Demant P, Rittner CA (1982) A molecular basis for the two locus model of human complement component C4. Nature 298:854—856

21 Fu, SM, Kunkel HG, Brusman HP et al. (1974) Evidence for linkage between HLA histocompatibility genes and those involved in the synthesis of the second component of complement. J Exp Med 140:1108

22 Teisberg B, Olaisen B, Gedde-Dahl T Jr. et al. (1975) On the localization of the Gb locus within the MHS region of chromosome no. 6. Tissue Antigens 5:257

23 Pariser KM, Raum D, Berkman EM et al. (1978) Evidence for a silent or null gene in hereditary C2 deficiency. J Immunol 121:2580

24 Glass D, Raum D, Balatvitch D (1978) Inherited deficiency of the sixth component: a silent or null gene. J Immunol 120:538—541

25 Weidinger S, Schwarzfischer F, Cleve H (1979) Properdin factor B-polymorphism. An indication for the existence of a Bf°allele. Z. Rechtsmed. 83:259

26 Brunn-Petersen G, Lamm LU, Sorensen IJ et al. (1981) Family studies of complement C4 and HLA in man. Hum Genet 58:269—267

27 Tokunaga K, Araki C, Juji T, Omoto K (1982) Polymorphism of properdin factor B in Japanese. Description of a rare variant and data of association with HLA and C2. Hum Genet. 60:42—45

28 O'Neill GJ, Yang SY, Tegoli J, et al. (1978) Chido and Rodgers blood groups are distinct antigenic components of human complement C4. Nature 273:668

29 Whitehead AS, Solomon E, Chambers D, et al. (1982) Assignment of the structural gene for the third component of human complement to chromosome 19. Proc. Natl. Acad. Sci. USA 79:5021—5025

30 McDuffie FC, Sams WM Jr, Maldona JE, et al. (1973) Hypocomplementemia with cutaneous vasculitis and arthritis. Possible immune complex syndrome. Mayo Clin Proc 48:340

31 Wara DW, Reiter EO, Doyle NE, et al. (1975) Persistent Clq deficiency in a patient with systemic lupus erythematosus-like syndrome. J Pediatr 86:743—745

32 Thompson RA, Haeney M, Reid KBM, et al. (1980) A genetic defect of the Clq subcomponent of complement associated with childhood (immune complex) nephritis. N. Engl. J. Med. 303:22–24

33 Nishino H, Shibuya K, Nishida Y, Mushimoto M (1981) Lupus erythematosus-like syndrome with selective complete deficiency of Clq. Ann Intern. Med. 95:322–324

34 Steinsson K, McLean RH, Merrow M, Rothfield NF, Weinstein A (1983) Selective complete Clq-deficiency associated with systemic lupus erythematosus. J Rheumatol 10:590–594

35 Hannema AJ, Kluin-Nelemans JC, Hack CE, Eerenberg-Belmer AJ, Malbe C, van Helden HP (1984) SLE-like syndrome and functional deficiency of Clq in members of a large family. Clin Exp Immunol 55:106–114

36 Voigtlaender V, Stach C, Haensch G (1982) Syndrome lupique avec déficit complet en Clq. Ann. Dermatol. Venereol. 109:823–824

37 Berkel AI, Loos M, Sanal O, et al. (1979) Clinical and immunological studies in a case of selective complete Clq deficiency. Clin. Exp. Immunol. 38:52–63

38 Arnaiz-Villena A, Lopez-Larrea C, Leyva-Cobian F, Bootello-Gil A (1981) Genetic independence between HLA and first component (Clq). Transplantation 31:139–140

39 Moncada B, Day NKB, Good RA, Windhurst DB (1972) Lupus-erythematosus-like syndrome with a familial defect of complement. N Engl J Med 286:689–693

40 Day NK, Geiger H, Stroud R, et al. (1972) Clr deficiency: an inborn error associated with cutaneous and renal disease. J Clin Invest 51:1102–1108

41 DeBracco MME, Windhorst D, Stroud RM, Moncada B (1974) The autosomal recessive mode of inheritance of Clr deficiency in a large Puerto Rican family. Clin. Exp. Immunol. 16:183–188

42 Rich KC, Hurley J, Gewurz H (1979) Inborn Clr deficiency with a mild lupus-like syndrome. Clin. Immunol. Immunopathol. 13:77–84

43 Lee SL, Wallace SL, Barone R (1978) Familial deficiency of two subunits of the first component of complement, Clr and Cls, associated with a lupus erythematosus-like disease. Arthritis Rheum. 21:958–967

44 Pickering RJ, Michael AF Jr., Herdman RC, et al. (1971) The complement system in chronic glomerulonephritis: three newly associated aberrations. J. Pediatr. 78:30–43

45 Pondman KW, Stoop JW, Cormane RH, Hannema AJ (1968) Abnormal C'l in a patient with systemic lupus erythematosus. J. Immunol. 101:811A (Abst.)

46 Chase PH, Barone R, Blum L, Wallace SL (1976) "Lupuslike" syndrome associated with deficiency of Cls: family studies. Ann R Coll Phys Surg 9:33

47 Kohler PF, Percy J, Campion WM, Smyth CJ (1974) Hereditary angioedema and "familial" lupus erythematosus in identical twin boys. Am J Med 56:406–411

48 Donaldson VH, Hess EV, McAdams AJ (1977) Lupus-erythematosus-like disease in three unrelated women with hereditary angioneurotic edema. Ann. Intern. Med. 86:312–313 (Letter to the editor)

49 Tuffanelli DL (1977) Discoid lupus erythematosus and the variant form of hereditary angioedema. Arch. Dermatol. 113:374–375 (Letter to the editor)

50 Rosenfeld GB, Partridge REH, Bartholomew W, Murphey WH, Singleton CM (1974) Hereditary angioneurotic edema (HANE) and systemic lupus erythematosus (SLE) in one of identical twin girls. J. Allergy Clin. Immunol. 53:68–69 (Abst.)

51 Young DW, Thompson RA, Mackie PH (1980) Plasmapheresis in hereditary angioneurotic edema and systemic lupus erythematosus. Arch Intern. Med. 140:127–128

52 Hory B, Panouse-Perrin J, Saint-Hyllier Y, Perot C (1983) Déficit héréditaire en inhibiteur de la Cl esterase. Lupus et glomerulonephrite. Rev Med Interne 4:57–63

53 Massa MC, Conolly SM (1982) An association between Cl esterase inhibitor deficiency and lupus erythematosus: report of two cases and review of the literature. J Acad Dermatol 7:255–264

54 Shiraishi S, Nara Y, Watanabe Y, Matsuda K, Miki Y (1982) Cl inhibitor deficiency simulating systemic lupus erythematosus. Br J Dermatol 106:455–460

55 Siegel M, Lee SL (1973) The epidemiology of systemic lupus erythematosus. Semin Arthritis Rheum 3:1–54

Complement and Complement Deficiencies **143**

56 Masse R, Youinou P, Dorval JC, Cledes J (1980) Reversal of lupus-erythematosus-like disease with danazol. Lancet 2:651 (Letter to the Editor)

57 Schreiber AD, Zweiman B, Atkins P et al. (1976) Acquired angioedema with lymphoproliferative disorder. Association of Cl inhibitor deficiency with cellular abnormality. Blood 48:567—580

58 Hauptmann G, Grosshans E, Heid E (1974) Lupus érythémateux aigu et déficits héréditaires en complément. A propos d'un cas par déficit complet en C4. Ann. Dermatol. Syph. (Paris) 101:479—496

59 Schaller JG, Gilliland BG, Ochs HD et al. (1977) Severe systemic lupus erythematosus with nephritis in a boy with deficiency of the fourth component of complement. Arthritis Rheum. 20:1519—1525

60 Ballow M, McLean RH, Einarson M, et al. (1979) Hereditary C4 deficiency-genetic studies and linkage to HLA. Transplant Proc. 11:1710—1712

61 Minta JO, Urowitz MB, Gladman DD (1980) Selective deficiency of the fourth component of complement in a patient with systemic lupus erythematosus (SLE): Immunochemical and biological studies. Clin. Exp. Immunol. 45:72—80

62 Tappeiner G, Wolff K (1980) Possible mediation of immune-complex vasculitis by C3 nephritic factor in hereditary C4 deficiency. In: Wolff K, Winkelmann RK (eds) Vasculitis. Major problems in dermatology. Lloyd-Luke, London, vol 10 pp 86—94

63 Tappeiner G, Hintner H, Scholz S, et al. (1982) Systemic lupus erythematosus in hereditary deficiency of the fourth component of complement. J Am Acad Dermatol 7:66—79

64 Kjellman M, Laurell AB, Loew B, Sjoeholm AG (1982) Homozygous deficiency of C4 in a child with a lupus erythematosus syndrome. Clin. Genet. 22,:331—339

65 Mascart-Lemone F, Hauptmann G, Goetz J, Duchateau J, Delespesse G, Kray B, Dab I (1983) Genetic deficiency of C4 presenting with recurrent infections and a SLE-like disease. Genetic and immunologic studies. Am J Med 75:295—304

66 Klein G, Tappeiner G, Hintner H, Scholz S, Wolff K (1984) Systemischer Lupus Erythematodes bei hereditärer Defizienz der vierten Komplementkomponente. Hautarzt 35:27—32

67 Giles CM, Swanson JL (1984) Anti-C4 in the serum of a transfused C4 deficient patient with systemic lupus erythematosus. Vox Sang. 46:291—299

68 Meyer O, Hauptmann G, Tappeiner G, Ochs HD, Mascart-Lemone F (1985) Genetic deficiency of C4, C2 or C1q and lupus syndromes. Association with anti-Ro (SS-A) antibodies. Clin. Exp. Immunol. 62:678—684

69 Jackson CA, Ochs HD, Wedgewood RJ, Immune response of a patient with deficiency of the fourth component of complement and systemic lupus erythematosus. N. Engl. J. Med 300:1124—1129

70 Ferrone S, Pellegrino MA, Cooper NR (1976) Expression of C4 on human lymphoid cells and possible involvement in immune recognition phenomena. Science 193:53—55

71 Berlin S, Weinberger A, Zamir R, Salomon F, Joohna HL, Pinkhas J (1981) Familial systemic lupus erythematosus and C4 deficiency. Scand. J. Rheumatol. 10:280—282

72 Muir WA, Hedrick S, Alper CA, Ratnoff OD, Schacter B, Wisnieski JJ (1984) Inherited incomplete deficiency of the fourth component of complement (C4) determined by a gene not linked to human histocompatibility leucocyte antigens. J. Clin. Invest. 74:1509—1514

73 Agnello V (1978) Complement deficiency states. Medicine 57:1—23

74 Agnello V, DeBracco MME, Kunkel HG (1972) Hereditary C2 deficiency with some manifestations of systemic lupus erythematosus. J. Immunol. 108:837—840

75 Guenther LC (1983) Inherited disorders of complement. J. Amer. Acad. Dermatol. 9:815—839

76 Provost TT, Arnett FC, Reichlin M (1983) Homozygous C2 deficiency, lupus erythematosus, and anti Ro (SSA) antibodies. Arthritis Rheum. 26:1279—1282

77 Levy SB, Pinnel SR, Meadows L, et al. (1979) Hereditary C2 deficiency associated with cutaneous lupus erythematosus: clinical, laboratory and genetic studies. Arch. Dermatol. 115:57

78 Nerl C, Grosse-Wilde H, Valet G (1978) Association of low C2 and C4 serum levels with the HLA-DW2 allele in healthy individuals. J. Exp. Med. 148:704—713

79 Hauptmann G, Tongio MM, Goetz J, et al. (1982) Association of the C2-deficiency gene (C2*Q0) with the C4A*4, C4B*2 genes. J. Immunogenet 9:127—132

80 Gibson DJ, Glass D, Carpenter CB, Schur PH (1976) Hereditary C2 deficiency: diagnosis and HLA gene complex associations. J. Immunol. 116:1065—1070
81 Glass D, Raum D, Gibson D, et al. (1971) Inherited deficiency of the second component of complement. Rheumatic disease associations. J. Clin. Invest. 58:853—861
82 McCarthy DJ, Tan EM, Zvaifler NJ, Koethe S, Duesnoy RJ (1981) Serologic studies in a family with heterozygous C2 deficiency. Am J Med 71:945—948
83 Sano Y, Nishimukai H, Kitamura H, Nayaki K, Inai S, Hamasaki Y, Maruyama I, Igata A (1981) Hereditary deficiency of the third component of complement in two sisters with systemic lupus erythematosus-like symptoms. Arthritis Rheum. 24:1255—1260
84 Miyarawa Y, Yamada A, Kosaka K, Tsuda F, Kosugi E, Mayumi M (1981) Defective immune-adherence (C3b) receptor on erythrocytes from patients with systemic lupus erythematosus. Lancet 2:493—493—497
85 Iida K, Mornaghi R, Nussenzweig V (1982) Complement receptor (CR1) deficiency in erythrocytes from patients with systemic lupus erythematosus. J Exp Med 155:1427—1438
86 Rosenfeld SI, Kelly ME, Leddy JP (1976) Hereditary deficiency of the fifth component of complement in man. I. Clinical, immunological, and family studies. J. Clin. Invest. 57:1626—1634
87 Tedesco F, Silvain CM, Agelli M, Giovanetti AM, Bombardier S (1981) A lupus-like syndrome in a patient with deficiency of the sixth component of complement. Arthritis Rheum 24:1438—1440
88 Zeitz HW, Miller GW, Lint TF, Ali MA, Gewurz H (1981) Deficiency of C7 with systemic lupus erythematosus: solubilization of immune complexes in complement-deficient sera. Arthritis Rheum 24:87—93
89 Jasin HE (1977) Absence of the eighth component of complement in association with systemic lupus erythematosus-like disease. J Clin Invest 60:709—715
90 Pickering RJ, Rynes RI, Lo Cascio N, Monahany JB, Sodetz JM (1982) Identification of the $\alpha - \gamma$ subunit of the eighth component of complement (C8) in a patient with systemic lupus erythematosus and absent C8 activity: patient and family studies. Clin. Immunol. Immunopathol. 23:323—334
91 Boyer JT, Gall EP, Norman ME, et al. (1975) Hereditary deficiency of the seventh component of complement. J. Clin. Invest. 56:905—913
92 Schifferli JA, NG YC, Peters DK (1986) The role of complement and its receptor in the elimination of immune complexes N Engl J Med 315:488—495
93 Woo P, Pereira RS, Lever AM (1984) Persistent immunoglobulin deficiency after prednisolone and antiepileptic therapy in a C2 deficient patient with a lupus-like syndrome. J Rheumatol. 11:828—831

The Role of Lymphokines in the Pathogenesis of Systemic Lupus Erythematosus

T. A. LUGER and J. S. SMOLEN

Lymphokines are lymphocyte-derived mediators which play an important role as regulators of inflammation and immunity. The term lymphokine [35] was introduced because the first mediators described were lymphocyte products that inhibited the motility of macrophages and therefore were true "kines" [11, 21]. More recently it was shown that factors similar to lymphokines are also produced by nonlymphocytic cells such as macrophages, fibroblasts, keratinocytes, and a variety of normal as well as transformed cells. Therefore the term cytokine was proposed for this class of substances [18]. Over recent years many different cytokines have been characterized which affect inflammatory cells such as lymphocytes, monocytes, natural killer cells, mast cells, and granulocytes but which can also act on noninflammatory cells, including fibroblasts, osteoblasts, osteoclasts, and epithelial as well as endothelial cells. Although cytokines at first were thought only to be responsible for the regulation of immunologic and inflammatory processes, they are now also known to participate in repair processes and to regulate normal cell growth and differentiation [19]. Moreover, the findings of even unicellular organisms producing hormonal peptide mediators and of the evolutionary conservation of similar cytokines in multicellular organisms suggest that they perform crucial biologic functions [146].

Soluble hormone-like mediators such as lymphokines or cytokines have a number of characteristics in common. They are actively synthesized and secreted in vitro by a number of different cells and are usually detectable in culture supernatants within 24 h following activation. Most, if not all, cytokines are proteins or glycoproteins with molecular weights varying from 1 kd to 70 kd. There is increasing evidence that many lymphokines have a subunit structure and may be assembled intracellularly in a precursor form, which is subsequently enzymatically converted to the extracellular biologically active form [87, 103]. A number of cytokines apparently affect their target cells by interacting with specific membrane receptors. In fact genes of some lymphokine receptors, e.g., interleukin 2 (IL 2) receptor, have been cloned and monoclonal antibodies directed against these proteins have been generated [94, 144, 145]. However, it has not yet been possible to demonstrate such receptors for all cytokines.

Cytokines can be divided according to their functions into inhibitory, stimulatory, or differentiation factors. The inhibitors in general, such as tumor necrosis factors (TNF) [54], are cytotoxic by lysing their target cells, or they inhibit cell proliferation, such as inhibitor of DNA synthesis or γ-interferon. Stimulatory lymphokines include growth factors (interleukin 2, B cell stimulatory factors) or differentiation factors (interleukin 3, colony stimulating factors).

146   T. A. Luger and J. S. Smolen

Cytokines or lymphokines are produced in minute amounts and are active at concentrations as low as 10^{-15} M. Therefore these regulatory proteins have been difficult to purify and isolate in larger quantities. Cytokines are still identified by various bioassays, which further complicates their characterization, since a single mediator may exhibit a multiplicity of effects but also distinct factors may be active in a given bioassay. Moreover, these mediators often act on cells in an additive, synergistic, or suppressive fashion, which again limits the capacity of bioassays to define these activities.

For many years it was difficult to prove that lymphokines produced and characterized in vitro actually played a role in vivo. Increasing evidence for an important in vivo regulatory function of cytokines is derived from several recent investigations. Various mediators have been isolated from tissues or body fluids during inflammatory diseases. For example, alterations in lymphokine production as well as serum lymphokine levels have been demonstrated in patients with septicemia, diabetes mellitus, systemic lupus erythematosus (SLE), rheumatoid arthritis, etc. [28, 82, 99, 108, 109. 111]. Intracutaneous injection of purified lymphokines will induce inflammatory skin reactions [52] and antibodies directed against lymphokines can also inhibit the appropriate in vivo biologic manifestation of lymphokines [26].

Systemic lupus erythematosus, the prototype of human autoimmune disease, is characterized by B-lymphocyte hyperactivity resulting in increased immunoglobulin and autoantibody formation. The early events responsible for this increased antibody formation are poorly understood (see pp. 6—20). Recent evidence suggests that the type of immunologic disturbance, which varies between individual patients, has a significant effect on the clinical expression of the disease [46, 159, 185]. Since lymphokines such as IL 1, IL 2, IL 3, and IFN are crucial immunomediators which may regulate lymphocyte proliferation and functions, we will discuss in this chapter studies on cytokine production in patients with SLE as well as their possible roles in the course of the pathogenesis of SLE.

Interleukin 1 (IL 1)

A monocyte product which stimulated the proliferation of murine thymocytes in conjunction with mitogens originally was defined as lymphocyte activating factor (LAF) [45]. Later it became clear that a multiplicity of amplifying effects on immunologic as well as inflammatory reactions could be ascribed to LAF, and this factor was renamed interleukin 1 (IL 1). Thus IL 1 enhances the release by T-lymphocytes of more of another lymphokine, namely interleukin 2 (IL 2), which induces the proliferation of activated T cells [163] but also stimulates T cells to an increased production of other cytokines such as γ-interferon or B-cell growth factor [32, 78, 198]. In addition IL 1 together with anti-μ-chain antibody also directly may costimulate B-lymphocytes to proliferate and to diferentiate to immunoglobulin-secreting cells [68, 101]. Thus the effect of IL 1 on the antibody response seems to be twofold: on the one hand, IL 1 directly causes B cell activation and proliferation; on the other, IL 1 affects B cells indirectly through its effects on T-helper and T-suppressor cells. IL 1 also has been shown to enhance the motility of mononuclear cells and polymorphonuclear granulocytes (PMN) in vitro as well as in vivo [52, 107, 117]. Moreover, IL 1 stimulates PMNs to release lysosomal enzymes and oxygen radicals [85, 86, 107] and elevated serum levels of IL 1 result in an increased release of PMNs from the bone marrow [73]. IL 1 has also been shown to stimulate the activity of osteoclasts and fibroblasts [49, 50, 151]. Aside from its mitogenic effect on fibroblasts or synovial cells, IL 1 also stimulates them to produce prostaglandins, collagen, and collagenase [115, 118, 135, 136]. According to a recent study, there is strong evidence that the biologic effects of IL 1 are mediated by plasma membrane receptors which have been shown to be expressed on a variety of different cell types and correlate with their capacity to respond to IL 1 [34].

Although not much is known of the in vivo effects of IL 1, there are some recent observations that this cytokine may have an important regulatory function during inflammation. Intravenous injection of IL 1 induces fever, owing to increased PGE_2 production in the hypothalamus [17, 27], and may also cause slow-wave sleep [89]. Moreover, increased serum levels of IL 1 are associated with increased levels of acute phase proteins such as serum amyloid A [172], C-reactive protein, fibrinogen, and haptoglobin [29, 76] and may also cause decreased levels of iron and zinc [74, 186], though at the same time copper levels are increased owing to an elevated hepatic synthesis of ceruloplasmin [75]. Another possible important in vivo role of IL 1 is the initiation of catabolic processes characterized by muscle wasting, protein degradation, and increased urea and amino acid excretion, as was observed when IL 1 was injected into animals [8, 160]. Strong evidence for a crucial in vivo role of IL 1 also comes from recent investigations demonstrating altered levels of IL 1 in different body fluids during various diseases. Thus, it was possible to detect significantly elevated IL 1 levels in serum, urine, synovial fluid, tears, and gingival fluid during inflammatory states [16, 82, 108, 124, 193].

A group of cytokines which were named according to their biologic effects are now also thought to be members of the IL 1 family. These include endogenous pyrogen, leukocytic endogenous mediator, mononuclear cell factor, catabolin, and proteolysis-inducing factor. Moreover, according to different recent investigations it is evident that IL 1 or IL 1-like moieties are not only synthesized by monocytes/macrophages but also by a variety of other cells such as keratinocytes (epidermal cell-derived thymocyte-activating factor) [105, 149], corneal epithelial cells [51], astrocytes [40], fibroblats [72], mesangial cells [104], natural killer cells [150], B cells [116], and granulocytes [195]. In fact it has not so far been possible to detect a cell which is not capable of producing IL 1. Since cDNA of murine IL 1 has recently been discovered [103] and cloning of two distinct human IL 1 complementary DNAs has also been reported [7, 14, 112], further studies will show whether all the different biologic effects of IL 1 are due to one and the same mediator or to a group of related molecules. Moreover, it is also quite conceivable that different active sites on the IL 1 molecule cause distinct biologic effects. This may be further elucidated by the use of a monoclonal antibody directed against the biologically active site of the IL 1 molecule, which causes thymocyte as well as fibroblast proliferation [87].

Because of this multiplicity of distinct effects of IL 1 on cells involved in immunity and inflammation and especially since IL 1 is considered essential for the regulation of T cell and B cell activity, it semed important to investigate IL 1 production in patients with SLE as well as the ability of T-lymphocytes to respond to IL 1. When adherent peripheral blood mononuclear cells (PBMCs) of patients with SLE were stimulated with phorbol myristic acetate (PMA) at different concentrations they consistently produced less IL 1 in comparison with PBMCs of healthy control persons [6, 99]. Similar results were obtained when PBMCs were stimulated with lipopolysaccharide (LPS). Whereas patients with active disease had significantly decreased production of IL 1, the capacity of monocytes of patients with inactive diseases to produce IL 1 upon stimulation with PMA or LPS was found to be normal in some cases [6]. Kinetic studies revealed that defective IL 1 production may not be explained by a lag in the onset of production [99].

Since IL 1 is an important amplifying signal for IL 2 dependent T cell proliferation, it might be assumed that deficient IL 1 production in patients with SLE could also be the cause of the low IL 2 activity described in this disease (see later). Thus, the effect of purified IL 1 on IL 2 production by T-lymphocytes in vitro was tested. When IL 1 was added to PBMCs of SLE patients only a slight increase in IL 2 was observed [99], whereas IL 1 greatly enhanced IL 2 production of lymphocytes from normal donors [106]. Moreover the response of T cells from SLE patients to IL 1 was decreased in comparison with lymphocytes of normal controls when tested for their capacity to form stable E rosettes or to increase their proliferation in an autologous mixed lymphocyte reaction [6].

IL 1 is produced by activated monocytes, B cells, and NK cells. However, it is not known whether there are subfractions of these cells responsible only for IL 1 production. Thus the decreased IL 1 production may be due to an intrinsic defect at the level of the interaction with the stimulant. On the other hand some adherent cells of SLE patients may inhibit producer cells. Since most IL 1 producer cells are Ia$^+$ and anti-Ia antibodies have been described in SLE [126], it is possible that circulating anti-Ia interfering with Ia$^+$ IL 1 producing cells is responsible for the IL 1 defect. From these data it may be concluded that monocytes from SLE patients have a defective capacity to produce or release the monokine IL 1 and also that T-lymphocytes respond poorly to this cytokine. Together with other observations showing defective phagocytic and enzymatic monocytic function in patients with SLE [80, 170], these findings of an additional monocyte dysfunction indicate that these cells may actively be involved in the immunoregulatory defect of SLE patients.

It should be noted in this context that there is also ample in vivo evidence for the postulated IL 1 defect in SLE: since IL 1 appears to be responsible for the production of acute phase proteins and leukocytosis, the failure to observe such changes (e.g. an increase in C-reactive protein or fibrinogen concentrations or leukocytosis in the course of lupus flares, see pp. 170—196) is compatible with a deficiency of IL 1.

Interleukin 2 (IL 2)

Interleukin 2 is a genetically unrestricted sialoglycoprotein which is synthesized and secreted by T-lymphocytes following stimulation with antigens or mitogens. Since this mediator is capable of sustaining long-term proliferation of activated T cells, it was originally designated T cell growth factor [47, 119]. In addition to activated T-lymphocytes, IL 2 has been shown to be produced by natural killer (NK) cells [79] as well as by a variety of different T cell lines or T—T hybridoma cell lines [58, 129, 156, 190]. The lymphocytotropic hormone IL 2 provides an essential signal for the transition of activated T cells from G1 to the S phase of the cell cycle [163], but also activates B-lymphocytes, leukemic B cell lines, and NK cells and enhances T cell production of other cytokines such as interferon and B cell growth factor [32, 78, 90, 198]. The mechanism of action of IL 2 involves binding to a high affinity cell surface receptor [15, 95, 189]. Although low affinity IL 2 binding sites have also been found on activated T- and B-lymphocytes and T cell lines, their physiologic role remains unclear [145]. The genes encoding for IL 2 [142] and its receptor [20], which are located on chromosome 10 [95], have been cloned, and in addition monoclonal antibodies against both IL 2 and IL 2 receptor are available [93, 157]. Therefore detailed biochemical studies on the control of DNA replication are now possible and may provide further insights into the mechanisms involved in diseases characterized by defective IL 2 production or responsiveness to IL 2.

Because of the crucial role IL 2 is believed to play in regulating T cell as well as B cell responses and in view of the immunoregulatory abnormalities in SLE, several investigations have been performed in IL 2 production and consumption of T cells of SLE patients. Some investigators report a marked defect in IL 2 production in response to allogeneic signals or mitogens such as concanavalin A (Con A) or phytohemagglutinin [5, 99, 100, 121]. The same is true for autologous mixed lymphocyte reactions [158]. Decreased IL 2 production was independent of the duration of the culture period or the dose of mitogen used and did not correlate with clinical stages of the disease [100, 121]. In a series of experiments we were able to demonstrate a deficiency in Con A-stimulated IL 2 production; however, the defect of IL 2 production was repaired by the addition of the tumor promoter PMA (unpublished observation). Similar results were obtained in murine SLE [147], indicating that lymphocytes from autoimmune mice as well as from patients with SLE are capable of producing normal levels of IL 2 and also of proliferating in response to Con A, provided the comitogen PMA is present. Since addition of exogenous IL 1 did not enhance IL 2 production in response to mitogens [99, 147], PMA does not correct the IL 2 defect by augmenting IL 1 production.

When the ability of PMA and Con A to induce normal IL 2 production and proliferation in autoimmune mice was investigated, it was demonstrated that PMA induced cells to enter the G_1 phase of the cell cycle. This allowed additional signals such as Con A to drive cells to later stages of G_1 in which IL 2 production occurred, with subsequent entry into the S phase and initiation of proliferation [147]. Depending on the length of time that cells are exposed to

150 T. A. Luger and J. S. Smolen

PMA, priming for proliferation or commitment to nonproliferation occurs. Priming by PMA allows autoimmune cells to progress through the cell cycle if subsequently stimulated by a second signal such as Con A [37]. In immunologically normal cells such PMA priming is not necessary and may be provided by IL 1 or an early Con A signal. Thus PMA renders T cells more receptive to Con A extending the G_1 phase of the cell cycle and reduces IL 2 adsorption by retarding the S phase [147, 148]. In addition PMA has recently been shown to induce both T and B cells to express functional IL 2 receptors [169]. Since lymphocytes, mainly CD4 cells, of SLE patients are deficient in IL 2 receptor expression [121], PMA may induce receptor expression in these cells and thereby correct a functional T cell defect. Thus the correction of the defect by PMA could be explained by the facts that only IL 2 receptor positive T cells proliferate in the presence of IL 2 and that T cells mainly produce IL 2 during the G_1 phase of the cell cycle.

There are several possible explanations for decreased IL 2 production in SLE patients. Since IL 2 production is macrophage dependent [36], a macrophage defect could be responsible for decreased IL 2 production in SLE patients. The defective macrophage IL 1 production observed in these patients does not appear to explain fully the failure of IL 2 synthesis, since addition of exogenous IL 1 was not able to restore the defect completely [101, 147]. Additionally, there is evidence that SLE patients have circulating monocytes producing high levels of prostaglandins [113] which in turn have been shown to inhibit IL 2 production [142], and SLE monocytes were only partially capable of inhibiting IL 2 production by normal 'T cells, suggesting that IL 2 deficiency in SLE patients may not solely be explained by a monocyte defect [121].

The issue of suppressor cells or suppressor factors causing decreased IL 2 production (Table 1) in SLE patients is controversial. Whereas some investigators were not able to detect suppressor cells or soluble inhibitors of IL 2 activity [121], other studies provide strong evidence that mononuclear suppressor cells are responsible for the decreased IL 2 production in SLE [105]. Thus removal of CD8 suppressor cells or natural killer cells (HNK -1^+) increased IL 2 production to normal levels in SLE patients [100]. In addition CD8 cells from SLE patients but not from normal donors decreased IL 2 production when added back to autologous CD8 depleted cells. The inhibiton of IL 2 production ap-

Table 1. Summary of studies on in vitro IL 1 and IL 2 in SLE patients

	Reference number	IL 1	IL 2	IL 2 receptor
1	100	Decreased	Decreased	—
2	5	—	Decreased	—
3	6	Decreased	—	—
4	101	—	Normal/decreased	Decreased
5	121	—	Decreased	Decreased
6	—[a]	Normal	Normal	—

[a] Luger et al. Unpublished observation

pears to be due to active suppression rather than to passive absorption of IL 2 since only a minor percentage of SLE lymphocytes expressed IL 2 receptors and they were unable to absorb exogenous IL 2. Moreover, culture supernatants derived from CD8 cells from SLE patients inhibited IL 2 production by normal T cells without inhibiting IL 2 activity [100], suggesting that the CD8 subset releases a soluble suppressor factor mediating this effect. In addition, IL 2 producer cells of SLE patients appear to be more sensitive to inhibitory signals, since CD8 cells from normal donors could significantly suppress IL 2 production in SLE but had no effect on autologous lymphocytes [90]. Whether or not this suppression involves interference with the cell cycle is not clear at present. However, SLE T cells have an increased RNA content without a proportional increase in DNA [4] and it is therefore conceivable that the corrective effects of PMA are due to its potential to lead to progression of the cell cycle to allow for DNA synthesis; the latter may be achieved by induction of appropriate IL 2 secretion. The observations in both autoimmune lupus mice and humans with SLE of a normal potential of T cells to proliferate and to secrete IL 2 in the pesence of PMA suggest however, that the IL 2 deficiency [174, 192] is not a genetic trait and thus not the main cause of SLE, as was initially believed, but rather a secondary manifestation.

Evidence for a regulatory function of large granular lymphocytes (LGLs, NK cells) in IL 2 production is provided by the finding that removal of LGLs enhances IL 2 production in normals as well as in SLE patients. Since about 30% of CD8 cells are also HNK^+, it is possible that this is one of the subsets responsible for the suppression of IL 2 production.

In addition to the suppressor T cell-derived inhibitor of IL 2 production [88], a serum inhibitor of IL 2 activity has been reported [31]. This 60—70 kd inhibitor is usually present in the sera of normal donors, whereas patients with SLE only have low or undetectable levels which do not correlate with disease activity. The decreased levels of this inhibitor, which may control IL 2 activity in normals, may represent a basic defect affecting the production of both IL 2 and its inhibitor or simply a reduced requirement of this protein due to decreased IL 2 production.

In order to explain the poor response to IL 2 of T cells from some SLE patients they were tested for their ability to absorb IL 2 and to express receptors for IL 2. It was found that T cells from these patients were able neither to absorb IL 2 nor to express Tac (IL 2 receptor) antigen, indicating a relative lack of surface receptors for IL 2 [121]. Furthermore this defect was only observed in CD4 cells, whereas CD8 cells from these patients had normal numbers of IL 2 receptors and proliferated normally in response to IL 2. However, there is another group of patients with SLE whose T cells, CD4 and CD8 cells, proliferate normally in response to IL 2 and express normal levels of IL 2 receptors. The defect observed in some SLE patients does not simply reflect disease activity and may represent the heterogeneity of this disorder ([159] and pp. 290—297).

Interferon

The interferons (IFNs) represent a family of distinct proteins which ware produced by different cells and all have antiviral and cell growth regulatory activities. Cells of every species make their own IFNs and even within one species a group of distinct IFNs is produced with different biologic and physicochemical properties. Recently, rapid progress has been made in knowledge of the primary structure of several human IFNs, since the amino acid compositions as well as the amino acid sequences have been reported and complementary DNAs encoding for different IFN activities have been isolated [133].

Thus three major classes of human IFN have been characterized [165]. Two species of type I IFN, IFNα and IFNβ, are mainly synthesized by leukocytes or fibroblasts after viral infection or treatment with synthetic polynucleotides, respectively. However, many other cell types as well as transformed cell lines have been shown to produce type I IFNs. Type II or immune IFN (IFNγ) is produced by antigen- or mitogen-stimulated lymphocytes, lymphocytic cell lines, and NK cells [79, 128], and its production may be regulated by other lymphokines such as IL 1 and IL 2 [78]. In comparison with IFNα and IFNβ, human IFNγ has a higher molecular weight and is sensitive to acidic pH (pH$_2$) and heat (56°C). In addition antigenic differences between the various IFNs have been detected using monoclonal antibodies [3]. Human IFNα represents a whole group of proteins that show about 70% homology at the level of their DNA. The IFNα gene family comprises at least 20 distinct members [48, 83] whereas IFNβ [22, 125] and IFNγ [53] are encoded by single genes. The genes for IFNα and IFNβ share 30%—95% sequence homology, are devoid of introns [48, 175], and are located at the short arm of chromosome 9 [127]. In contrast there is no homology between IFNγ and the other IFNs, and the gene of IFNγ is localized on chromosome 12 [122].

Interferons initially were discovered as antiviral agents; however, during recent years it became evident that they have a multiplicity of effects on different cells; these are termed "non-antiviral" or "cellular" effects. Among the numerous cellular effects of IFNs, the antiproliferative effect [55] and cell surface alteration [41] are particularly important. Most interesting are the effects of IFNs on both humoral and cellular aspects of the immune response [162]. Some of these activities are mediated by all three IFN types, but IFNγ is effective at much lower doses than IFNα and IFNβ [161]. For instance, IFN treatment acts differently on antibody forming B cells. Thus IFN added at the time of sensitization inhibits B cell activation and maturation into antibody secreting plasma cells. In contrast, low concentrations of IFN added after antigen sensitization may not act on B cells directly, but may enhance T-helper cell activity or inhibit suppressor T cells, both of these effects resulting in increased antibody formation [12, 161, 166]. Recent studies show that IFN, if added before antigen, results in enhanced antibody production, whereas IFN added after antigen depresses antibody synthesis [97, 131].

The effects of IFN on cell-mediated immunity are again multiphasic. If IFN is given before the antigen, inhibition of delayed hypersensitivity reactions, probably due to inhibition of blast formation, is observed. The augmentation of delayed hypersensitivity which is seen when the antigen is given later may be attributed to the inhibition of suppressor T cells [24, 98]. IFN may also be involved in the pathogenesis of allergic diseases since it may augment the motility of basophils [96], and the interaction of antigens or allergens with IgE on the surface of basophils in the presence of IFN may result in increased release of pharmacologic mediators of anaphylaxis [65, 70].

Another possibly important immunoregulatory function of IFNγ is the induction of the high affinity Fc receptor on myelomonocytic cells [132]. All three types of IFN enhance the expression of class I MHC antigens, although IFNγ is again more efficient [14, 187]. Moreover it has been amply documented that IFNγ enhances the expression of class II (Ia) antigens or induces their de novo synthesis in a wide variety of ontogenetically diverse cell types [67, 81, 134, 164, 172, 188]. This may have important immunologic implications, since the spontaneous loss and IFN-dependent augmentation of HLA D antigens by macrophages correlates directly with the antigen-presenting function of these cells [10]. In addition to its capacity to induce class I and II antigens, IFNγ may also induce differentiation of myeloid cells [132], inhibit prostaglandin synthesis in mononuclear cells [33], and activate mature myelocytic cells such as neutrophilic granulocytes and monocytes/macrophages [183]. Recently it has also been demonstrated that macrophage-activating factor and IFNγ appear to be identical and enhance cytotoxicity of human monocytes against tumor cells [110, 152].

Several cell types with cytotoxic function have been described, including cytotoxic T cells, killer cells in antibody-dependent cell-mediated cytotoxicity, and natural killer (NK) cells, and IFN may enhance their cytotoxic activity [61, 98, 182]. IFN enhances NK activity by augmenting the cytotoxic capacity of mature NK cells and stimulates pre-NK cells to differentiate, acquire NK surface markers, and become active killer cells [61, 182].

Since the IFN system appears to be involved in many aspects of the immune response, it was thought to play a crucial role in the pathogenesis of autoimmune diseases such as SLE. Indeed, many patients with SLE have been reported to have high levels of circulating IFN [64, 66, 138, 167, 196]. Originally, increased levels of pH 2 labile IFN (which is regarded to be IFNγ) were found. However, recently pH 2 stable IFNα as well as an unusual acid-labile form of IFNα was detected in the sera of SLE patients (Table 2) [138, 167]. Similarly, increased IFN levels were also found in the sera of patients with other autoimmune diseases such as rheumatoid arthritis, scleroderma, Sjögren's syndrome, and autoimmune vasculitis [66, 137]. In contrast, no IFN could be detected in the sera of drug-induced lupus erythematosus [137].

When SLE patients were divided into those with active disease and those with inactive disease, sera of patients with active SLE mostly contained IFN whereas only a few patients with inactive disease had circulating IFN. In addition to the correlation with disease activity, the presence of IFN in SLE also correlated positively with serum anti-DNA antibodies and complement consumption [64, 65]. There are several possible explanations for high IFN levels in SLE. For instance, chronic viral infection could induce leukocytes to produce IFN or antigens, immune complexes, and antilymphocytic antibodies (which are frequently found in the sera of these patients) might cause IFN synthesis.

Several studies have been performed to investigate the capacity of peripheral blood leukocytes of SLE patients to produce IFN. Although peripheral blood leukocytes of SLE patients made conventional IFNα, β, or γ in response to the appropriate stimulus, none of the cultures specifically produced acid-labile IFNα spontaneously in response to different stimuli. Thus peripheral lymphocytes appear not to be the source of this acid-labile IFNα found in the circulation of SLE patients [139] and tissue-bound lymphocytes may be responsible for serum IFN. This is also supported by another observation demonstrating intrathecal synthesis of acid-labile IFNα in SLE patients during the occurrence of neurologic complications [92]. In addition, the in vitro production of acid-stable IFNα and IFNγ in response to various stimuli was deficient in most SLE patients [123, 139, 167, 168, 184]. However, an increase in IFN-induced 2'—5'-adenylate synthetase in these cells was observed [139]. There appears to be an inverse correlation between serum IFN and in vitro produced IFN. Moreover, serum IFN was found more frequently in patients with active SLE who were also unable to produce IFN in vitro [64, 137, 138]. In contrast, patients with inactive disease only occasionally have circulating IFN associated with deficient in vitro IFN production [123, 139].

The discrepancy between in vivo and in vitro production of IFN (Table 2) resembles that of immunoglobulin secretions: increased in vivo production is paralleled by decreased in vitro synthesis after stimulation. Although this could obviously be explained by in vitro exhaustion of in vivo-hyperactive IFN-producing cells, it is more challenging to interpret the observations as helper defects for the stimuli employed for IFN induction and/or increased suppressive effects, as has been observed for PWM-induced B cell activation [9]. Furthermore, the discrepancy may also indicate that the mechanisms leading to IFN activation in vivo differ from those employed in vitro in the investigations quoted.

The increased IFN production may be important with regard to some pathogenetic events: application of IFN increases disease severity [2, 62], whereas inhibition of IFN (e.g., by antibodies) inhibits the development of nephritis in

Table 2. Summary of studies on IFN activity in SLE patients

	Reference number	IFN activity in vitro	Serum IFN	Type of serum IFN
1	64	—	Increased	γ
2	138	—	Increased	Acid-labile α
3	66	—	Increased	α, γ
4	139	Decreased	Increased	Acid-labile α
5	168	Decreased	—	—
6	167	Decreased α, γ	Increased	Acid-labile and -stabile α
7	123	Decreased γ	—	—
8	196	—	Increased	α, γ
9	184	Decreased γ	—	—

The Role of Lymphokines in the Pathogenesis 155

some murine strains with SLE [56]. The exact mechanisms responsible for these events are not known as has been discussed above.

Natural killer cells are considered to be important in the host immune surveillance against tumors and virus-infected cells [42, 60, 114]. IFN plays a crucial role in the augmentation of NK cell activity [61, 182]. Several studies have been performed to investigate NK cell activity as well as effects of IFN on NK cells in SLE patients. Patients with SLE apparently have significantly decreased NK activity in comparison with controls [63, 77, 154, 167, 184]. Although there was no correlation with other laboratory parameters, according to some investigators a correlation exists between clinical activity of the disease and decreased NK cell function [154, 184]. Moreover exacerbation of the disease may be associated with a further impairment of NK cell function. This decreased NK activity is the result of several factors, such as immune aggregates, antilymphocyte antibodies and anti-NK autoantibodies [155, 184]. In contrast, the number of cells responsible for NK activity may be not decreased in SLE patients, nor the effector target cell binding impaired [154]. Another possible explanation for impaired NK cell function in some SLE patients is the lack of NK enhancement by IFN or IFN inducers [39, 154, 167, 184]. Interestingly, cells of SLE patients which failed to respond to IFN had a significantly lower baseline NK activity than those responding to IFN [184].

In addition, PBMCs of the group of SLE patients unresponsive to exogenous IFN failed to produce significant levels of IFNγ after stimulation with mitogens [184]. Since NK cells appear capable of producing IFN [30], there might exist a self-regulatory circuit which may be disrupted in SLE, possibly by anti-NK cell antibodies. Moreover the defective response of SLE NK cells seems to be a primary abnormality and not due to previous priming with endogenous IFN. Recently a soluble cytotoxic factor released by NK cells that mediates lysis of NK cell sensitive tumor targets (NKCF) has been described [194]. Since a decrease in NKCF release has been noted in SLE patients, the impaired NK cell function in SLE may be based on a cellular defect resulting in diminished synthesis and release of this factor [154]. Beside their cytotoxic properties NK cells have also been shown to suppress granulocytes [57] and antibody production [181]. Thus NK cell dysfunction may result in increased antibody formation and autoantibody production.

These data regarding impaired IFN production as well as impaired response to IFN in SLE indicate the importance of IFN in the regulation of lymphocyte function in SLE. Since it is well documented that IFN increases the severity of disease in autoimmune mice [2, 62, 153], some of the patghologic changes in SLE could also be related to the presence of IFN in serum and other body fluids, which is probably produced by organ-bound lymphocytes activated by foreign antigens or modified cell membranes of damaged tissue.

Other Mediators

The main feature of SLE is B cell hyperactivity with hypergammaglobulinemia, and antibodies against a variety of autoantigens [38, 143, 178, 179]. It has recently been shown that a resting B cell requires multiple signals to undergo activation, proliferation, and differentiation. B cells may be activated by T independend antigens binding to the B cell antigen receptor. However, most antigens are T dependent, requiring a second signal consisting of an antigen-specific, Ia-restricted T cell—B cell interaction [198]. Once activated, B cells are capable of responding to different lymphokines which may mediate proliferation (interleukin 1, interleukin 2, and B cell growth factors) and differentiation (T cell replacing factor, TRF, and multiple B cell differentiation factors, BCDFμ, BCDFγ, BCDFα, and BCDFϵ [69, 84, 91, 119, 171, 197].

The role of B cell growth and differentiation factors in lupus erythematosus has mainly been investigated in murine models of SLE. Accordingly, a T-lymphocyte subset of autoimmune mice (C$_3$H/HeJ *lpr/lpr*) spontaneously (i.e., in the absence of mitogenic stimulation) produces a BCDF-like factor which enhances IgM and IgG production in LPS-activated B cells [180]. In contrast, no other B cell activity or differentiation-influencing factors such as BCGF, TRF, or IFN are detectable in culture supernatant of spleen cells from autoimmune mice without mitogenic stimulation. Thus the increased production of this antigen-nonspecific BCDF secreted by T cells of the helper-inducer phenotype could be responsible for B cell hyperactivity in SLE [140, 141, 180].

According to other investigations, a polyclonal B cell activator (PBA), which appears to be associated with α_2 macroglobulins may serve as an accelerator of autoimmunity. PBA activates B cells, followed by hypergammaglobulinemia and autoantibody production [177]. Patients with autoimmune disease such as rheumatoid arthritis or SLE were found to have PBA in their serum. In contrast, normal individuals do not have circulating PBA. Furthermore PBA from patient serum induces in vitro B cell activation, which may be blocked by another serum-derived low-molecular-weight protease inhibitor (LOMPIN) [177].

Another T cell-derived lymphokine, which regulates differentiation of hematopoietic stem cells and recently has been shown to play a role in early T and B cell differentiation, is interleukin 3 (IL 3). IL 3 has recently been cloned and appears to be identical to one of the colony-stimulating factors [43, 44, 71, 191]. Results regarding IL 3 activity in spleen cell cultures of autoimmune mice are controversial. Some authors report an increased spontaneous as well as mitogen-induced IL 3 production, which may account for B cell hyperactivity in MRL/1 mice [130]. According to other investigations no spontaneous IL 3 production is detected in MRL/1 mice and mitogen-induced IL 3 release is significantly decreased in comparison with normal mice [59]. However, these differences may also be explained by the use of different IL 3 dependent cell lines as an indicator system.

Conclusion

In this report we have tried to review the present status of the role of different cytokines (Fig. 1) in view of immune dysfunction in patients with SLE. PBMCs of most SLE patients with active disease fail to produce normal levels of lymphokines such as IL 1, IL 2, and IFN in response to mitogens or autoantigens, and expression if IL 2 receptors in T cells appears to be impaired. Deficient IL 2 activity may lead to impaired expansion of suppressor (and helper) T cells and subsequently to unregulated autoantibody synthesis. In contrast, T cell production of BCDF, at least in murine models of LE, has been shown to be increased. Additionally, sera of patients with SLE contain significant levels of pH-stable IFNα, migration inhibitory factor, lymphotoxin, and PBA. Such multiple abnormalities of cytokine production in SLE reflect multiple defects of cellular as well as humoral immune functions. Since the precise role of all cytokines is not yet

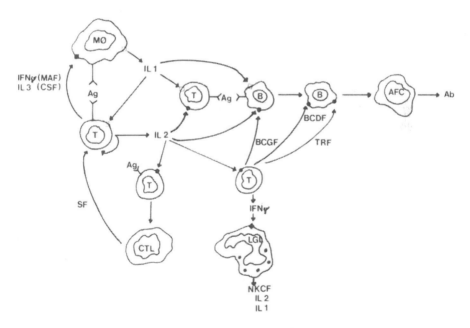

Fig. 1. The role of lymphokines in the regulation of antigen-specific T cell *(T)* and B cell *(B)* responses. In response to antigenic *(Ag)* stimulation, Ia[+] macrophages *(MØ)* interact with T-lymphocytes and produce interleukin 1 *(IL 1)*. Subsequently T cells produce a variety of distinct cytokines such as interleukin 2 *(IL 2)*, interleukin 3 *(IL 3)*, or colony-stimulating factor *(CSF)*, and B cell growth and differentiation factors *(BCGF, BCDF, and TRF)*. This results in (a) T cell activation, (b) IL 2 receptor expression (●), (c) differentiation into cytotoxic T-lymphocytes *(CTL)* which may release suppressor factors, (d) activation of large granular lymphocytes *(LGL)* which secrete IL 1, IL 2, and a natural killer cell cytotoxic factor *(NKCF)*, and (e) activation, proliferation, and differentiation of B cells into antibody *(Ab)* forming cells *(AFC)*

158 T. A. Luger and J. S. Smolen

fully elucidated and since the lymphokine cascade may be even more complex, involving as yet unknown mediators, it is not surprising that there is no strong correlation between defective lymphokine secretion and disease activity. However, some of the cellular defects in SLE patients might be explained by the defective lymphokine production.

Thus the cardinal pathologic findings in SLE — excessive antibody formation and autoantibody production by B cells as well as regulatory cell abnormalities (see pp. 6—20) may at least in part be mediated by dysregulated lymphokine synthesis and release. Although this hypothesis may be rather speculative in some respects, it points toward the important role that regulatory factors such as lymphokines and cytokines play in immune surveillance.

References

1. Abdou NI, Sagawa A, Pascual E, Herbert J, Sadeghee S (1976) Suppressor T cell abnormality in idiopathic systemic lupus erythematosus. Clin Immunol Immunopathol 6:192—199
2. Adam C, Thoua Y, Ronco P, Verroust P, Tovey M, Morel-Maroger L (1980) The effect of exogenous interferon: acceleration of autoimmune and renal diseases in NZB/W F1 mice. Clin Exp Immunol 40:373—382
3. Adolf GR, Bodo G, Swetly P (1982) Production of monoclonal antibodies to human IFN-α and their use for analysis of the antigenic composition of various natural interferons. J Cell Physiol 2 [Suppl]:61—68
4. Alarcon-Segovia D, Llorente L, Fishbein E, Diaz-Jouanen E (1982) Abnormalities in the content of nucleic acids of peripheral blood mononuclear cells from patients with systemic lupus erythematosus: relationship to DNA-antibodies. Arth Rheum 25:304—317
5. Alcocer-Varela J, Alarcon-Segovia D (1982) Decreased production of and response to interleukin-2 by cultured lymphocytes from patients with systemic lupus erythematosus. J Clin Invest 69:1388
6. Alcocer-Varela J, Laffon A, Alarcon-Segovia D (1983) Defective monocyte production of, and T lymphocyte response to, interleukin-1 in the peripheral blood of patients with systemic lupus erythematosus. Clin Exp Immunol 54:125—132
7. Auron PE, Webb AC, Rosenwasser LJ, Mucci SF, Rich A, Wolff SM, Dinarello CA (1984) Nucleotide sequence of human monocyte interleukin 1 precursor cDNA. Proc Natl Acad Sci USA 81:7907
8. Baracos V, Rodemann HP, Dinarello CA, Goldberg AL (1983) Stimulation of muscle protein degradation and prostaglandin E2 release by leukocytic pyrogen (interleukin 1). A mechanism for the increased degradation of muscle proteins during fever. N Engl J Med 308:553—558
9. Beale MG, Nash GS, Bertovich MJ, McDermott R (1982) Similar disturbances in B cell activity and regulatory T cell function in Henoch-Schönlein purpura and systemic lupus erythematosus. J Immunol 128:486—491
10. Beller DI, Ho K (1982) Regulation of macrophage populations. V. Evaluation of the control of macrophage Ia expression in vitro. J Immunol 129:971—976
11. Bloom BR, Bennett B (1966) Mechanism of a reaction in vitro associated with delayed-type hypersensitivity. Science 153:180—182
12. Booth RJ, Booth JM, Marbrook J (1976) Immune conservation: a possible consequence of the mechanism of interferon-induced antibody suppression. Eur J Immunol 6:769—772
13. Burrone OR, Milstein C (1982) Control of HLA-A, B, C synthesis and expression in interferon-treated cells. Eur Mol Biol Organ 1:345—349

The Role of Lymphokines in the Pathogenesis 159

14. Cameron P, Limjuco G, Rodkey J, Bennett C, Schmidt JA (1985) Amino acid sequence analysis of human interleukin 1 (IL-1). J Exp Med 162:790—801
15. Cantrell DA, Smith KA (1984) The interleukin-2 T-cell system: a new cell growth model. Science 224:1312—1316
16. Charon JA, Luger TA, Oppenheim JJ, Mergenhagen SE (1982) Increased thymocyte activating factor in human gingival fluid during gingival inflammation. Infect Immun 38:1190—1195
17. Coceani F, Bishai I, Dinarello CA, Fitzpatrick FA (1983) Prostaglandin E2 and thromboxane B2 in cerebrospinal fluid of afebrile and febrile cat. Am J Physiol 244:R785—R793
18. Cohen S (1977) The role of cell-mediated immunity in the induction of inflammatory responses. Am J Pathol 88:501—528
19. Cohen S, Yoshida T (1983) Physiological and pathological roles of lymphokines. In: Yamamura Y, Hayashi H, Honjo T, Kishimoto T, Muramatsu M, Osawa T (eds) Humoral factors in host defense. Academic, Washington, pp 245—256
20. Cosman D, Cerretti DP, Larsen A, Park L, March C, Dower S, Gillis S, Urdal D (1984) Cloning, sequence and expression of human interleukin-2 receptor. Nature 312:768—771
21. David JR (1966) Delayed hypersensitivity in vitro: its mediation by cell-free substances formed by lymphoid-cell-antigen interactions. Proc Natl Acad Sci USA 56:73—77
22. Degrave W, Derynck R, Tavernier J, Haegeman G, Fiers W (1981) Nucleotide sequence of the chromosomal gene for human fibroblast (β1) interferon and of the flanking regions. Gene 14:137
23. Delfraissy JF, Segond P, Galanaud P, Wallon C, Massias P, Dormont J (1980) Depressed primary in vitro antibody response in untreated systemic lupus erythematosus (T helper cell defect and lack of defective suppressor cell function). J Clin Invest 66:141—148
24. De Maeyer E, De Maeyer-Guignard J (1980) Effects of interferon on sensitization and expression of delayed hypersensitivity in the mouse. In: De Weck AL (ed) Biochemical characterization of lymphokines, Academic, New York, pp 383—391
25. DeStefano E, Friedman RM, Friedman-Kien AE, Goedert JJ, Henricksen D, Preble OT, Sonnabend JA, Vilcek J (1982) Acid-labile leukocyte interferon in homosexual men with Kaposi's sarcoma and lymphadenopathy. J Infect Dis 146:451
26. Dinarello CA, Renfer L, Wolff SM (1977) Human leukocytic pyrogen: purification and development of a radioimmunoassay. Proc Natl Acad Sci USA 74:4624
27. Dinarello CA, Wolff SM (1982) Molecular basis of fever in humans. Am J Med 72:799—819
28. Dinarello CA, Clowes Jr GHA, Gordon HH, Sarvis CA, Wolff SM (1984) Cleavage of human interleukin 1: isolation of a peptide fragment from plasma of febrile humans and activated monocytes. J Immunol 133:1332—1338
29. Dinarello CA (1984) Interleukin-1. Rev Infect Dis 6:51—83
30. Djeu JY, Timonen T, Herberman RB (1981) Augmentation of natural killer cell activity and induction of interferon by tumor cells and other biological response modifiers. In: Chirigos MA, Michell M, Mastrangelo MJ, Kvein M (eds) Mediation of cellular immunity in cancer by immune modifiers. Raven, New York, pp 161
31. Djeu JY, Kashahara T, Balow JE, Tsokos GC (1983) An interleukin (IL-2) inhibitor is present in normal sera and is decreased in patients with connective tissue disorders. Clin Res 31:343A
32. Domzig W, Stadler BM, Herberman RB (1983) Interleukin 2 dependence of human natural killer (NK) cell activity. J Immunol 130:1970—1973
33. Dore-Duffy P, Perry W, Kuo HH (1983) Interferon-mediated inhibition of prostaglandin synthesis in human mononuclear leukocytes. Cell Immunol 79:232—239
34. Dower SK, Kronheim SR, March CJ, Conlon PJ, Hopp TP, Gillis S, Urdal DL (1985) Detection and characterization of high affinity plasma membrane receptors for human interleukin 1. J Exp Med 162:501—515
35. Dumonde DC, Wolstencroft RA, Panayi GS, Mathew M, Morley J, Howson WT (1969) Lymphokines: nonantibody mediators of cellular immunity generated by lymphocyte activation. Nature 224:38—42
36. Farrar JJ, Mizel SB, Fuller-Farrar J, Farrar WL, Hilfiker ML (1980) Macrophage-independent activation of helper T cells. I. Production of interleukin 2. J Immunol 125:793

37. Farrar JJ, Benjamin WR, Hilfiker ML, Howard M, Farrar WL, Fuller-Farrar J (1982) The biochemistry, biology, and role of sinterleukin 2 in the induction of cytotoxic T cell and antibody-forming B cell responses. Immunol Rev 63:129—166
38. Fauci AS (1980) Immunoregulation and auto-immunity. J Allergy Clin Immunol 66:5
39. Fitzharris P, Lacocer J, Stephens HAF, Knight RA, Snaith ML (1982) Insensitivity to interferon of NK cells from patients with systemic lupus erythematosus. Clin exp Immunol 47:110—115
40. Fontana A, Kristensen F, Dubs R Gemsa D, Weber E (1982) Production of prostaglandin E and interleukin 1 like factor by cultured astrocytes and C_6 glioma cells. J Immunol 129:2413—2419
41. Friedman RM (1977) Antiviral activity of interferons. Bacteriol Rev 41:543—567
42. Fijimiya Y, Babiuk LA, Rouse BT (1978) Direct lymphocytotoxicity against herpes simplex virus-infected cells. Can J Microbiol 24:1076—1081
43. Fung MC, Hapel AJ, Ymer S, Cohen DR, Johnson RM, Campbell HD, Young IG (1984) Molecular cloning of cDNA for murine interleukin 3. Nature 307:233
44. Garland JM (1984) Involvement of interleukin 3 in lymphocyte biology and leukemogenesis. In Pick E (ed) Lymphokines, Vol 9. Academic, New York, pp 154—196
45. Gery I, Gershon RK, Waksman BH (1972) Potentiation of the T-lymphocyte response to mitogens. I. The responding Cell. J Exp Med 136:128—142
46. Gilliam JN (1981) Immunopathology and pathogenesis of cutaneous lupus erythematosus. In: Safai B, Good RA (eds) Comprehensive immunology. Immunodermatology, vol 7. Plenum Med, New York, pp 323—343
47. Gillis S, Smith KA (1977) Long-term culture of cytotoxic T-lymphocytes. Nature 268:154
48. Goeddel DV, Leung DW, Dull TJ, Gross M, Lawn RM, McCandliss R, Seeburg PH, Ullrich A, Yelverton E, Gray PW (1981) The structure of eight distinct cloned human leukocyte interferon cDNAs. Nature 290:20
49. Gowen M, Wood DD, Ihrie EJ, McGuire MKB, Russell GG (1983) An interleukin 1 like factor stimulates bone resorption in vitro. Nature 306:378—380
50. Gowen M, Wood DD, Russell RGG (1985) Stimulation of the proliferation of human bone cells in vitro by human monocyte products with interleukin-1 Activity. J Clin Invest 75:1223—1229
51. Grabner G, Luger TA, Smolin G, Oppenheim JJ (1982) Corneal epithelial cell thymocyte activating factor (CETAF). Invest Ophthalmol Vis Sci 23:757
52. Granstein RD, Margolis RJ, Mizel SB, Sauder DN (1985) In vivo chemotactic activity of epidermal cell-derived thymocyte activating factor (ETAF) and interleukin-1 (IL-1) in the mouse. J Leukocyte Biol 37:709
53. Gray PW, Goeddel DV (1982) Structure of the human immune interferon (IFN-γ) gene. Nature 298:859
54. Gray PW, Aggarwal BB, Benton CV, Bringman TS, Henzel WJ, Jarrett JA, Leung DW, Moffat B, Ng P, Svedersky LP, Palladino MA, Nedwin GE (1984) Cloning and expression of cDNA for human lymphotoxin, a lymphokine with tumour necrosis activity. Nature 312:721—724
55. Gresser I, Tovey MG, Maury C, Bandu MT (1976) Role of interferon in the pathogenesis of virus diseases in mice as demonstrated by the use of anti-interferon serum. II. Studies with herpes simplex, Maloney sarcoma, vesicular stomatitis, Newcastle disease, and influenza viruses. J Exp Med 144:1316—1323
56. Gresser I, Morel-Maroger L, Verroust P (1978) Anti-interferon inhibits the development of glomerulonephritis in mice infected at birth with lymphocytic choriomeningitis virus. Proc Natl Acad Sci USA 75:3413—3416
57. Hansson M, Kiessling R (1982) Natural killing of hematopoietic cells. In: Herberman RB (ed) NK cells and other natural effector cells. Academic, New York, pp 1077—1084
58. Harwell L, Skidmore B, Marrack P, Kappler J (1980) Concanavalin A-inducible interleukin 2 producing T cell hybridoma. J Exp Med 152:893
59. Hefeneider SH, Conlon PJ, Dower SK, Henney CS, Gillis S (1984) Limiting dilution analysis of interleukin 2 and colony stimulating factor producer cells in normal and autoimmune mice. J Immunol 132:1863

The Role of Lymphokines in the Pathogenesis **161**

60. Heberman RB, Holden HT (1979) Natural killer cells as antitumor effector cells. J Natl Cancer Inst 62:441—444
61. Herberman RR, Ortaldo JR, Bonnard GD (1979) Augmentation by interferon of human natural and antibody-dependent cell-mediated cytotoxicity. Nature 277:222—223
62. Heremans H, Biliau A, Colombatti A, Hilgers J, DeSomer P (1978) Interferon treatment of NZB mice: accelerated progression of autoimmune disease. Infect Immun 21:925
63. Hoffman T (1980) Natural killer function in systemic lupus erythematosus. Arthritis Rheum 23:30—35
64. Hooks JJ, Moutsopoulos HM, Geis SA, Stahl NI, Decker JL, Notkins AL (1979) Immune interferon in the circulation of patients with autoimmune diseases. N Engl J Med 301:5
65. Hooks JJ, Moutsopoulos HM, Notkins AL (1980) The role of interferon in immediate hypersensitivity and autoimmune disease. Ann NY Acad Sci 350:21—32
66. Hooks JJ, Jordan GW, Gupps T, Moutsopoulos HM, Fauci AS, Notkins AL (1982) Multiple interferons in systemic lupus erythematosus and vasculitis. Arth Rheum 25:396—400
67. Houghton AN, Thomson TM, Gross D, Oettgen HF, Old LJ (1984) Surface antigens of melanoma and melanocytes. Specificity of induction of Ia antigen by human γ-interferon. J Exp Med 160:255—269
68. Howard M, Mizel SB, Lachman L, Ansel J, Kohnson B, Paul WE (1983) Role of interleukin 1 in anti-immunglobulin-induced B cell proliferation. J Exp Med 157:1529—1543
69. Howard M, Nakanishi K, Paul WE (1984) B cell growth and differentiation factors. Immunol Rev 78:185—210
70. Ida S, Hooks JJ, Siraganian RP, Notkins AL (1980) Enhancement of IgE-mediated histamine release from human basophils by immune-specific lymphokines. Clin Exp Immunol 41:380—387
71. Ihle JN, Rebar L, Keller J, Lee JC, Hapel AJ (1982) Interleukin 3: possible roles in the regulation of lymphocyte differentiation and growth. Immunol Rev 63:5
72. Iribe H, Hoga T, Kotani S, Kusumoto S, Shiba T (1982) Stimulating effect of MDP and its adjuvant active analogous on guinea pig fibroblasts for the production of thymocyte activating factor. J Exp Med 157:2190—2195
73. Kampschmidt RF, Long RD, Upchurch HF (1972) Neutrophil releasing activity in rats injected with endogenous pyrogen. Proc Soc Exp Biol Med 139:1224—1226
74. Kampschmidt RF, Pulliam LA (1978) Effect of human monocyte pyrogen on plasma iron, plasma zinc, and blood neutrophils in rabbits and rats. Proc Soc Exp Biol Med 158:32—35
75. Kampschmidt RF (1981) Leukocytic endogenous mediator/endogenous pyrogen. In: Powanda MC, Canonico PG (eds) The physiologic and metabolic responses of the host. Elsevier, North-Holland, pp 55—74
76. Kampschmidt RF, Upchurch HF, Worthington ML (1983) Further comparisons of endogenous pyrogens and leukocytic endogenous mediators. Infect Immunity 41:6—10
77. Karsh J, Dorval G, Osterland CK (1981) Natural cytotoxicity in rheumatoid arthritis and systemic lupus erythematosus. Clin Immunol Immunopathol 19:437—446
78. Kasahara T, Hooks JJ, Dougherty SF, Oppenheim JJ (1983) Interleukin 2-mediated immune interferon (IFN-γ) production by human T cells and T cell subsets. J Immunol 130:1784—1789
79. Kasahara T, Djeu JY, Dougherty SF, Oppenheim JJ (1983) Capacity of human large granular lymphocytes (LGL) to produce multiple lymphokines: interleukin 2, interferon, and colony stimulating factor. J Immunol 131:2379—2385
80. Kavai M, Lukacs K, Sonkoly I, Paloczi K, Szegedi G (1979) Circulating immune complexes and monocyte Fc function in autoimmune diseases. Ann Rheum Dis 38—79
81. Kelley VE, Fiers W, Strom TB (1984) Cloned human interferon-γ, but not interferon-β or -α, induces expression of HLA-DR determinants by fetal monocytes and myeloid leukemic cell lines. J Immunol 132:240—245
82. Kimball ES, Pichard SF, Oppenheim JJ, Rosio JL (1984) Interleukin 1 activity in normal human urine. J Immunol 133:256—260
83. Kirchner H (1984) Interferon gamma research. In: Progress in clinical biochemistry and medicine. Springer, Berlin Heidelberg New York Tokyo, vol 1, pp 169—203

162 T. A. Luger and J. S. Smolen

84. Kishimoto T, Yoshizaki K, Okada M, Kuritani T, Kikutani H, Skaguchi N, Miki Y, Kishi H, Nakagawa T, Shimizu K, Fukunaga K, Taga T (1985) Growth and differentiation factors and activation of human B cells. In: Schreier MH, Smith KA (eds), Lymphokines, vol 10. Academic, New York, pp 15—30
85. Klempner MS, Dinarello CA, Gallin JI (1978) Human leukocytic pyrogen induces release of specific granule contents from human neutrophils. J Clin Incest 61:1330—1336
86. Klempner MS, Dinarello CA, Henderson WR, Gallin JI (1979) Stimulation of human neutrophil oxygen metabolism by leukocytic pyrogen. J Clin Invest 64:996—1002
87. Köck A, Danner M, Stadler BM, Luger TA (1986) Characterization of a monoclonal antibody directed against the biologically active site of human interleukin 1. J Exp Med 163:463—468
88. Kramer M, Koszinowski U (1982) T cell-specific suppressor factors(s) with regulatory influence of interleukin 2 production and function. J Immunol 128:784—790
89. Krueger J, Dinarello CA, Chedid L (1983) Promotion of slow-wave sleep by a purified interleukin-1 preparation. Fed Proc 42:356
90. Lantz O, Grillot-Courvalin C, Schmitt C, Fermand JP, Brouet JC (1985) Interleukin 2-induced proliferation of leukemic human B cells. J Exp Med 161:1225—1230
91. Leanderson T, Pettersson S, Ruuth E, Lundgren E, Coutinho A (1985) Lymphokine participation in B cell responses. In: Schreier MH, Smith KA (eds) Lymphokines, vol 10. Academic, New York, pp 165—173
92. Lebon P, Lenoir GR, Fischer A, Lagrue A (1983) Synthesis of intrathecal interferon in systemic lupus erythematosus with neurological complications. Br Med J 287:1165—1167
93. Leonard WJ, Depper JM, Cuhiyama T, Smith KA (1982) A monoclonal antibody, anti-Tac, blocks the membrane binding and action of human T-cell growth factor. Nature 300:267
94. Leonard WJ, Depper JM, Uchiyama T, Smith KA, Waldmann TA, Greene WC (1982) A monoclonal antibody that appears to recognize the receptor for human T-cell growth factor: partial characterization of the receptor. Nature 300:267
95. Leonard WJ, Depper JM, Robb RJ, Waldmann TA, Grenne WC (1983) Characterization of the human receptor for T-cell growth factor. Proc Natl Acad Sci USA 80:6957
96. Leonard WJ, Donlan T, Lebo RV, Greene WC (1985) The gene encoding the human interleukin-2 (IL-2) receptor is located on chromosome 10. Clin Res 33:381A
97. Lett-Brown MA, Aelvoet M, Hooks JJ, Georgiades JA, Tueson DO, Grant JA (1981) Enhancement of basophil chemotaxis in vitro by virus-induced interferon. J Clin Invest 67:547—552
98. Levinson P, Leary P, Gresser I (1972) Human leukocyte (alpha) interferon modulates lymphocyte proliferation and B-cell differentiation. Arth Rheum 24[Suppl]:93
99. Lindahl P, Leary P, Greser I (1972) Enhancement by interferon of the specific cytotoxicity of sensitized lymphocytes. Proc Soc Exp Biol Med 69:721—725
100. Linker-Israeli M, Bakke AC, Kitridou RC, Gendler S, Gillis S, Horwitz DA (1983) Defective production of interleukin 1 and interleukin 2 in patients with systemic lupus erythematosus (SLE). J Immunol 130:2651—2655
101. Linker-Israeli M, Bakke AC, Quismorio FP, Horwitz D (1985) Correction of interleukin-2 production in patients with systemic lupus erythematosus by removal of spontaneously activated suppressor cells. J Clin Invest 75:762—768
102. Lipsky PE, Thompson PA, Rosenwasser LJ, Dinarello CA (1983) The role of interleukin 1 in human B cell activation: inhibition of B cell proliferation and the generation of immunoglobulin-secreting cells by an antibody against human leukocytic pyrogen. J Immunol 130:2708—2714
103. Lomedico PT, Gubler U, Hellmann CP, Dukovich M, Giri JC, Pan YE, Collier K, Semionow R, Chua AO, Mizel SB (1984) Cloning and expression of murine interleukin-1 cDNA in *Escherichia coli*. Nature 312:458
104. Lovett DH, Ryan JL, Sterzl RB (1983) A thymocyte activating factor derived from glomerular mesangial cells. J Immunol 130:1796—1801
105. Luger TA, Stadler BM, Katz SI, Oppenheim JJ (1981) Epidermal cell (keratinocyte) derived thymocyte activating factor (ETAF). J Immunol 127:1493—1498

The Role of Lymphokines in the Pathogenesis 163

106. Luger TA, Smolen JS, Chused TM, Steinberg AD, Oppenheim JJ (1982) Human lymphocytes with either the OKT4 or OKT8 phenotype produce interleukin 2 in culture. J Clin Invest 70:470
107. Luger TA, Charon JA, Colot M, Micksche M, Oppenheim JJ (1983) Chemotactic properties of partially purified human epidermal cell-derived thymocyte-activating factor (ETAF) for polymorphonuclear and mononuclear cells. J Immunol 131:816—820
108. Luger A, Graf H, Schwarz HP, Stummvoll HK, Luger TA (1986) Decreased serum interleukin 1 activity and monocyte interleukin 1 production in patients with fatal sepsis. Crit Care Med 14:458—464
109. Luger A, Schernthaner G, Urbanska A, Luger TA (1985) Altered production of interleukin 1 and interleukin 2 in patients with insulin-dependent diabetes mellitus. Europ J Clin Invest 15, A 1
110. Männel DN, Falk W (1983) Interferon-γ is required in activation of macrophages for tumor cytotoxicity. Cell Immunol 79:396—402
111. Maluish AE, Ortaldo JR, Sherwin SA, Oldham RK, Herberman RB (1983) Changes in immune function in patients receiving natural leukocyte interferon. J Biol Resp Mod 2:418—427
112. March CL, Mosley B, Larsen A, Cerretti DP, Braedt G, Price V, Gillis S, Henny CS, Kronheim SR, Grabstein K, Conlon PJ, Hopp TP, Cosman D (1985) Cloning, sequence and expression of two distinct human interleukin-1 complementary DNAs. Nature 315:641—647
113. Markenson JA, Morgan JW, Lochshin MD, Joachim C, Winfield JB (1978) Responses of fractionated cells from patients with systemic lupus erythematosus and normals to plant mitogen: evidence for a suppressor population of monocytes. Proc Soc Exp Biol Med 158:5
114. Marx J (1980) Natural killer cells help defend the body. Science 7:624—626
115. Matsushima K, Bano M, Kidwell WR, Oppenheim JJ (1985) Interleukin 1 increases collagen type IV production by murine mammary epithelial cells. J Immunol 134:904—909
116. Matshushima K, Procopio A, Abe H, Scala G, Ortaldo JR, Oppenheim JJ (1985) Production of interleukin 1 activity by normal human peripheral blood B lymphocytes. J Immunol 135:1132—1136
117. Miossec P, Yu CL, Ziff M (1984) Lymphocyte chemotactic activity of human interleukin 1. J Immunol 133:2007—2011
118. Mizel SB, Dayer JM, Krane SM, Mergenhagen SE (1980) Stimulation of rheumatoid synovial cell collagenase and prostaglandin production by partially purified lymphocyte-activating factor (interleukin 1). Proc Natl Acad Sci USA 78:2474
119. Morgan DA, Ruscetti FW, Gallo RC (1976) Selective in vitro growth of T lymphocytes from normal human bone marrows. Science 193:1007
120. Muraguchi A, Kehrl JH, Fauci AS (1985) Activation, proliferation and differentiation of human B lymphocytes. In: Schreier MH, Smith KA (eds) Lymphokines, vol 10. Academic, New York, pp 33—53
121. Murakawa Y, Takada S, Ueda Y, Suzuki N, Hoshino T, Sakane T (1985) Characterization of T lymphocyte subpopulations responsible for deficient interleukin 2 activity in patients with systemic lupus erythematosus. J Immunol 134:187—195
122. Nayloer SL, Sakaguchi AY, Shows TB, Law ML, Goeddel DV, Gray PW (1983) Human immune interferon gene is located on chromosome 12. J Exp Med 57:1020—1027
123. Neighbour PA, Grayzel AI (1981) Interferon production in vitro by leucocytes from patients with systemic lupus erythematosus and rheumatoid arthritis. Clin Exp Immunol 45:576
124. Nouri AME, Panayi GS, Goodman SM (1984) Cytokines and the chronic inflammation of rheumatic disease. I. The presence of interleukin-1 in synovial fluids. J Exp Immunol 55:295—302
125. Ohno S, Taniguchi T (1981) Structure of a chromosomal gene for human interferon β. Proc Natl Acad Sci USA 78:5305
126. Okudaira K, Searles RP, Ceuppens JL, Goodwin JS, Williams RC (1982) Anti-Ia reactivity in sera from patients with systemic lupus erythematosus. J Clin Invest 69:17

127. Owerbach D, Rutter WJ, Shows TB, Gray P, Goeddel DV, Lawn RM (1981) Leukocyte and fibroblast interferon genes are located on human chromosome 9. Proc Natl Acad Sci USA 78:3123

128. Palladino MA, VonWussow P, Pearlstein KT, Welte K, Scheid MP (1983) Characterization of interleukin 2-dependent cytotoxic T-cell clones. Cell Immunol 81:313—322

129. Palacios R (1982) Clones of interleukin 2 producer human T lymphocytes. J Immunol 129:2586

130. Palacios R (1984) Spontaneous production of interleukin 3 by T lymphocytes from autoimmune MRL/Mp-*lpr/lpr* mice. Eur J Immunol 14:599

131. Parker MA, Mandel AD, Wallace JH, Sonnefeld H (1981) Modulation of the human in vitro antibody response by human leukocyte interferon preparations. Cell Immunol 58:464—469

132. Perussia B, Dayton ET, Lazarus R, Fanning V, Trincheri G (1983) Immune interferon induces the receptor for monomeric IgG1 on human monocytic and myeloid cells. J Exp Med 158:1092—1113

133. Pestka S, Maeda S (1983) The human interferons: their purification and sequence cloning and expression in bacteria, and biological properties. In: Yamamura Y, Hayashi H, Honjo T, Kishimoto T, Muramatsu M, Osawa T (eds) Humoral factors in host defense. Academic, Tokyo, pp 191—244

134. Pober JS, Gimbrone MA, Cotran RS, Reiss CS, Burakoff SJ, Fiers W, Ault KA (1983) Ia expression by vascular endothelium is inducible by activated T cells and by human γ-interferon. J Exp Med 157:1339—1353

135. Postlethwaite AE, Kang AH (1982) Characterization of fibroblast proliferation factors elaborated by antigen- and mitogen-stimulated guinea pig lymph node cells: differentiation from lymphocyte-derived chemotactic factor for fibroblasts, lymphocyte mitogenic factor, and interleukin-1. Cell Immunol 73:169—178

136. Postlethwaite AE, Lachman LB, Mainardi CL, Kang AH (1983) Interleukin 1 stimulation of collagenase production by cultured fibroblasts. J Exp Med 157:801—806

137. Preble OT, Black RJ, Klippel JH, Friedman RM, Vilcek J (1982) Interferon in systemic lupus erythematosus. In: Merigan C, Friedman RM, Fox CF (eds) Interferons. Academic, New York, p 219 (UCLA Symp molec cell biol, vol 25)

138. Preble OT, Black RJ, Friedman RM, Klippel JH, Vilcek J (1982) Systemic lupus erythematosus: presence in human serum of an unusual acid-labile leukocyte interferon. Science 216:429

139. Preble OT, Rothko K, Klippel JH, Friedman RM, Johnston MI (1983) Interferon-induced 2'—5'adenylate synthetase in vivo and interferon production in vitro by lymphocytes from systemic lupus erythematosus patients with and without circulating interferon. J Exp Med 157:2140—2146

140. Prud'homme GJ, Park CL, Fieser TM, Kofler R, Dixon FJ, Theofilopoulos AN (1983) Identification of a B-cell differentiation factor(s) spontaneously produced by proliferating T cells in murine lupus strains of *lpr/lpr* genotype. J Exp Med 157:730

141. Prud'homme GJ, Fieser TM, Dixon FJ, Theofilopoulos AN (1984) B cell-tropic interleukins in murine systemic lupus erythematosus (SLE) 1. Immunol Rev 78:159—183

142. Rappaport RS, Dodge GR (1982) Prostaglandin E inhibits the production of human interleukin 2. J Exp Med 155:943

143. Raveche ES, Steinberg AD, DeFranco AL, Tijo JH (1982) Cell cycle analysis of lymphocyte activation in normal and autoimmune strains of mice. J Immunol 129:1219

144. Robb RJ, Kutny RM, Panico M, Morris HR, Chowdry V (1984) Amino acid sequence and post-translational modification of human interleukin 2. Proc Natl Acad Sci USA (in press)

145. Robb RJ, Greene WG, Rusk CM (1984) Low and high affinity cellular receptors for interleukin 2. Implications for the level of Tac antigen. J Exp Med 160:1126—1146

146. Roth J, LeRoith D, Shiloach J, Rosenzweig JL, Lesniak MA, Havrankova J (1982) The evolutionary origins of hormones, neurotransmitters, and other ectracellular chemical messengers. Implications for mammalian biology. N Engl J Med 306:523—527

The Role of Lymphokines in the Pathogenesis **165**

147. Santoro TJ, Luger TA, Ravache ES, Smolen JS, Oppenheim JJ, Steinberg AD (1983) In vitro correction of the interleukin 2 defect of autoimmune mice. Eur J Immunol 13:601—604

148. Santoro TJ, Malek TR, Rosenberg YJ, Oppenheim JJ, Steinberg AD (1984) The induction of interleukin 2 (IL 2) responsiveness in autoimmune MRL-*lpr/lpr* mice. Fed Proc Fed Am Soc Exp Biol 43:1736

149. Sauder DN, Carter C, Katz SI, Oppenheim JJ (1982) Epidermal cell production of thymocyte activating factor (ETAF). J Invest Derm 79:34

150. Scala G, Allavena P, Djeu JY, Kasahara T, Ortaldo JR, Herbermann RB, Oppenheim JJ (1984) Human granular lymphocytes are potent producers of interleukin-1. Nature 309:56—59

151. Schmidt JA, Mizel SB, Cohen D, Green I (1982) Interleukin 1, a potential regulator of fibroblast proliferation. J Immunol 128:2177—2182

152. Schultz RM, Kleinschmidt WJ (1983) Functional identity between murine γ-interferon and macrophage activating factor. Nature 305:239—240

153. Sergiescu D, Cerutti I, Efthymiou E, Kahan A, Chany C (1979) Adverse effects of interferon treatment on the life span of NZB mice. Biomedicine 31:48—51

154. Sibbitt WL, Mathews PM, Bankhurst AD (1983) Natural killer cell in systemic lupus erythematosus. J Clin Invest 71:2130—2139

155. Sibbitt WL, Froelich CJ, Bankhurst AD (1983) Natural cytotoxicity in systemic lupus erythematosus: mechanisms of suppression by inhibitory serum factors. Clin Exp Immunol 53:363—370

156. Smith KA (1980) T cell growth factor. Immunol Rev 51:337

157. Smith KA, Favata MF, Oroszlan S (1983) Production and characterization of monoclonal antibodies to human interleukin-2: strategy and tactics. J Immunol 131:1808—1815

158. Smolen JS, Siminovitch K, Luger TA, Steinberg AD (1983) Responder cells in the human autologous mixed lymphocyte reaction (AMLR). Characterization and interactions in healthy individuals and patients with SLE. Behring Inst Mitt 72:135—142

159. Smolen JS, Morimoto CH, Steinberg AD, Wolf A, Schlossman SF, Steinberg RT, Penner E, Reinherz E, Reichlin M, Chused TM (1985) Systemic lupus erythematosus: delineation of subpopulations by clinical, serologic, and T cell subset analysis. Am J Med Sci 289:139—146

160. Sobrado J, Moldawer LL, Dinarello CA, Blackburn GL, Bistrian BR (1983) Continuous infusion of human leukocytic pyrogen in the guinea pig. Fed Proc 42:699

161. Sonnenfeld G, Mandel AD, Merigan TC (1977) The immunosuppressive effect of type II mouse interferon preparations on antibody production. Cell Immunol 34:193—206

162. Sonnenfeld G (1980) Modulation of immunity by interferon. In: Pick E (ed) Lymphokine reports, vol I. Academic, New York, pp 113—131

163. Stadler BM, Dougherty SF, Farrar JJ, Oppenheim JJ (1981) Relationship of cell cycle to recovery of IL 2 activity from human mononuclear cells, human and mouse T cell lines. J Immunol 127:1936—1940

164. Steeg PS, Moore RN, Johnson HW, Oppenheim JJ (1982) Regulation of murine macrophage Ia antigen expression by a lymphokine with immune interferon activity. J Exp Med 156:1780—1793

165. Stewart WE II, Blalock JE, Burke DC, Chaney C, Dunnick JK, Falcoff E, Friedman RM, Galasso GJ, Joklik WK, Vilcek JT, Youngner JS, Zoon KC (1980) Interferon nomenclature. Nature 286:110

166. Strannegard O, Larsson I, Lundgren E, Miorner H, Persson H (1978) Modulation of immune responses in newborn and adult mice by interferon. Infect Immuno 20:334—339

167. Strannegard Ö, Hermodsson S, Westberg G (1982) Interferon and natural killer cells in systemic lupus erythematosus. Clin Exp Immunol 50:246—252

168. Suzuki H (1978) Studies on the assay procedures for immune interferon and its determination on lymphocytes from patients with systemic lupus erythematosus (SLE). Ryumachi 18:5

169. Suzuki T, Cooper MD (1985) Comparison of the expression of IL 2 receptors by human T and B cells: induction by the polyclonal mitogens, phorbol myristate acetate, and anti-μ antibody. J Immunol 134:1311—3119

170. Svensson B (1975) Serum factors causing impaired macrophage function in systemic lupus erythematosus. Scan J Immunol 4:145
171. Swain SL, Wetzel GD, Dutton RW (1985) B cell growth and differentiation factors. In: Schreier MH, Smith KA (eds) Lymphokines, vol 10. Academic, New York, pp 1—13
172. Sztein MB, Vogel SN, Sipe JD, Murphy PA, Mizel SB, Oppenheim JJ, Rosenstreich DL (1981) The role of macrophages in the acute-phase response: SAA inducer is closely related to lymphocyte activating factor and endogenous pyrogen. Cell Immunol 63:164—176
173. Sztein MB, Steeg PS, Johnson HM, Oppenheim JJ (1984) Regulation of human peripheral blood monocyte DR antigen expression in vitro by lymphokines and recombinant interferons. J Clin Invest 73:556—565
174. Talal N, Dauphinee MJ, Wofsy D (1982) Interleukin-2 deficiency, genes, and systemic lupus erythematosus. Arth Rheum 25:838—842
175. Taniguchi T, Mantei N, Schwarzstein M, Nagata S, Muramatsu M, Weissmann G (1980) Human leukocyte and fibroblast interferons are structurally related. Nature 285:547
176. Taniguchi T, Matsui H, Fujita T, Takaoka C, Kashima N, Yoshimoto R, Hamuro J (1983) Structure and expression of a cloned cDNA for human interleukin-2. Nature 302:305—310
177. Theodorescu M (1983) A polyclonal B-cell activating lymphokine and its natural inhibitor: possible role in antibody formation and autoimmune disease. In: Pick E (ed) Lymphkine, vol 8. Academic, New York, pp 81—138
178. Theofilopoulus AN, Shawler DL, Eisenberg RA, Dixon FJ (1980) Splenic immunoglobulin-secreting cells and their regulation in auto-immune mice. J Exp Med 151:446
179. Theofilopoulos AN, Dixon FJ (1981) Etiopathogenesis of murine SLE. Immunol Rev 44:179
180. Theofilopoulos AN, Dixon FJ (1985) Murine models of systemic lupus erythematosus. In: Kunkel HG, Dixon FJ (eds) Advances in immunology, vol 37. Academic, New York, pp 269—390
181. Tilden AB, Abo T, Balch CM (1983) Suppressor cell function of human granular lymphocytes identified by the HNK-1 (Leu 7) monoclonal antibody. J Immunol 130:1171—1175
182. Trinchieri D, Santoli D, Koprowski H (1978) Spontaneous cell-mediated cytotoxicity in humans: role of interferon and immunoglobulins. J Immunol 120:1849—1855
183. Trinchieri G, Perussia B (1985) Immune interferon: a pleiotropic lymphokine with multiple effects. Immunol Today 6:131—136
184. Tsokos GC, Rook AH, Djeu JY, Balow JE (1982) Natural killer cells and interferon responses in patients with systemic lupus erythematosus. Clin Exp Immunol 50:239—245
185. Tsokos GC, Balow JE (1984) Cellular immune responses in systemic lupus erythematosus. In: Schwartz RS (ed) Progress in allergy. Karger, Basel, pp 93—161
186. VanSnick JL, Masson PL, Heremans JF (1974) The involvement of lactoferrin in the hyposideremia of acute inflammation. J Exp Med 140:1068—1084
187. Vignaux S, Gresser I (1978) Enhanced expression of histocompatibility antigens on interferon-treated mouse embryonic fibroblasts. Proc Soc Exp Biol Med 157:456—460
188. Volc-Platzer B, Leibl H, Luger T, Zahn G, Stingl G (1985) Human epidermal cells synthesize HLA-DR alloantigens in vitro upon stimulation with γ-interferon. J Invest Derm 85:16—19
189. Waldmann TA, Goldman CK, Robb RJ, Depper JM, Leonard WJ, Sharrow SO, Bongiovanni KF, Korsmeyer SJ, Greene WC (1984) Expression of interleukin 2 receptors on activated human B cells. J Exp Med 160:1450—1466
190. Watson J, Mochizuki D (1980) Interleukin 2: a class of T cell growth factors. Immunol Rev 51:257
191. Watson JD, Prestidge (1983) Interleukin 3 and colony stimulating factors. Immunol Today 4:278
192. Wofsy D, Murphy ED, Rothe JB, Dauphinee MJ, Kipper SB, Talal N (1981) Deficient interleukin 2 activity in MRL/Mp and C57BL/6J mice bearing the *lpr* gene. J Exp Med 154:1671

193. Wood DD, Ihrie EJ, Dinarello CA, Cohen PL (1983) Isolation of an interleukin 1-like factor from human joint effusions. Arth Rheum 26:978—983
194. Wright SC, Bonavida B (1982) Studies on the mechanism of natural killer (NK) cell-mediated cytotoxicity (CMC). J Immunol 129:433—439
195. Yoshinaga M, Goto F, Goto K, Nakamura S, Ohokawara S, Kitamura M (1985) A large-scale production and purification of IL 1-like factor from PMN of rabbits with tumor-induced granulocytosis. J Leukocyte Biol 37:754
196. Ytterberg SR, Schnitzer TJ (1982) Serum interferon levels in patients with systemic lupus erythematosus. Arthritis Rheum 25:401—406
197. Zubler RH, Lowenthal JW, Erard F, Hashimoto N, Davos R, MacDonald R (1984) Activated B cells express receptors for and proliferate in response to, pure interleukin 2. J Exp Med 160:1170—1183
198. Zubler RH (1985) Signal Requirements for T-dependent and T-independent B cell activation. In: Schreier MH, Smith KA (eds) Lymphokines, vol 10. Academic, New York, pp 89—105

Part IV:
Clinical Aspects of Human SLE

Clinical and Serologic Features: Incidence and Diagnostic Approach

J. S. SMOLEN

The Spectrum

Systemic lupus erythematosus (SLE) is a nonspecific autoimmune disorder which may involve any organ. Although its etiology is still unclear, some of its pathogenetic aspects as well as the spectrum of its clinical manifestations and a variety of indicators of disease activity have become increasingly known over the past decades. In conjunction with improved diagnostic modalities, this knowledge has lately made possible (a) earlier recognition, (b) an increase in diagnostic accuracy, and (c) improved therapeutic approaches. At present, SLE may therefore be considered a well controllable disease provided it is recognized early and treated appropriately.

SLE has always been regarded as a rather rare disease. However, with recent reports of a population incidence of 4—7 per 100 000 per year [1, 2] this is no longer the case. Moreover, the incidence appears to be rising as a consequence of better diagnostic approaches, a true increase, or both [1].

Which organs are involved, what is the risk of their involvement, and how can we diagnose their involvement? First of all, it should be recalled that SLE has no single "target organ." However, some patients may have circulating autoantibodies directed against certain target cell types (such as anti-red cell antibodies), while others may have autoantibodies to specific intracellular proteins which might interfere with cell cycle kinetics and cell function [3, 4, and p. 105 ff.]. Nevertheless, the majority of the clinical symptoms are the consequence of immune complex deposition in blood vessels and kidneys. The size and composition of these immune complexes appear to determine the preferential site of their deposition and their inflammatory and thus tissue-destructive potential [5—8]. These few facts, well known to clinicians and immunologists, suffice to indicate that heterogeneity of clinical as well as immunologic features is a distinct characteristic of SLE, a characteristic that might adhere to certain rules currently not well understood (see pp. 290—297).

Table 1 provides an overview of a variety of clinical and serologic features of SLE and includes the incidence of organ involvement obtained from the study of almost 200 patients. It does not divide these features into specific clinical subentities, since this will be done in subsequent chapters. It simply reflects the spectrum of SLE and is meant to provide a basis for the analyses to follow. It also indicates that the disease itself, and even more so lupus therapy and its side-effects, challenges the entire field of internal medicine.

Table 1. Clinical and serologic features in SLE (Figures are percentages)[a]

Male patients	7
Family history of autoimmune disease	31
Age of onset < 20	35
Age of onset 20—40	51
Age of onset > 40	14
Renal involvement	62
Severe renal involvement	50
Hypertension	36
Central nervous system involvement	40
Thrombocytopenia	19
Leukocytopenia	50
Anemia	64
Lymphadenopathy	45
Joint involvement	91
Muscle involvement	40
Raynaud's phenomenon	36
Oral ulcers	23
Cutaneous vasculitis	32
Alopecia	53
Lung involvement (parenchymal)	25
Serositis	57
Sjögren's syndrome	33
DNA binding	95
Anti-Ro (SS-A)	37
Anti-La (SS-B)	6
Anti-Sm	9
Anti-RNP	16
Anti-Laux	3
Nonidentified precipitins	10
False-positive STS	13
Positive Coombs test	30

[a]) Data are based on analysis of 194 patients with SLE [81]

Clinical Manifestations

General Symptoms

Fatigue, fever, malaise, loss of weight, and nausea may occur in SLE patients (in decreasing incidence) at the onset and during flares of the disease. Fatigue is often one of the earliest symptoms of an imminent flare. Moreover, patients with SLE tend to develop drug allergies, especially to sulfonamides [9]. Some patients may be prone to exacerbation of their disease after sun exposure; in others SLE may flare (or occasionally be first diagnosed) in the course of infection, during exposure to certain drugs, after operations, or during pregnancy [10—14].

Joints

Arthralgia or frank arthritis is present in up to 90% of patients. Pain upon motion, tenderness, effusion, and morning stiffness may all occur and may mimic rheumatoid arthritis. Most commonly, arthritis is polyarticular and predominantly involves the proximal interphalangeal and metacarpophalangeal joints, less often the wrist joints and knee joints, and only rarely other joints. As in rheumatoid arthritis (RA), distal interphalangeal joints are usually spared. The majority of the patients have nondeforming and nonerosive joint disease, although 10%—15% may have deformities, such as ulnar deviation and swan-neck deformities. Moreover, erosions may be present later in the course of lupus arthritis, and the vast majority of these patients appear to have serologic and genetic features that make concomitant RA rather unlikely (see p. 276). Occasional patients, however, may have SLE/RA overlap disease [15]. Aseptic necrosis (especially of the hip) is not uncommon in SLE patients, predominantly occurring in those on corticosteroids.

Differential diagnosis: RA, juvenile arthritis, rheumatic fever, viral, bacterial and neoplastic syndromes, sarcoidosis.

Muscle Involvement

Myalgia occurs in approximately 40% of SLE patients. Frank myositis is observed in only about 8% [16]. The predominant symptom is shoulder- or pelvicgirdle weakness, usually insidious in onset. Occasional patients may develop myositis abruptly. Rarely there is muscle tenderness. CPK and/or aldolase levels and urinary creatine excreation may be significantly elevated. Electromyographic investigations may reveal abnormalities (membrane irritability, polyphasic potentials, etc.). Approximately 10% of SLE patients have abnormal muscle enzyme levels and/or EMG abnormalities. Upon muscle biopsy, interstitial inflammatory infiltrates (often perivascular), fiber atrophy or degeneration, and occasionally vacuolization may be seen. Although "vacuolar myopathy" may be induced by certain drugs used for the treatment of SLE (such as hydroxychloroquine and corticosteroids), this form of myopathy can also be observed in lupus patients who have not received these agents [16a and our own observations]. Vacuolar myopathy not only constitutes a severe form of lupus muscle involvement, it is usually also relatively therapy-resistant and may require application of immunosuppressive agents to become controllable. Cytotoxic drugs may also be necessary in occasional patients with other forms of myositis (especially if cricopharyngeal or intercostal muscles are involved).

Differential diagnosis: polymyositis, dermatomyositis, mixed connective tissue disease, polymyalgia rheumatica, corticosteroid and chloroquine myopathy, viral and neoplastic syndromes.

Cutaneous Manifestations (see pp. 227—250)

Vascular Manifestations

Vasculitis most often affects the skin and the muscles but may be present in any organ system. Involvement of the coronary arteries may lead to myocardial infarction; involvement of mesenteric arteries may lead to an abdominal emergency situation; and involvement of cerebral arteries may lead to a cerebrovascular accident. *Raynaud's phenomenon* is present in 35% of the patients and is probably also associated with vasculitis. Although Raynaud's phenomenon is no longer considered a criterion in the revised ARA criteria for SLE classification because of its insensitivity as a feature distinguishing between SLE and other connective tissue disorders [17], its presence must still be regarded an additional diagnostic "hint" in many patients with oligosymptomatic lupus.

Thrombophlebitis is seen in approximately 5% of individuals with SLE and often constitutes a symptom present early in the course of the disease. Interestingly, such patients and occasional patients with other thrombotic complications may have circulating anticoagulants [18, 19].

Hypertension, present in approximately 35%, may accompany renal lupus, but may also occur in the absence of nephritic disease manifestations. It should be rigorously controlled to avoid the additional risk that it imposes on patients prone to develop kidney and coronary heart disease [20]. Moreover, especially in young patients with SLE, even blood pressure values generally regarded as borderline should be tightly controlled and treated if repeatedly present [21].

Cardiac Manifestations

Pericarditis is quite common in SLE (25%—30%), although often asymptomatic. Occasionally, large pericardial effusions may be seen.

Myocarditis is observed in less than 10% of SLE patients. Its manifestations may be reflected by conduction abnormalities (such as first degree AV block) or arrhythmias and tachycardia; however, occasionally dilatation of the heart and congestive heart failure may occur and be life threatening. Obviously, in elderly lupus patients differentiation between cardiac abnormalities as a consequence of coronary heart disease and lupus myocarditis may be difficult, and care must be taken to evaluate the disease activity in such patients. In addition, *"coronary heart disease"* in lupus patients may be due to underlying vasculitis of coronary arteries, and accelerated coronary atherosclerosis as well as a tendency to develop myocardial infarction at a relatively young age are well documented in SLE [22—24].

The classic endocardial lupus lesion, namely Libman-Sacks *endocarditis,* is not only rarely diagnosed but also usually does not lead to significant valvular disease. In the corticosteroid era, Libman-Sacks endocarditis (verrucous endocarditis) has become an autoptic diagnosis rather than a clinical one [25]. Although systolic murmurs may often be heard in SLE patients, they reflect fever, tachycardia, anemia or cardiac dilatation rather than valvular disease. Diastolic murmurs have been reported to occur in less than 1% of the patients [10]. However, bacterial endocarditis may develop in occasional patients as a consequence of immunosuppression, Libman-Sacks type changes of the endocardium, or both.

Differential diagnosis: arteriosclerosis, viral carditis, bacterial endocarditis, rheumatic fever, rheumatoid arthritis, other connective tissue disorders.

Pulmonary Manifestations

Pleuritic chest pain may be present in up to 50% of the patients in the course of their disease; together with arthritis, skin rash, and leukopenia, pleurisy is one of the most common presenting symptoms in SLE, and it tends to recur in the course of flares. Pleural effusion can be demonstrated in only about half of these patients. Rarely there is massive pleural effusion. Since thrombotic complications are not uncommon in SLE (see below), pleuritis can be due to pulmonary embolism and thus should not be generally attributed to the underlying disease.

About 5% of lupus patients develop *acute pneumonitis* characterized by dyspnea and rales, and hemoptysis may be occasionally present; x-ray reveals diffuse infiltrates (usually in the basal region) [26]. Despite the recognition of acute pneumonitis as a feature of SLE, the majority of SLE patients with pulmonary infiltrates have infection or congestive heart failure [27].

Up to 25% of the patients suffer from *chronic pneumonitis*; these patients may be asymptomatic but can also develop dyspnea, frank cyanosis, and clubbing [28]. Physical examination may reveal rales or crepitation. Upon x-ray examination, linear or reticular interstitial infiltrates may be seen, and characteristically, plate atelectases are present (see p. 270). Pulmonary artery pressures may be elevated. Lung biopsy (transbronchial or open) may be necessary for diagnosis.

Lung function test abnormalities are seen far more often than clinically manifest lung involvement and are an indication of subclinical pulmonary disease. Such abnormalities are restriction, decreased vital capacity, hypocapnia, and occasionally reduction of diffusion capacity [29, 30].

Vasculitis of the upper respiratory tract can lead to nasal ulcerations (up to 10%), and rarely to ulcerations of the epipharynx, larynx, or trachea; hemoptysis may be present. Pulmonary vasculitis may be associated with pneumonitis [31].

Differential diagnosis: scleroderma, MCTD, lung fibrosis due to nonrheumatologic disorders; Goodpasture's syndrome. In patients on immunosuppressive therapy: respiratory tract infections (bacterial, viral, opportunistic).

Hematopoietic System

Anemia occurs in approximately 65% of the patients. Most frequently, SLE patients suffer from "anemia of chronic diseases" [32], which is usually normocytic and normochromic despite hypoferremia; the latter is due to increased iron uptake by the reticuloendothelial system. Ferritin levels are normal. Thus, iron therapy is not necessary and would only induce further increase in iron stores. In lupus patients with end-stage kidney disease, anemia can be aggravated by factors involved in uremia, such as decreased erythropoietin production. Iron deficiency anemia may occur in patients with gastrointestinal or other chronic blood losses; in these patients there is usually a decreased serum ferritin level, and control of the blood loss or other causes as well as iron substitution are necessary.

A positive *Coombs test* can be observed in 30% of the patients. Coombs positivity does not necessarily indicate the presence of antierythrocyte antibodies, since immune complexes containing C3b can bind to the erythrocyte C3b receptor [33] and may induce a positive Coombs test (even though SLE patients have a deficiency in C3b receptors [34]). Moreover, Coombs positivity does not always go along with hemolysis. In fact, only about 20% of the patients with positive Coombs tests have signs of hemolysis. When hemolytic anemia is present, it is often only mild, but in occasional patients severe hemolytic crises may occur, and we have seen patients with hemoglobin lower than 4 g/100 ml. Such patients obviously may be comatous in the absence of central nervous system disease. The therapeutic response (to corticosteroids with or without additional immunosuppressive agents) can be well controlled by the reticulocyte count.

The most common leukocyte abnormalitiy is *leukocytopenia* (white blood cell counts < 4000/mm³), which can be observed in 50% of untreated SLE patients. It is often due to granulocytopenia (< 3000/mm³) which may be induced by autoantibodies or by elimination by the reticuloendothelial system after coating with preformed immune complexes or activated complement components and aggregation [35]. Lymphopenia (< 1000/mm³) is also common in SLE and is usually due to anti-T cell antibodies; these may be directed against different T cell subsets [36, 37]. Severe leukopenia is rare, but leukocyte counts around or less than 2500/mm³ may often be observed. Neutropenia may occasionally lead to increased susceptibility to infections. Drug effects, such as allergic reactions (e.g., to nonsteroidal anti-inflammatory agents) or toxic effects of immunosuppressive substances, have to be excluded in all these instances. Lymphopenia, on the other hand, may be seen in the course of corticosteroid therapy.

In contrast to other rheumatic disorders (such as RA) *leukocytosis* (granulocytosis) is rarely observed in SLE unless in the course of infections or corticosteroid therapy.

Thrombocytopenia (< 100 000/mm³) is found in 20% of SLE patients and may be due to autoantibodies or to coating of thrombocytes by immune complexes and splenic elimination. Rarely thrombocytopenia leads to bleeding episodes in SLE. However, thrombocytopenia (often presenting as idiopathic thrombocytop-

176   J. S. Smolen

enic purpura) may precede SLE by years [38]. Idiopathic thrombocytopenic purpura in conjunction with autoimmune hemolytic anemia (Evan's syndrome) may be associated with (or be a feature of) SLE. Thrombotic thrombocytopenic purpura very rarely complicates SLE [38a].

Thrombocytosis, in contrast to other rheumatic diseases such as RA, is only very rarely observed in lupus.

In 5%—10% of SLE patients, *circulating anticoagulants* (antibodies to coagulation factors) can be found. These may be directed against factors VIII—XIII or against the prothrombin activator complex. The vast majority of these patients have no increased bleeding tendency, although partial thromboplastin time and prothrombin time are increased. These patients often have an associated false-positive serologic test for syphilis (cross-reactivity of the antigens involved), and — as compared with other SLE patients — an increased incidence of thrombocytopenia and thromboembolic complications (requiring heparin administration) [18, 18a, 19]. Moreover, the incidence of cerebro-vascular accidents is increased in these patients [38b].

Gastrointestinal Abnormalities

Oral ulceration can be seen in approximately 20% of the patients; these ulcers, often associated with ulcers of the nasal mucosa, are usually not painful and therefore easily missed; they only rarely exulcerate deeply (e.g., gingivitis).

Dysphagia can be an occasional problem in SLE. In our experience, it is only rarely due to involvement of the lower esophagus (similar to but much milder than in scleroderma) as indicated by esophageal manometry. Much more often it is a sequela of associated sicca syndrome. Occasionally, lupus myositis or vasculitis and ulceration of the esophagus may be the underlying cause of dysphagia.

Much more common than SLE-related abnormalities are *drug-induced lesions of the stomach and duodenum,* such as gastroduodenitis or ulcers in the course of therapy with aspirin, nonsteroidal anti-inflammatory agents, or high dose cortcosteroids. *Anorexia, nausea, and vomiting* may accompany the patient during flares as nonspecific signs or may be due to the abnormalities mentioned above and below.

Mesenteric vasculitis is a rare but very serious intestinal manifestation of SLE leading to abdominal emergency situations which require immediate surgical intervention.

Pancreatitis has been observed in 5%—10% of SLE patients; the underlying cause is not quite clear. Vasculitis can be one cause, but it should be noted that pancreatitis may also be a feature of concomitant Sjögren's syndrome [39]. Finally, we have recently seen a lupus patient with evidence of pancreatitis who was found to have mumps virus infection.

Peritonitis has been observed in approximately 10% of the patients and may also be a cause of abdominal pain in SLE. (The relatively low incidence as compared with pleuritis may be due to the fact that it is easily missed in asymptomatic patients.)

Finally, *hepatitis* is seen in up to 15% of SLE patients. The spectrum varies from mild elevation of liver enzymes detected only upon routine laboratory examinations to significant hepatomegaly and chronic active hepatitis-like disease. Liver biopsy may reveal fatty degeneration, mesenchymal activation, vasculitis, or chronic hepatitis. Subclinical liver disease is the rule in SLE [40]. However, we have seen two female patients who did not fulfill four ARA criteria for the classification of SLE but had high titer antibodies to double-stranded DNA and absent antibodies to smooth muscle or mitochondria as well as biopsy-proven chronic hepatitis. Especially, these patients did not have clinically proven kidney or CNS involvement, which is in accordance with observations by Rothfield [41]. Thus, there may be a subset of patients with features similar to "lupoid" (chronic active) hepatitis and SLE serology, constituting a link between these two disorders.

In the context of hepatic abnormalities, it should be noted that liver enzyme elevations and liver disease may obviously be *drug-induced* or due to a concomitant *viral infection*.

Immunocompetent Organs

Lymphadenopathy is seen in 45% of SLE patients and represents "nonspecific" lymphadenitis, usually with follicular hyperplasis and sometimes with additional signs of vasculitis. Upon physical examination, lymph nodes are not tender and often rather small (0.5—1.0 cm), but massive lymphadenopathy (up to 5 cm) can be observed in some patients. Lymphadenopathy vanishes with treatment, but may recur early in the course of flares.

In SLE, *malignant lymphoid neoplasia* seem to be a rare, though reported event [42—45]. It appears from studying the literature that patients with SLE have a much lower incidence of lymphoid malignancies than patients with RA and, especially, primary Sjögren's syndrome [46—48], but comparative studies have not been performed. It should be noted in this context that the different mouse strains with lupus all have enlarged lymph nodes (and spleens) and that one strain, MRL-*lpr/lpr*, has massive lymphadenopathy due to expansion of an abnormal T cell population; nevertheless, the incidence of lymphoma was recently reported to be about 1% taking all strains together [49]. Immunosuppressive agents have been implicated as a risk factor for lymphoid malignancies [50]. Nevertheless, there is indirect evidence against a role of such agents in the occasional development of lymphoma in SLE patients:

1. Primary Sjögren's syndrome, which may have a similar pathogenesis to SLE (see pp. 197—203), has a much higher incidence of lymphomas than SLE, irrespective of the therapeutic modalities applied [39].
2. In rheumatoid arthritis the risk of developing lymphoma may be associated with the concomitant presence of Sjögren's syndrome [39] and appears to be independent of the use of cytotoxic agents [46, 51]; it has not been investigated whether or not the few SLE patients reported to suffer from lymphoma had the sicca complex.
3. Patients with SLE who usually receive some kind of therapy, including cytotoxic agents, develop lymphoma less often than untreated lupus-prone mice [49, 52, 53].
4. Immunosuppressive agents are quite widely used in SLE and more often than in RA or Sjögren's syndrome, but still the incidence of malignant lymphoma appears to be lower in SLE.

Thus, not only is there little evidence for the association of SLE with lymphoid malignancy, but immunosuppressive therapy might decrease rather than increase the risk of development of lymphoma in SLE. Since immunosuppressive drugs interfere with the immune response and since lymphoid malignancy in Sjögren's syndrome may be a consequence of long-term antigenic stimulation [39], there is even a rationale behind this assumption. Nevertheless, with the new immunosuppressive protocols, such as high-dose pulse corticosteroids or cyclophosphamide, we may have to reevaluate this issue as soon as more and longer experience with these regimens has been gained.

It should finally be mentioned that there is one (primary?) lymphadenopathy mimicking many features of SLE (but usually lacking antibodies to double-stranded DNA), namely *angioimmunoblastic lymphadenopathy* [54, 55, 55a], which is regarded as semimalignant and necessitates vigorous therapy.

The *spleen* is enlarged in 10%—20% of the patients, usually only mildly. "Onion skin arterioles," which represent a vasculitic end-stage, may be found upon histologic examination.

The *thymus* appears to be a crucial organ in the pathogenesis of SLE, because neonatal thymectomy may "cure" or "worsen" murine lupus depending upon the strain studied and the development of immunologic tolerance appears to depend upon the presence of a "normal" thymus [56]. Early thymic atrophy has been also observed in lupus mice. In man, abnormalities of the thymus have not been noted [11]; however, this does not exclude the possibility that thymic function is deranged in a similar way as in lupus-prone mice. Adult thymectomy does not alter the course of human SLE [57, 58]. Coexistence of SLE and myasthenia gravis is more common than should be expected [59, 60], and development of SLE after thymectomy for myasthenia has been observed by ourselves and others [61]. Malignant thymoma may occur rarely [45].

Ocular Manifestations

The *eyelids* may occasionally be involved in cutaneous manifestations (see p. 227), or may be edematous when nephrotic syndrome or angioneurotic edema is present.

Conjunctivitis, scleritis, and *subconjunctival hemorrhages* can be observed in up to 10% of patients.

Retinal abnormalities, such as retinal exudates ("cytoid bodies") or optic atrophy (due to vasculitis), are occasionally seen, especially in patients with CNS lupus, and such patients may also have papilledema.

Finally, although *xerophthalmia* and abnormal Schirmer tests may be found in up to 25% of SLE patients as an indication of concomitant Sjögren's syndrome (secondary Sjögren's syndrome), *keratoconjunctivitis sicca* — in contrast to patients with primary Sjögren's syndrome — has only rarely been observed in our own and other series [62].

Renal Manifestations

Although glomerular involvement — including mild mesangial hypercellularity (upon light microscopy) or mesangial immune complex deposits (upon electron microscopy) — can be seen in virtually all patients with SLE [63], clinically manifest *glomerulonephritis* occurs in only 50%—60% of the patients. There is a broad spectrum of manifestations: proteinuria (minimal to nephrotic range), hematuria (not present to macrohematuria), and cylindruria (none, hyaline casts, cellular casts) may occur in any combination, and kidney function may be normal to severely impaired. The pathohistologic basis of these clinical abnormalities is immune-complex deposition in different glomerular sites and in different quantities (see p. 204).

Less than 10% of in-hospital SLE patients have significant renal insufficiency (creatinine > 1.8 mg%) at the time of diagnosis. Thus, if uremia occurs, it develops in the course of clinically recognized disease in the vast majority of these lupus patients; therefore indications for kidney involvement by urinalysis may necessitate vigorous treatment even in the early stages of SLE. Since mild urinary abnormalities and normal kidney function may be present not only in patients with minimal glomerular involvement but also in the initial stages of severe forms of lupus nephritis, we try to obtain kidney biopsies in every lupus patient with abnormal urinalysis (although opinions vary with regard to the value of renal biopsy in SLE, [64]). The result of kidney biopsy influences our therapeutic approach. Serial biopsies may be necessary in some patients, since a high rate of transformation from one histologic type to another has been observed, often with minimal predictive clinical basis [65—69]. Histologic gradings of activity and sclerosis have been described by several authors [68, 69] and are discussed on pp. 204—221. Their importance is their prognostic significance.

180 J. S. Smolen

Urinary sediment usually but not always represents a good indicator of the "activity" and/or "severity" of lupus nephritis; the presence of cellular casts and/or more than 30 erythrocytes per high power field, or an increase in these elements after periods of stability, indicates severe nephritis or a flare and is rarely found in milder forms of SLE nephritis. Proteinuria (and hyaline casts) may be present to different degrees in mild and severe nephritis, although proteinuria in the nephrotic range (<3.5 g/day) usually indicates severe kidney involvement (diffuse proliferative, membranoproliferative, or mebranous glomerulonephritis). However, even profuse proteinuria does not necessarily reflect active nephritis, since it may be a consequence of past severe kidney involvement.

Persistent high titer antibodies to ds-DNA and low serum complement have been found to be associated with disease activity and poorer prognosis by some [70—73] but not all investigators [69, 73]. It is conceivable that the different histologic types are due to deposition of different types of immune complexes; this has been suggested by several authors on the basis of histologic and immunologic studies [74—81]. Some histologic studies indicate that — despite a limited, albeit not rare, transition potential between certain histologic types of nephritis (such as diffuse proliferative and focal proliferative) — there is rarely transition between histologic types with basic differences in immune-complex localization (such as the proliferative forms and the membranous one) [74]. These findings together would indicate a pathogenetic heterogeneity of glomerulonephritis in SLE.

With increasing renal insufficiency patients may require dialysis, although with successful therapy kidney function can be regained [82, 83]. Such patients only rarely continue to have active disease. Lupus patients with kidney transplants tend to remain inactive (most likely because of the immunosuppressive therapy in the posttransplant period), but the disease may occasionally recur [84, 85].

In the context of glomerulonephritis, it is necessary to bear in mind that a sudden rise in creatinine levels does not necessarily reflect a flare of nephritis but may be due to side-effects of therapy: aspirin and other nonsteroidal anti-inflammatory agents (probably with the exception of sulindac) may reversibly reduce kidney function, especially in hyperreninemic states (such as congestive heart failure or nephritis, even if mild), due to inhibition of the synthesis of vasodilatory renal prostaglandins [86, 87]. Increased creatinine levels have also been observed with cimetidine therapy [88]. Obviously, application of nephrotoxic drugs, such as cephalosporins and aminoglycosides, can also be responsible for impairment of renal function.

Hypertension, which can be a consequence of glomerulonephritis, has been discussed above.

The issue of *interstitial nephritis,* in our view, is still controversial. Although there is no doubt that a small numer of patients with lupus have interstitial infiltrates and interstitial immune complex deposition ([89—92] and p. 215), the implications of this pathohistologic finding are not quite clear. In particular, there have been no detailed investigations on the concomitant presence of Sjögren's syndrome in the patients reported to have interstitial nephritis [89—92]. It is well known that in primary Sjögren's syndrome interstitial nephritis is the nephrologic hallmark and that many of these patients have tubular abnormalities leading to features of Fanconi's syndrome [39, 93]. Therefore, we have recently evaluated SLE patients with interstitial nephritis in the absence of marked glomerular involvement and have found that these patients (1%—2% of SLE patients) have Sjögren's syndrome associated with their lupus, have keratoconjunctivitis sicca, and have antibodies to Ro and La in their circulation, which are also characteristic for primary Sjögren's syndrome [94]. Thus, we believe that severe tubulointerstitial disease is not a manifestation of SLE but rather one of concomitant primary Sjögren's syndrome, and that these patients suffer from an overlap between the two disorders.

Neuropsychiatric Manifestations (see pp. 251—269)

SLE and Association with Other Autoimmune Disorders

The most commonly associated abnormality is *sicca syndrome* (25% of lupus patients) (see also pp. 197—203). This may lead to xerostomia and dry eyes and may be detected by Schirmer test, radionuclide scanning of the salivary glands, or lip biopsy. These patients only rarely present with anti-La/SSB antibodies ([63] our own observations, and pp. 197—203). Their clinical and serologic features are similar to those observed in sicca syndrome associated with RA and other connective tissue disorders [63], and therefore it is appropriate to term it *secondary* Sjögren's syndrome [95, 96]. Occasional patients also have other clinical and serologic features of primary Sjögren's syndrome and thus suffer from an overlap type disease (see above).

Myasthenia gravis is observed in 1%—2% of SLE patients (and SLE in about 1% of myasthenia patients).

SLE can be a part of several *overlap diseases:* Features of SLE can be seen in so-called mixed connective tissue disease (MCTD), and SLE may occasionally be associated with RA [15] and, as mentioned before, with primary Sjögren's syndrome.

Although abnormalities of *thyroid function* are rare in SLE, antibodies to thyroid antigens are commonly observed.

Finally, SLE or SLE-like disorders can be seen in the context of *complement deficiencies* (see p. 126).

Lupus and Pregnancy

Systemic lupus erythematosus represents a high risk for the *fetus*. Early abortion, late abortion, and prematurity are significantly increased in SLE patients as compared with the normal population, and in many patients repeated early abortion is the first symptom of underlying disease (for review see [14]). Abortion is often associated with the lupus anticoagulant (38b), and in such patients corticosteroids and aspirin may have a favourable effect upon the outcome of pregnancy [96b], also according to our own experience. Congenital heart block is a complication in children born to anti-Ro positive patients (even in the absence of SLE) (see p. 110f.), and children of SLE patients may have "congenital" lupus or thrombocytopenia due to crossing of the placenta by maternal antibodies [14]. Finally, the risk of developing SLE is significantly increased in the offspring of SLE patients [97, 98].

With regard to the *mother,* disease exacerbations during pregnancy and especially in the early postpartum period have been observed. In some patients SLE is diagnosed for the first time in the course of pregnancy. There are several theoretical reasons why SLE may flare in the context of pregnancy [14]. However, the issue of disease exacerbations due to pregnancy is still controversial, since Lockshin et al. recently failed to found a significant association [99]; nevertheless, even these authors have observed deterioration of proteinuria, thrombocytopenia, and hypocomplementemia in some of their patients during pregnancy [99, 100], and pre-eclampsia and fetal distress were common. In 1 of the 28 patients studied, SLE was first diagnosed during pregnancy; moreover, very few patients investigated appeared to have active disease, indicating that patients with rather inactive disease may be relatively safe during pregnancy. In our view SLE is a particular risk for the pregnant mother if kidney, CNS, or heart are involved. Therefore, SLE patients with major organ involvement, if not inactive for at least 1 year, should not become pregnant (and use birth control pills with very little or, better still, no estrogene). In all other patients pregnancy is not contraindicated as long as careful monitoring is performed by an obstetrician and a rheumatologist [14].

Serologic Features

Antinuclear Antibodies (ANAs)

If SLE is suspected, the first diagnostic test should be determination of ANAs, since this test, which can be performed by indirect immunofluorescence methods on rat or mouse liver cryostat sections or on commercially available cell lines (such as HEp2 cells), approaches 99% positivity in SLE. The sensitivity of the tissue culture cell lines is somewhat higher. In the vast majority of SLE patients, ANA titers at the time of diagnosis are over 1:320; the maximal titer we have ever observed was 1:40 960. Low-titer ANAs, however, do not exclude SLE, and occasional patients may be ANA-negative (see pp. 110f.). ANAs, as tested by indirect immunofluorescence, are by no means specific for SLE, since they can occur in many other inflammatory rheumatologic conditions, including RA, in other autoimmune disorders, in some infectious diseases, and occasionally in healthy individuals. Finally, indirect immunofluorescence allows for the recognition of "ANA" patterns (homogeneous, speckled, peripheral, and nucleolar pattern). These patterns may vary with the dilution of the serum. Homogeneous patterns can be observed with sera from all kinds of connective tissue diseases. The speckled pattern is observed when the sera contain antibodies to Sm, RNP, Ro/SSA, and/or La/SSB (see below and p. 110ff.); the peripheral ("rim") pattern is found with sera containing anti-ds-DNA antibodies; and the nucleolar pattern is only very rarely seen in SLE. Determination of the patterns is less helpful than definition of ANA subspecificities.

Once ANAs have been detected, analysis of their *specificity* should be attempted. In this respect, sera should be screened for the presence of antibodies to ds-DNA, antibodies to ss-DNA, and precipitating antibodies to nuclear subsets (Ro/SS-A, La/SS-B, Sm, n-RNP, etc.), as well as antibodies to histones.

Antibodies to ds-DNA as determined by radioimmunoassay or indirect immunofluorescence employing *Crithidia luciliae* occur in up to 90% of the patients with SLE, but only very rarely in other diseases. Thus, determination of anti-ds-DNA antibodies represents a powerful diagnostic tool for SLE. These antibodies have been demonstrated to participate in the formation of circulating and deposited immune complexes [77], and their presence, amount, and avidity correlates well with kidney involvement [70—72, 74, 75, 81]. Titers of anti-ds-DNA usually reflect the clinical activity of the disease [70—72, 101]. The absence of anti-ds-DNA antibodies, however, does not exclude the diagnosis of SLE, especially if other antinuclear autoantibody subsets are present.

Antibodies to ss-DNA have little diagnostic power. They occur in sizeable proportions of patients with different types of connective tissue diseases. Nevertheless, determination of these antibodies by radioimmunoassay (or hemagglutination) should be routinely performed in the patients, since their absence in a patient with suspected SLE makes this diagnosis highly unlikely (unless the disease has been quiescent for a long time).

Determination of antibodies to other *nuclear subsets* is an important addition to the serologic test profile obtainable nowadays. Anti-Sm antibodies, although not as sensitive as anti-ds-DNA, are quite specific for SLE. Anti-Ro/SSA antibodies allowed for the detection and definition of SLE disease subgroups, and anti-RNP antibodies appear to be associated with a favorable prognosis. Details on the molecular biology, immunobiology, and clinical importance of these autoantibodies are presented on pp. 105—123.

184 J. S. Smolen

Other Autoantibodies

Aside from ANAs and their subsets, other autoantibodies can be found in SLE. Thus, rheumatoid factor (RF) occurs in up to 30% of the patients, albeit usually in much lower titers than in RA. Moreover, the presence of RF does not correlate with severity of arthritic disease in SLE (unpublished observations). Anti-leukocyte antibodies can be found in patients with leukopenia, antineuronal antibodies in patients with CNS lupus, and anti-red cell antibodies in patients with associated hemolytic anemia. A list of autoantibody specificities observed in SLE is provided in Table 2. It should be kept in mind in this context that the number of epitope specificities involved is much smaller than would appear from this table, since many of these specificities are shared and there is cross-reactivity of the autoantibodies ([102, 103] and pp. 88—104).

Immune Complexes

Immune complexes can be analyzed with several methods; most reliable are the solid-phase C1q assay, the C1q binding assay, and the Raji cell assay [104]. Immune complex levels tend to reflect disease activity; however, increased levels can be observed for prolonged periods even after institution of vigorous therapy and clinical improvement [105]. Since SLE is the prototype immune complex disease and since most of the tissue injuries are due to immune complex deposition, determination of immune complexes is a good serologic tool for follow-up. Nevertheless, presence of immune complexes is by no means of diagnostic val-

Table 2. Autoantibody specificities observed in SLE

a) *Antibodies to nuclear antigens*
   DNA: ds-DNA, ss-DNA, Z-DNA
   Histones
   Small nuclear ribonucleoproteins ("snurps"): Sm, n-RNP, Ro/SSA, La/SSB
   Other: proliferating cell nuclear antigen (PCNA), Sjögren/Lupus antigen (SL), MA antigen, undefined antigens

b) *Antibodies to cytoplasmic antigens*
   RNA: single-stranded RNA, t-RNA, ribosomal ribonucleoprotein (r-RNP), undefined antigens
   Microsomes (thyroid)

c) *Antibodies to cell membrane-associated antigens*
   Erythrocytes, granulocytes, lymphocytes (helper and suppressor T cells, B cells, NK cells, monocytes, lymphoblasts), thrombocytes, neurons and glial cells, trophoblastic antigens, β_2-microglobulin, HLA antigens, Ia antigens

d) *Antibodies to soluble and other non-cellmembrane-associated proteins*
   Immunoglobulin (rheumatoid factor), collagen (types I—III), tubular basement membrane (very rare), phospholipids (anticoagulant, anticardiolipin, false-positive test for syphilis), thyroglobulin

For references see pp. 88 ff. and 105 ff. and [111]

ue, since they can occur in a large number of disorders, including infectious and neoplastic diseases. In SLE, immune complexes may contain nuclear antigens, such as DNA, Ro/SSA [77, 78, 106], and probably others as well.

Complement

Analysis of total hemolytic complement (CH50) or complement compoments (especially C3 and C4) reveals reduced values (as a consequence of activation by immune complexes) in active SLE. In very active disease, complement measurements may reveal very low levels. A CH50 of 0 may be due to a congenital complement deficiency (usually C2 deficiency, but C4 or C1q deficiency are also possible in association with SLE). Further details are given on pp. 124—144.

Miscellaneous

Electrophoresis may reveal polyclonal hypergammaglobulinemia, but α- and β-globulins are usually within the normal range unless there is infection or nephrotic syndrome. Hypergammaglobulinemia, which may vary with disease activity, is reflected by increased immunoglobulin levels, which often include high levels of IgA. C-reactive protein (CRP) is only mildly elevated in active SLE; however, in the course of infections its levels are more consistently raised; thus CRP determination may potentially serve as a helpful differentiating tool [107, 108].

Diagnostic Assessment

In patients with suspected SLE, the initial laboratory studies should be ANA and complement levels. If one or both of these tests reveal results compatible with the diagnosis, further clinical and laboratory investigations should follow. The latter should include anti-ds-DNA antibodies, precipitating antibodies to nuclear subsets (RNA-protein antigens), determination of other autoantibodies (e.g., rheumatoid factor, antierythrocyte antibodies) and immune complexes. Regular control of most of these measures (especially anti-DNA antibodies, complement levels, and immune complexes), in addition to routine laboratory examinations, should be performed at intervals (weekly to every 3 months) which depend upon the state of disease activity.

The clinical analyses should attempt to assess the whole spectrum of organ involvement in an individual patient. This is important for three reasons: (a) as a prognostic and therapeutic guide; (b) to uncover subclinical manifestations that may require specific therapy; and (c) to obtain a basis for comparison and differential diagnosis when future flares or other complications (e.g., infections, side-effects of drugs) occur.

186 J. S. Smolen

Table 3. Revised criteria for the classification of SLE (1982)[a] [109]

Criterion	Definition
1. Malar rash	Fixed erythema, flat or raised, over the malar eminences, tending to spare the nasolabial folds
2. Discoid rash	Erythematous raised patches with adherent keratotic scaling and follicular plugging; atrophic scarring may occur in older lesions
3. Photosensitivity	Skin rash as a result of unusual reaction to sunlight, by patient history or physician observation
4. Oral ulcers	Oral or nasopharyngeal ulceration, usually painless, observed by a physician
5. Arthritis	Nonerosive arthritis involving 2 or more peripheral joints, characterized by tenderness, swelling, or effusion
6. Serositis	a) Pleuritis — convincing history of pleuritic pain or rub heard by a physician or evidence of pleural effusion *OR* b) Pericarditis — documented by ECG or rub or evidence of pericardial effusion
7. Renal disorder	a) Persistent proteinuria greater than 0.5 g per day or greater than 3+ if quantitation not performed *OR* b) Cellular casts — may be red cell, hemoglobin, granular, tubular, or mixed
8. Neurologic disorder	a) Seizures — in the absence of offending drugs or known metabolic derangements; e.g., uremia, ketoacidosis, or electrolyte imbalance *OR* b) Psychosis — in the absence of offending drugs or known metabolic derangements, e.g., uremia, ketoacidosis, or electrolyte imbalance
9. Hematologic disorder	a) Hemolytic anemia — with reticulocytosis *OR* b) Leukopenia—less than $4000/mm^3$ total on 2 or more occasions *OR* c) Lymphopenia — less than $1500/mm^3$ on 2 or more occasions *OR* d) Thrombocytopenia — less than $100\,000/mm^3$ in the absence of offending drugs
10. Immunologic disorder	a) Positive LE cell preparation *OR* b) Anti-DNA: antibody to native DNA in abnormal titer *OR* c) Anti-Sm: presence of antibody to Sm nuclear antigen *OR* d) False positive serologic test for syphilis known to be positive for at least 6 months and confirmed by *Treponema pallidum* immobilization or fluorescent treponemal antibody absorption test
11. Antinuclear antibody	An abnormal titer of antinuclear antibody by immunofluorescence or an equivalent assay at any point in time and in the absence of drugs known to be associated with "drug-induced lupus" syndrome

[a] The proposed classification is based on 11 criteria. For the purpose of identifying patients in clinical studies, a person shall be said to have systemic lupus erythematosus if any 4 or more of the 11 criteria are present, serially or simultaneously, during any interval of observation.

Clinical and Serologic Features 187

Table 4. Preliminary criteria for the classification of SLE (1971) [110]

Manifestation

1. Facial erythema (butterfly rash). Diffuse erythema, flat or raised, over the malar eminence(s) and/or bridge of the nose; may be unilateral.
2. Discoid lupus. Erythematous raised patches with adherent keratotic scaling and follicular plugging; atrophic scarring may occur in older lesions; may be present anywhere on the body.
3. Raynaud's phenomenon. Requires a two-phase color reaction, by patient's history or physician's observation.
4. Alopecia. Rapid loss of large amount of the scalp hair, by patient's history or physician's observation.
5. Photosensitivity. Unusual skin reaction from exposure to sunlight, by patient's history or physician's observation.
6. Oral or nasopharyngeal ulceration.
7. Arthritis without deformity. One or more peripheral joints involved with any of the following in the absence of deformity: (a) Pain on motion. (b) Tenderness. (c) Effusion or periarticular soft tissue swelling (peripheral joints are defined for this purpose as feet, ankles, knees, hips, shoulders, elbows, wrists, metacarpophalangeal, proximal interphalangeal, terminal interphalangeal, and temporomandibular joints).
8. LE cells. Two or more classic LE cells seen on one occasion or one cell seen on two or more occasions, using an accepted published method.
9. Chronic false-positive STS. Known to be present for at least 6 months and confirmed by TPI or Reiter's tests.
10. Profuse proteinuria. Greater than 3.5 g per day.
11. Cellular casts. May be red cell, hemoglobin, granular, tubular, or mixed.
12. One or both of the following: (a) Pleuritis, good history of pleuritic pain; or rub heard by a physician; or X-ray evidence of both pleural thickening and fluid. (b) Pericarditis, documented by EKG or rub.
13. One or both of the following: (a) Psychosis. (b) Convulsions, by patient's history or physician's observation in the absence of uremia and offending drugs.
14. One or more of the following: (a) Hemolytic anemia. (b) Leukopenia. WBC less than 4000 per cubic millimeter on two or more occasions. (c) Thrombocytopenia, platelet count less than 100000 per cubic millimeter

"A person shall be said to have systemic LE if any 4 or more of the above 14 manifestations are present, serially or simultaneously, during any period of observation."

The American Rheumatism Association (ARA) has recently revised the criteria for the classification of SLE ([109]; Table 3). These revised criteria weight the serologic advances made since the original preliminary criteria ([110]; Table 4) were described. Thus, two clinical and two serologic criteria or three clinical and one serologic criterion now allow for the classification of a rheumatic disorder as SLE. Nevertheless, the revised ARA criteria do not include all possible clinical features of SLE (because of their insensitivity in differentiating SLE from other diseases); in particular, the features "Raynaud's phenomenon" and "alopecia," which commonly occur in SLE, have now been omitted. Thus, occasional patients who meet no or only one or two clinical "revised" ARA criteria (but who may have other features compatible with SLE) should, in our opinion, still be suspected of suffering from SLE, especially if anti-DNA and/or anti-Sm antibodies are present. These patients may acquire additional features in the

188 J. S. Smolen

course of their disease and should be carefully monitored with regard to the development of SLE or other rheumatic diseases. However, they will only rarely require vigorous therapy during this observation period.

Assessment of Disease Activity and Severity

A final important question relates to the definition of disease activity in SLE. Clinically active disease has been associated with high levels of anti-DNA antibodies and low complement levels. However, the reverse does not always hold true, i.e., patients with high titers of anti-DNA antibodies and hypocomplementemia may have clinically quiescent disease or only minor disease manifestations and do not necessarily require therapeutic changes. Since vigorous therapy (which includes the use of corticosteroids) can be associated with profound side-effects and since we should attempt to treat disease and not serologic abnormalities, such patients should be carefully monitored clinically and serologically on a short-term basis. New therapeutic regimens should be instituted only if warranted by the clinical situation or by detailed knowledge of the patient's past disease history, such as the occurrence of major clinical exacerbations shortly after deterioration of serologic parameters.

Thus, especially with regard to the therapeutic approach to SLE and the management of SLE patients, the use of an activity or severity index seems necessary. There has not been widespread application of such indices. The reason is that an index would have to reflect overall disease activity (or severity), but should not lead to underestimation of the state of a single, albeit vital, organ. Thus, different clinical features ought to be differently weighted (e.g., renal involvement more than arthritis).

At present, different authors tend to define their own activity indices on the basis of the ARA criteria or by attempting to include "well accepted" signs of disease activity (fever, CNS involvement, nephritis, arthritis, pleuritis, anti-DNA and complement levels, etc.) [e.g., 70, 79—81, 86, 99, 101, 104—110]. But what is "severe" proteinuria to to one physician may be "mild" proteinuria to an other (where is the borderline?), and what is "arthritis" to one may be "arthralgia" to an other, and so forth. In order to obviate such differences in perception, we have recently started to employ a weighted SLE activity index scoring system which is shown in Table 5.

Obviously, even a weighted scoring system may have its limitations when applied to a disease like SLE since many of its symptoms require exclusion of other causes: Is pleuritis due to the underlying disease, to an infection, or to pulmonary infarction? Is an organic brain syndrome due to SLE or to corticosteroids? Is fever due to a flare of the disease or a consequence of an infection? Does an increased creatinine level reflect lupus kidney involvement or is it a side-effect of nonsteroidal anti-inflammatory agents? These few of many possible examples indicate that (rather than making life easier) a scoring system, just like the care of the individual patient with SLE, represents a challenge to the

Clinical and Serologic Features **189**

Table 5. Preliminary SLE activity index scoring system[a]

Clinical		Laboratory	
1. Fatigue	1	22. Sed. rate 25—50 mm/h	1
2. Temperature $> 38\,^{\circ}$C	1	Sed. rate > 50 mm/h	2
3. Arthralgia	1	23. DNA binding $< 50\%$	1
4. Arthritis (joint effusion)	1	DNA binding $> 50\%$	2
5. Myalgia	1	24. CH50 80—150 U/ml	1
6. Muscle weakness	2	CH50 < 80 U/ml	2
7. Serositis — pain	1	25. CPK > 100/aldolase > 10 U/ml	2
8. Serositis — friction Rub/X-ray/Sono	2	26. LE anticoagulant	1
9. Vasculitis — minor[b]	1	27. Proteinuria/24 h < 1.5 g	1
10. Vasculitis — major[c]	3	Proteinuria/24 h > 1.5 g	2
11. Bullous skin lesions	3	28. 5—15 RBC or 1—3 casts/HPF	1
12. Active LE rash	1	> 15 RBC or > 3 casts/HPF	2
13. Active alopecia	1	29. Hemolytic anemia (> 8 g Hb)	1
14. Mucosal ulcers	1	Hemolytic anemia (< 8 g Hb)	2
15. CNS — minor[d]	2	30. Thrombopenia (40—100000)	1
16. CNS — major[e]	3	Thrombopenia (< 40000)	2
17. Cranial nerve palsy	2	31. Neutropenia (< 3000)	1
18. Blood pressure $> 150/90$	1	32. Lymphopenia (< 1000)	1
19. Lymphadenopathy	1		
20. Noninfectious pulmonary infiltrates	3		
21. Active thromboembolic event	1		
Maximal	33	Maximal	19

Total SLE index score: _____ (maximum: 52)

Physician's assessment of activity: _____

          0 1 2 3 4 5 6 7 8 9 10

          none   severe

Working hypothesis for SLE index score (SIS):
SIS 0—4: inactive disease
SIS 5—8: mildly active disease $(+)^{f}$
SIS 9—12: moderately active disease $(+ +)^{f}$
SIS 13—15: active disease $(+ + +)$
SIS > 15: very active disease $(+ + + +)$

[a] The selection of features is partly based upon an activity index designed at the Arthritis Branch, NIADDK, NIH, by Drs. J. Decker, J. Klippel, P. Plotz, A. Steinberg, and J. Balow. Selection of other clinical and laboratory features is partly based upon an index designed at the Arthritis Branch by Drs. H. Smith, J. Smolen, and A. Steinberg
[b] Raynaud's phenomenon, periungual infarcts, purpura
[c] Ulcerations, cytoid bodies, mononeuritis
[d] Confusion, depression, organic brain syndrome
[e] Stupor, coma, seizures, cerebrovascular accident
[f] There will virtually never be very active manifestations in vital organs without concomitant involvement of other organ systems and/or abnormal laboratory findings

physician and requires his whole attention and differential diagnostic as well as combinatory capabilities. Even then, it has to be admitted that it is inconceivable that an activity index will be helpful in determining the "correct" therapeutic

Table 6. Diagnostic and differential diagnostic assessment in SLE

	Clinical evaluation	Laboratory tests
General	Consultation of specialists (e.g. dermatologist, neurologist, etc.)	Routine laboratory evaluation (CBC, blood chemistry, electrophoresis, urinanalysis coagulation tests); ANA, anti-ds-DNA, anti-ss-DNA, anti-Sm, anti-RNP, anti-Ro/SSA, anti-La/SSB, LE cells, C3, C4, CH50, IgG, IgA, IgM, CRP, VDRL
Joints	X-ray, radionuclide joint scanning	RF
Muscle	Electromyography, biopsy	CPK, aldolase, creatinuria
Skin	Biopsy of lesional and nonlesional skin	
Vasculitis	Acral thermometry, phlebography, arteriography, nerve conduction time, biopsy	Occult blood in stool
Cardiac	Chest X-ray, EKG, echocardiography, coronary angiography, pericardiocentesis	
Pulmonary	Chest X-ray, lung function test, thoracocentesis, lung biopsy	Sputum cultures and stains, analysis of pleural fluid, blood gas analysis
Hematologic	Bone marrow aspirate	Coombs' test, occult blood in stool, ferritin, antileukocyte antibodies, clotting tests, haptoglobin
Gastrointestinal	Endoscopy, large and small bowel series, sonography, liver biopsy	Test for occult blood, antibodies to mitochondria and smooth muscle, amylase, lipase
Lymph nodes	Biopsy	
Ocular	Funduscopy, Schirmer's test	
Renal	Sonography, radionuclide imaging, (pyelography), biopsy	24-h urinary protein excretion, urinary protein electrophoresis, blood gases
Neuropsychiatric	Brain scan, ECHO-flow, funduscopy, nerve conduction time, psychological testing, lumbar puncture, CT scan, NMR	CSF analyses including C4, anti-DNA, antineuronal ab

approach, since this will still depend upon the type and degree of organ involvement (see pp. 300–343). However, a unified activity score may be of some help in the assessment of therapeutic responses or with regard to the imminence of a flare, and, more importantly, it may allow for better comparison between individual patients and improved exchange of experience between individual physicians and centers.

Finally, the term disease "activity" is not necessarily synonymous with disease "severity." Often, activity and severity go hand in hand; however, there are exceptions: A patient with impaired renal function as a consequence of lupus nephritis suffers from severe disease although his nephritis may be inactive at the time of assessment; pulmonary fibrosis as a consequence of lupus pneumonitis represents severe organ damage, but the patient may already have quiescent disease after appropriate therapy; a patient who has had life-threatening CNS involvement in the past but has never again experienced CNS symptoms will still be regarded as having severe SLE; etc. Thus, whereas activity describes the patient's actual condition, severity reflects the overall state (past and present) of the patient, primarily taking into account the degree of involvement of vital organs. This should be kept in mind when comparing individual patients or groups of patients with SLE.

Summary

Successful management of SLE disease depends upon optimal evaluation of involvement of the patient's organs and continuous clinical and serologic monitoring. Table 6 summarizes potentially necessary investigations in SLE patients. It is not meant to imply that all these examinations ought to be performed in every patient with SLE. Rather, they should be selectively applied according to their necessity in assessing an individual patient's disease. Detailed past history, physical examination, the results of a few initial tests, and consultation of other specialists will indicate such necessities.

The patient should be informed about the disease and told that successful management depends greatly upon compliance with therapy, keeping appointments for control examinations, and submitting reports of physical or psychological changes. If these preconditions are fulfilled, the way is paved for optimal management of SLE.

References

1. Hochberg MC (1985) The incidence of systemic lupus erythematosus in Baltimore, Maryland, 1970–1977. Arthritis Rheum 28:80–86
2. Fessel EJ (1974) Systemic lupus erythematosus in the community: incidence, prevalence, outcome and first symptoms; the high prevalence in black women. Arch Intern Med 134:1027–1035

3. Hardin JA, Rahn DR, Shen C, Lerner EM, Steitz JA (1982) Antibodies from patients with connective tissue diseases bind specific subsets of cellular RNA-protein particles. J Clin Invest 70:141–147
4. Alarcon-Segovia D, Lloerente L, Fishbein E, Diaz-Jouanen E (1982) Abnormalities in the content of nucleic acids of peripheral blood mononuclear cells from patients with systemic lupus erythematosus: relationship to DNA-antibodies. Arthritis Rheum 25:304–317
5. Cochrane CG, Hawkins D (1968) Studies on circulating immune complexes. III. Factors governing the ability of circulating immune complexes to localize in blood vessels. J Exp Med 127:137
6. Winfield JB, Faiferman I, Koffler D (1977) Avidity of anti-DNA antibodies in serum and IgG glomerular eluates from patients with systemic lupus erythematosus. Association of high-avidity anti-native DNA antibody with glomerulonephritis. J Clin Invest 59:90
7. Aarden L, Lakmaker F, DeGroot E, Feltkamp TEW (1979) Avidity of antibodies to DNA in relation to SLE. Behring Institute Mitteilungen 64. Die Medizinische Verlagsgesellschaft mbH, Marburg
8. Johnson KJ, Ward PA (1982) Biology of disease: newer concepts in the pathogenesis of immune complex-induced tissue injury. Lab Invest 17:218–226
9. Becker LC (1973) Allergy in systemic lupus erythematosus. Johns Hopkins Med J 133:38
10. Dubois EL, Tuffanelli DL (1964) Clinical manifestations of systemic lupus erythematosus. Computer analysis of 520 cases. JAMA 190:104–111
11. Ropes MW (1976) Systemic lupus erythematosus. Harvard University Press, Cambridge
12. Louis PA, Lambert PH (1979) Lipopolysaccharides: from immune stimulation to autoimmunity. Springer Semin Immunopathol 2:215–228
13. Alarcon-Segovia D (1975) Drug-induced systemic lupus erythematosus and related syndromes. Clin Rheum Dis 1:573
14. Smolen JS, Steinberg AD (1981) Systemic lupus erythematosus and pregnancy: clinical, immunological, and theoretical aspects. Prog Biol Res 67:283–302
15. Fischman AS, Abeles M, Zanetti M, Weinstein A, Rothfield NF (1981) The coexistence of rheumatoid arthritis and systemic lupus erythematosus: a case report and review of the literature. J Rheumatol 8:405–415
16. Tsokos GC, Moutsopoulos HM, Steinberg AD (1981) Muscle involvement in systemic lupus erythematosus. JAMA 246:766–768
16a. Sibrans DF, Holley HL (1967) Vacuolar myopathy in a patient with a positive LE cell preparation. Arthritis Rheum 10:141–146
17. Tan EM, Cohen AS, Fries JF, Masi AT, McShane DJ, Rothfield NF, Schaller JG, Talal N, Winchester RJ (1982) The 1982 revised criteria for the classification of systemic lupus erythematosus. Arthritis Rheum 25:1271–1277
18. Much JR, Herbst KD, Rapaport SI (1980) Thrombosis in patients with lupus anticoagulant. Ann Intern Med 92:156–159
18a. Lechner K, Pabinger-Fasching I. (1985) Lupus anticoagulants and thrombosis. A study of 25 cases and review of the literature. Hemostasis 15:254–262
19. Carreras LO, Defreyn G, Machin SJ, Vermylen J, Deman R, Spitz B, Asche AV (1981) Arterial thrombosis, intrauterine death and "lupus" anticoagulant: detection of immunoglobulin interfering with prostacyclin formation. Lancet 1:244–246
20. Budman DR, Steinberg AD (1976) Hypertension and renal disease in systemic lupus erythematosus. Arch Intern Med 136:1003–1007
21. Steinberg AD (1985) Management of systemic lupus erythematosus. In: Kelley WN, Harris ED, Ruddy S, Sledge CB (eds) Textbook of rheumatology, 2nd edn. Saunders, Philadelphia, pp 1098–1115
22. Haider YS, Roberts WC (1981) Coronary arterial disease in systemic lupus erythematosus: quantification of degrees of narrowing in 22 necropsy patients (21 women) aged 16 to 37 years. Am J Med 70:755–781
23. Korbet SM, Schwartz MM, Lewis EJ (1984) Immune complex deposition and coronary vasculitis in systemic lupus erythematosus. Report of two cases. Am J Med 77:141–146
24. Hosenpude JD, Montanaro A, Hart MV, Haines JE, Specht HD, Bennett RM, Kloster FE (1984) Myocardial perfusion abnormalities in asymptomatic patients with systemic lupus erythematosus. Am J Med 77:286–292

25. Bulkley BH, Roberts WC (1975) The heart in systemic lupus erythematosus and the changes induced in it by corticosteroid therapy. Am J Med 58:243–264
26. Matthay RA, Schwarz MI, Petty TL, Stanford RE, Gupta RC, Sahn SA, Steigerwald JC (1975) Pulmonary manifestations of systemic lupus erythematosus: a review of 12 cases of acute pneumonitis. Medicine (Baltimore) 54:347–409
27. Haupt HM, Moore GW, Hutchins GM (1981) The lung in systemic lupus erythematosus: analysis of the pathologic changes in 120 patients. Am J Med 71:791–798
28. Eisenberg H, Dubois EL, Sherwin RP, Balchum OJ (1973) Diffuse interstitial lung disease in systemic lupus erythematosus. Ann Intern Med 79:37–45
29. Huang CT, Hennigar GR, Lyons HA (1965) Pulmonary dysfunction in systemic lupus erythematosus. N Engl J Med 272:288–293
30. Scherak O, Hofner W, Haber P, Kummer F, Kolarz G, Seidl G (1979) Zur Diagnose und Differentialdiagnose pulmonaler Manifestationen bei Kollagenosen. Prax Pneumol 33:1168–1177
31. Gross M, Easterly JR, Earle RH (1972) Pulmonary alterations in systemic lupus erythematosus. Am Rev Respir Dis 105:572–577
32. Budman DR, Steinberg AD (1977) Hematologic aspects of systemic lupus erythematosus. Ann Intern Med 86:220–229
33. Fearon DT (1980) Identification of the membrane glycoprotein that is the C3b receptor of the human erythrocyte, polymorphonuclear leukocyte, B lymphocyte and monocyte. J Exp Med 152:20–30
34. Iida K, Mornaghi R, Nussenzweig V (1982) Complement receptor (CR1) deficiency in erythrocytes from patients with systemic lupus erythematosus. J Exp Med 155:1427–1438
35. Abramson SB, Given WP, Edelson HS, Weissmann G (1983) Neutrophil aggregation induced by sera from patients with active systemic lupus erythematosus. Arthritis Rheum 26:630–636
36. Okudaira K, Nakai H, Hayakawa T, Kashiwado T, Tanimoto K, Horiuchi Y, Tuji T (1979) Detection of antilymphocyte antibody with two-color method and its heterogeneous specificities against human T cell subsets. J Clin Invest 64:1213
37. Winfield JB, Cohen PL, Litvin DA (1982) Antibodies to activated T cells and their soluble products in systemic lupus erythematosus. Arthritis Rheum 25:814–819
38. Rabinowitz Y, Dameshek W (1960) Systemic lupus erythematosus after "idiopathic" thrombocytopenic purpura: a review. Ann Intern Med 52:1–28
38a. Dixit R, Krieg AM, Atkinson JP (1985) Thrombotic thrombocytopenic purpura developing during pregnancy in a C2-deficient patient with a history of systemic lupus erythematosus. Arthritis Rheum 28:341–344
38b. Hughes GRV (1983) Thrombosis, abortion, cerebral disease, and the lupus anticoagulant. Br Med J 287:1088–1089
39. Whaley K, Alspaugh MA (1985) Sjögren's syndrome. In: Kelley WN, Harris ED, Ruddy S, Sledge CB (eds) Textbook of rheumatology. Saunders, Philadelphia, pp 956–978
40. Miller MH, Urowitz MB, Gladman DD, Blendis LM (1984) The liver in systemic lupus erythematosus. Q J Med 211:401–409
41. Rothfield N (1981) Clinical features of systemic lupus erythematosus. In: Kelley WN, Harris ED, Ruddy S, Sledge CB (eds) Textbook of rheumatology. Saunders, Philadelphia, p 1119
42. Green JA, Dawson AA, Walker W (1978) Systemic lupus erythematosus and lymphoma. Lancet 2:753–758
43. Agudelo CA, Schumacher HR, Glick JH, Molina J (1981) Non-Hodgkin's lymphoma in systemic lupus erythematosus. Report of 4 cases with ultrastructural studies in 2. J Rheumatol 8:69–78
44. Butler RC, Thomas SM, Thompson JM, Keat ACS (1984) Anaplastic myeloma in systemic lupus erythematosus. Ann Rheum Dis 43:653–655
45. Steven MM, Westedt ML, Eulderink F, Hazevoet HM, Dijkman JH, Cats A (1984) Systemic lupus erythematosus and invasive thymoma: report of two cases. Ann Rheum Dis 43:825–828
46. Symmons DPM (1985) Neoplasms of the immune system in rheumatoid arthritis. Am J Med 78[Suppl 1A]:22–28

47. Talal N, Bunim JJ (1964) The development of malignant lymphoma in the course of Sjögren's syndrome. Am J Med 36:529—540
48. Zulman J, Jaffe R, Talal N (1978) Evidence that the malignant lymphoma of Sjögren's syndrome is a monoclonal B-cell neoplasm. N Engl J Med 229:1215—1220
49. Andrews BS, Eisenberg RA, Theofilopoulos AN, Izui S, Wilson CB, McConahey PJ, Murphy ED, Roths JB, Dixon FJ (1978) Spontaneous lupus-like syndromes. Clinical and immunopathological manifestations in several strains. J Exp Med 148:1198—1215
50. Kinlen LJ, Sheil AGR, Peto J, Doll R (1979) A collaborative UK—Australasian study of cancer in patients treated with immunosuppressive drugs. Br Med J 2:1461
51. Prior P (1985) Cancer and rheumatoid arthritis: epidemiologic considerations. Am J Med 78[Suppl 1A]:15—21
52. Canoso JJ, Cohen AS (1974) Malignancy in a series of 70 patients with systemic lupus erythematosus. Arthritis Rheum 17:383—388
53. Lewis RB, Castor CW, Kinsley RE, Bole GG (1976) Frequency of neoplasia in systemic lupus erythematosus and rheumatoid arthritis. Arthritis Rheum 19:1256—1260
54. Forster G, Moeschlin S (1954) Extramedulläres leukämisches Plasmocytom mit Dysproteinämie und erworbener hämolytischer Anämie. Schweiz Med Wochenschr 84:1106—1110
55. Cullen MH, Stansfeld AG, Oliver RTD, Lister TA, Malpas JS (1979) Angioimmunoblastic lymphadenopathy: report of ten cases and review of literature. Q J Med 48:151—176
56. Steinberg AD, Smith HR, Laskin CA, Steinberg BJ, Smolen JS (1982) Studies of immune abnormalities in systemic lupus erythematosus. Am J Kidney Dis 2[Suppl 1]:101—110
57. Mackay IR, Goldstein G, McConchie IH (1963) Thymectomy in systemic lupus erythematosus. Br Med J 2:792
58. Milne JA, Anderson JR, MacSween RN, Fraser K, Short I, Stevens J, Shaw GB, Tankel HI (1967) Thymectomy in acute systemic lupus erythematosus and rheumatoid arthritis. Br Med J 1:461
59. Makela TE, Ruosteenoja R, Wager O, Wallgren GR, Jokinen EJ (1964) Myasthenia gravis and systemic lupus erythematosus. Acta Med Scand 175:777
60. Chan MK, Britton M (1980) Comparative clinical features in patients with myasthenia gravis with systemic lupus erythematosus. J Rheumatol 7:838—842
61. Alarcon-Segovia D, Galbraith RF, Maldonado JE, Howard FM (1963) Systemic lupus erythematosus following thymectomy for myasthenia gravis. Lancet 2:662
62. Klippel JH (1980) Sjögren's syndrome and systemic lupus erythematosus, pp 217—219. In: Moutsopoulos HM (moderator) (1980) Sjögren's syndrome (sicca syndrome): current issues. Ann Intern Med 92:212—226
63. Mahajan SK, Ordonez NG, Feitelsen PJ, Lim KS, Spargo BH, Katz AI (1977) Lupus nephropathy without clinical renal involvement. Medicine (Baltimore) 56:493—501
64. Fries JF, Porta J, Liang MH (1978) Marginal benefit of renal biopsy in systemic lupus erythematosus. Arch Intern Med 138:1386—1389
65. Lee HS, Mujais SK, Kasinath BS, Spargo BH, Katz AI (1984) Course of renal pathology in patients with systemic lupus erythematosus. Am J Med 77:612—620
66. Appel GB, Silva FG, Pirani CL, Meltzer JI, Estes D (1978) Renal involvement in systemic lupus erythematosus (SLE): a study of 56 patients emphasizing histologic classification. Medicine 57:371—410
67. Baldwin DS, Gluck MC, Lowenstein J, Gallo GR (1977) Lupus nephritis. Clinical course as related to morphologic forms and their transitions. Am J Med 62:12—30
68. Morel-Maroger L, Mery JPH, Droz D, Godin M, Verroust P, Kourilsky O, Richet G (1976) The course of lupus nephritis: contribution of serial renal biopsies. Adv Nephrol 6:79
69. Balow JE (1979) Clinicopathologic correlations in lupus nephritis. In: Decker JL (moderator) Systemic lupus erythematosus: evolving concepts. Ann Intern Med 91:587—604
70. Schur PH, Sandsor J (1968) Immunologic factors and clinical activity in systemic lupus erythematosus. N Engl J Med 278:533—538
71. Tron F, Bach JF (1977) Relationships between antibodies to native DNA and glomerulonephritis in systemic lupus erythematosus. Clin Exp Immunol 28:426—432
72. Hecht B, Siegel NJ, Adler M, Kashgarian M, Hayslett JP (1976) Prognostic indices in lupus nephropathy. Medicine (Baltimore) 55:163—181

Clinical and Serologic Features 195

73. Cameron JS, Lessof MH, Ogg CS, Williams BD, Williams DG (1976) Disease activity in the nephritis of systemic lupus erythematosus in relation to serum complement concentrations, DNA-binding capacity and precipitating anti-DNA antibody. Clin Exp Immunol 25:418—427

74. Leon SA, Green A, Ehrlich GE, Poland M, Shapiro B (1977) Avidity of antibodies in SLE: relationship to severity of renal involvement. Arthritis Rheum 20:23—29

75. Gershwin ME, Steinberg AD (1974) Qualitative characteristics of anti-DNA antibodies in lupus nephritis. Arthritis Rheum 17:947—954

76. Clough JD, Valenzuela R (1980) Relationship of renal histopathology in SLE nephritis to immunoglobulin class of anti-DNA. Am J Med 68:80—85

77. Winfield JB, Faiferman I, Koffler D (1977) Avidity of anti-DNA antibodies in serum and IgG glomerular eluates from patients with systemic lupus erythematosus. Association of high avidity antinative DNA antibody with glomerulonephritis. J Clin Invest 59:90—96

78. Maddison PJ, Reichlin M (1979) Deposition of antibodies to a soluble cytoplasmic antigen in the kidneys of patients with systemic lupus erythematosus. Arthritis Rheum 22:858—863

79. Smolen JS, Chused TM, Leiserson WM, Reeves JP, Alling D, Steinberg AD (1982) Heterogeneity of immunoregulatory T cell subsets in systemic lupus erythematosus. Correlation with clinical features. Am J Med 72:783—790

80. Bakke AC, Kirkland PA, Kitridou RC, Horwitz DA (1983) T lymphocyte subsets in systemic lupus erythematosus. Arthritis Rheum 26:745—750

81. Smolen JS, Morimoto Ch, Steinberg AD, Wolf A, Schlossman SF, Steinberg RT, Penner E, Reinherz E, Reichlin M, Chused TM (1985) Systemic lupus erythematosus: delineation of subpopulations by clinical, serologic, and T cell subset analysis. Am J Med Sci 289:139—146

82. Kimberly RP, Lockshin MD, Sherman RL, Beary JF, Mouradian J, Cheigh JS (1981) "End-stage" lupus nephritis: clinical course to and outcome on dialysis. Medicine 60:277—287

83. Kimberly RP, Lockshin MD, Sherman RL, Mouradian J, Saal S (1983) Reversible "end-stage" lupus nephritis. Analysis of patients able to discontinue dialysis. Am J Med 74:361—368

84. Coplon NS, Diskin CJ, Peterson J, Swenson RS (1983) The long-term clinical course of systemic lupus erythematosus in end-stage renal disease. N Engl J Med 308:186—90

85. Amend WJC, Vincenti F, Feduska NJ, Salvatierra O, Johnston WH, Jackson J, Tilney N, Garovoy M, Burwell EL (1981) Recurrent systemic lupus erythematosus involving renal allografts. Ann Intern Med 94:444—448

86. Kimberly RP, Plotz PH (1977) Aspirin-induced depression of renal function. N Engl J Med 296:418—428

87. Ciabattoni G, Cinotti GA, Pierucci A, Simonetti B, Manzi M, Pugliese F, Barsotti P, Pecci G, Taggi F, Patrono C (1984) Effects of sulindac and ibuprofen in patients with chronic glomerular disease. N Engl J Med 310:279—283

88. Haggie SJ, Fermont DC, Wyllie JH (1976) Treatment of duodenal ulcers with cimetidine. Lancet 1:983—984

89. Brentjens JR, Sepulveda M, Baliah T, Bentzel C, Erlanger BF, Elwood G, Mantes M, Hsu KD, Andres GA (1975) Interstitial immune complex nephritis in patients with systemic lupus erythematosus. Kidney Int 7:342—350

90. Cunningham E, Provost T, Brentjens J, Reichlin M, Venuto RC (1978) Acute renal failure secondary to interstitial lupus nephritis. Arch Intern Med 138:1560—1561

91. Tron F, Ganval D, Droz D (1979) Immunologically-mediated acute renal failure of non-glomerular origin in the course of systemic lupus erythematosus (SLE). Report of two cases. Am J Med 67:529—532

92. Clinicopathologic Conference (1980) Interstitial nephritis in a patient with systemic lupus erythematosus. Am J Med 69:775—781

93. Tu WH, Shearn MA, Lee JC, Hopper J (1968) Interstitial nephritis in Sjögren's syndrome. Ann Intern Med 69:1163—1170

94. Smolen JS, Zielinski CC, Penner E, Syre G, Steinberg AD (1985) Interstitial nephritis with renal tubular acidosis in SLE: A feature of concomitant primary Sjögren's syndrome? Report of 2 cases and review of literature. (Submitted for publication)

95. Moutsopoulos HM, Webber BL, Vlagolopoulos TP, Chused TM, Decker JL (1979) Differences in the clinical manifestations of sicca syndrome in the presence and absence of rheumatoid arthritis. Am J Med 66:733—736
96. Talal N (1985) Sjögren's syndrome and connective tissue disease with other immunologic disorders. In: McCarty DJ (ed) Arthritis and allied conditions, 10th edn. Lea and Febiger, Philadelphia, pp 1037—1051
96b. Lubbe WF, Butler WS, Palmer SJ, Liggins GC (1983) Fetal survival after prednisone suppression of maternal lupus-anticoagulant. Lancet i: 1461—1462
97. Estes D, Christian CL (1971) The natural history of systemic lupus erythematosus by prospective analysis. Medicine (Baltimore) 50:85—95
98. Arnett FC, Shulman LE (1976) Studies in familial systemic lupus erythematosus. Medicine 55:313
99. Lockshin MD, Reinitz E, Druzin ML, Murrman M, Estes D. Lupus pregnancy (1984) Case-control prospective study demonstrating absence of lupus exacerbation during or after pregnancy. Am J Med 77:893—898
100. Lockshin MD, Harpel PC, Druzin ML, Becker CG, Klein RF, Watson RM, Elkon KB, Reinitz E (1985) Lupus pregnancy. II. Unusual pattern of hypocomplementemia and thrombocytopenia in the pregnant patient. Arthritis Rheum 28:58—66
101. Swaak AJG, Aarden LA, Statius van Eps LW, Feltkamp TEW (1979) Anti-dsDNA and complement profiles as prognostic guides in SLE. Arthritis Rheum 22:226
102. Shoenfeld Y, Rauch J, Massicotte H, Datta SK, Andre-Schwartz J, Stollar BD, Schwartz RS. Polyspecificity of monoclonal lupus autoantibodies produced by human—human hybridomas. N Engl J Med 1983; 308:414—20
103. Jacob L, Lety MA, Louvard D, Bach JF (1985) Binding of a monoclonal anti-DNA autoantibody to identical protein(s) present at the surface of several human cell types involved in lupus pathogenesis. J Clin Invest 75:315—17
104. Lambert PH et al. (1978) A WHO collaborative study of the evaluation of eighteen methods for detecting immune complexes in serum. J Clin Lab Immunol 1:1—16
105. Menzel EJ, Smolen JS, Knapp W, Scherak O, Steffen C (1979) Klinische Relevanz zirkulierender Immunkomplexe bei Patienten mit systemischem Lupus erythematodes und chronischer Polyarthritis. Acta Med Austriaca 6:212—214
106. Harbeck RJ, Bardana EJ, Kohler PG, Carr RI (1973) DNA-anti-DNA complexes: their detection in systemic lupus erythematosus sera. J Clin Invest 52:789—795
107. Becker GJ, Waldburger M, Hughes GRV, Pepys MB (1980) Value of C-reactive protein measurements in the investigations of fever in systemic lupus erythematosus. Ann Rheum Dis 39:50—52
108. Bravo MG, Alarcon-Segovia D (1981) C-reactive protein in the differential diagnosis between infection and disease reactivation in SLE. J Rheumatol 8:291—294
109. Tan EM, Cohen AS, Fries JF, Masi AT, McShane DJ, Rothfield NF, Schaller JG, Talal N, Winchester RJ (1982) The 1982 revised criteria for the classification of systemic lupus erythematosus. Arthritis Rheum 25:1271—77
110. Cohen AS, Reynolds WE, Franklin EC, Kulka JP, Ropes MW, Shulam LE, Wallace SL (1971) Preliminary criteria for classification of systemic lupus erythematosus. Bull Rheum Dis 21:643—48
111. Zvaifler NJ, Woods VL (1985) Etiology and pathogenesis of systemic lupus erythematosus. In: Kelley WN, Harris Ed, Ruddy S, Sledge CB (eds) Textbook of rheumatology, 2nd edn. Saunders, Philadelphia, p 1042—1070

Immunologic Similarities and Differences Between Systemic Lupus Erythematosus and Sjögren's Syndrome

H. M. MOUTSOPOULOS

Introduction

Sjögren's syndrome is a chronic autoimmune disorder which primarily affects females and has a diverse clinical spectrum expanding from an organ (exocrine glands) specific autoimmune disorder to systemic (extraglandular) disease and finally to lymphoid neoplasia [1].

The glandular manifestations — xerostomia, xerophthalmia, and recurrent parotid gland enlargement — are mediated through a lymphocytic invasion and subsequent destruction of the glands that leads to diminished or absent secretions and mucosal dryness. Extraglandular disease may result from direct lymphocytic invasion and destruction of nonexocrine tissue or from the deposition of immune complexes. It may affect the lungs, kidneys, muscles, reticuloendothelial organs, nervous system, and/or blood vessels [1]. Despite the involvement of many organs in the extraglandular form of Sjögren's syndrome, none of these patients fulfill the classification criteria for systemic lupus erythematosus (SLE) [1].

Sjögren's syndrome can also be a part of another autoimmune disease, most commonly rheumatoid arthritis (RA) and SLE. Clinical, serologic, and immunogenetic studies have shown similarities and differences between patients with Sjögren's syndrome alone and patients with Sjögren's syndrome and RA, allowing the term "primary" to be applied to patients with Sjögren's syndrome alone and "secondary" to those with Sjögren's syndrome and RA [2, 4]. Careful studies of primary Sjögren's syndrome and Sjögren's syndrome in SLE have not been performed. This review will summarize the immunologic similarities and differences between primary Sjögren's syndrome and SLE, and will compare these with the data available regarding patients with SLE and Sjögren's syndrome.

Incidence of Sjögren's Syndrome in SLE

The overlap of Sjögren's syndrome and SLE has been recognized for many years [5, 6]. Systematic studies evaluating the evidence of Sjögren's syndrome in patients with SLE have revealed histologic or functional impairment of lacrimal

H. M. Moutsopoulos

and salivary glands in one-fourth to all SLE patients studied [6, 7]. In contrast, studies of patients with Sjögren's syndrome have discovered SLE in only 5%—10% of patients examined [8].

Autoantibody Profile

Both Sjögren's syndrome and SLE are characterized by a polyclonal B-lymphocyte hyperreactivity leading to multiple organ- and non-organ-specific autoantibodies and immune complex formation.

Antibodies directed at nuclear antigens and particularly native DNA predominate in SLE, a finding which is observed very rarely or not at all in primary Sjögren's syndrome [1]. In contrast, rheumatoid factors or antibodies against γ-globulins are found more often in patients with primary Sjögren's syndrome than in SLE patients [1].

Antibodies to cellular antigens Ro(SSA) and La(SSB) were initially described as specific antibodies for primary Sjögren's syndrome [4]. Subsequent studies have shown that antibodies to Ro(SSA) are found in many subgroups of SLE patients, namely seronegative lupus, subacute cutaneous lupus, and SLE with Sjögren's syndrome [7, 9, 10]. Antibodies to La(SSB) are found predominantly in primary Sjögren's syndrome as well as in patients with SLE and Sjögren's syndrome. This finding contrasts with the fact that anti-La(SSB) antibodies are rarely present in the sera of patients with rheumatoid arthritis and Sjögren's syndrome [11]. In Table 1 the incidence of these autoantibodies in SLE and primary and secondary Sjögren's syndrome is shown. Assuming that histologic abnormalities in exocrine glands are the most indicative feature if Sjögren's syndrome, these findings imply that Sjögren's syndrome in patients with SLE is, from a serologic standpoint, related to primary Sjögren's syndrome more than Sjögren's syndrome in RA.

A.possible explanation for the serologic similarities of SLE and primary Sjögren's syndrome is the similarity of the HLA antigens in the two diseases [3, 12]. Increased occurrences of HLA-DR3 and B-lymphocyte alloantigen MT-2 are found in both. With the finding of increases in the occurrence of HLA-DR2 in SLE and increases in B-lymphocyte alloantigen MT-1 in primary Sjögren's syn-

Table 1. Incidence of autoantibodies in different autoimmune diseases

Disease	Antibodies (% positive) to			
	ds-DNA	Ig (RF)	Ro (SSA)	La (SSB)
SLE	60—80	10—20	20—30	3— 5
Primary Sjögren's syndrome	0— 5	60—80	40—60	30—50
Sjögren's syndrome and SLE	40—60	20—30	30—40	0—30
Sjögren's syndrome and rheumatoid arthritis	0— 5	60—80	5—15	0— 5

drome, some differences are evident as well. An attractive hypothesis, therefore, is that the presence of one or more of these sicca B-lymphocyte alloantigens (DR3 and MT-2) in a patient with SLE might confer an increased risk for the development of Sjögren's syndrome.

Immunoregulatory Abnormalities

B-lymphocyte Hyperreactivity

The etiology of the B-lymphocyte hyperreactivity observed in the human autoimmune diseases remains obscure. There is evidence from the mouse models of autoimmunity [NZB and (NZB·NZW)F$_1$ hybrid mice] that the B cell hyperreactivity is a polyclonal process [13, 14]. The B cell hyperreactivity is directed against multiple self- and non-self-determinants and cannot be explained solely by the activation of self-reactive clones. Beside the hyperreactivity of B cells, abnormalities of immunoregulatory T cell subpopulations have been shown in murine models, usually in the form of deficiencies of suppressor T cell subsets [15, 16]. Although it was originally believed that B cell hyperreactivity resulted from defective suppressor cell immunoregulation, recent studies have provided evidence that B cell hyperreactivity may be present in murine models from as early as the first week of life, before aberrations of immunoregulatory T cell subsets are evident [14]. This is compatible with the hypothesis that one of the consequences of antilymphocyte antibodies is specific for suppressor cells [17]. Removal of suppressor cells may perpetuate the hyperreactivity of B cells and thus intensify the underlying defect of B cells leading to autoimmunity.

The analogy between the immunologic abnormalities in human SLE and the mouse model is quite clear. There is now ample evidence in SLE that the well recognized B cell hyperreactivity is polyclonal, in that circulating B cells spontaneously secrete antibodies against multiple non-cross-reacting hapten determinants [18]. Further, patients with SLE have deficiencies of subsets of suppressor T cells [19—21] in the face of lymphocytotoxic antibodies directed against T cell subsets with suppressor capability [22, 23]. Additional pathogenetic aspects of SLE are discussed on pp. 6—20. Due to the obvious constraints of the human system in which disease mechanisms are observed only after they develop, it is difficult to ascertain the sequential evolution of the B cell hyperreactivity in relation to the defect in suppressor cell immunoregulation. Nonetheless, the end result is pathologic autoimmunity of a severe degree.

With regard to spontaneous B-lymphocyte hyperreactivity, unlike patients with SLE, patients with primary Sjögren's syndrome do not have increased numbers of circulating or homed in the bone marrow B cells spontaneously secreting polyclonal antibody [24, 25] (Table 2). Thus, the activated B cell in Sjögren's syndrome patients must be homed in other organs such as the exocrine glands or the spleen. In this regard, it has previously been demonstrated that the lympho-

200 H. M. Moutsopoulos

Table 2. Polyclonally activated B cells in the peripheral blood and bone marrow of patients and normal controls

Patients	Direct plaque-forming cells per 10^6 lymphocytes	
	Peripheral blood, anti-TNP	Bone marrow, anti-TNP
Primary Sjögren's syndrome (n = 5)	17± 3.9	14± 5.2
SLE (n = 5)	135±42	145±30
Normal control (n = 7)	4± 1.5	7± 2.4

Table 3. Intracytoplasmic Ig class in patients with primary Sjögren's syndrome, patients with SLE without Sjögren's syndrome, and one healthy volunteer

Patients	Percent of plasma cells staining for				
	κ	λ	μ	γ	α
Primary Sjögren's syndrome (n = 13)	52±5	48±5	14±3	53±7	34±6
SLE (n = 3)	55±5	48±5	6±2	17±6	76±6
Normal control (n = 1)	50	50	5	5	90

cytes infiltrating accessory salivary glands in lip biopsies of Sjögren's syndrome patients synthesize immunoglobulins in a much higher amount than found in normal salivary glands [26]. Furthermore, we have demonstrated that the lip biopsies contain an increased number of plasmacytoid cells. The cells have shifted towrd production of IgG compared with the IgA production in normals, as determined by staining for intracytoplasmic immunoglobulins [27] (Table 3).

These findings contrast with results of B-lymphocyte study in patients with SLE. The activated B cells in lupus patients are circulating in the peripheral blood as well as in the bone marrow [17]. The lack or circulating or homed in the bone marrow activated B cells in Sjögren's syndrome may reflect a more restrictive range of triggering polyclonal B cell activation. Patients with glandular Sjögren's syndrome had levels of pokeweed motogen-induced antisheep erythrocyte plaque-forming cell responses generally within the normal range. Patients with extraglandular disease, however, had markedly suppressed pokeweed mitogen-induced plaque-forming cell responses [24]. The reason for this defect is uncertain. As has been speculated with similar findings in the mouse model [17] and in human SLE [21], however, the refractoriness to in vitro mitogen stimulation may reflect previous ongoing in vivo polyclonal activation of B cells.

Immunoregulatory T Cells

With regard to immunoregulatory T cells, patients with primary Sjögren's syndrome have normal absolute numbers of lymphocytes, T cells, and B cells [24]. In addition, when relative proportions of T cell subsets were examined, there were no significant differences among normal subjects with glandular or extraglandular primary Sjögren's syndrome [24]. When relative proportions of T_G cells (T suppressor) were examined in individual patients, however, a striking difference was noted. Of the seven patients with glandular Sjögren's syndrome, five had proportions of T suppressor cells within the normal range, whereas six of eight patients with extraglandular Sjögren's syndrome had proportions of T suppressor cells that were markedly decreased [24]. This deficiency of T suppressor cells is similar to findings in patients with SLE [19, 28]. Unlike this defect in Sjögren's syndrome, the selective T suppressor defect in SLE was associated with an absolute T-lymphocytopenia and was not reversible by preincubation of T cells or trypsin treatment to remove potential blocking factors of the Fc receptor expression. Although it has been shown that there are heterogeneous types of human suppressor cells in a humber of in vitro systems, the T_G subset has clearly been shown to be the suppressor cell in at least one system of pokeweed mitogen-induced Ig production by human B cells [29].

Because a deficiency of T suppressor cells may be due to an absolute deficiency ot these cells, as in SLE, or alternatively to a blocking of modulation or expression of the Fc receptor by immune complexes [30], we ascertained whether the T suppressor defect in Sjögren's syndrome was reversible. Indeed, trypsinization of T cells before determination of T suppressor proportions resulted in a normalization of the relative proportion of these cells [24]. Further preincubation of normal T cells with sera from patients with Sjögren's syndrome with low T suppressor levels, but not sera from patients with normal T suppressor cells, resulted in reversible blockage of the expression of the T_G Fc receptor [24].

In contrast to patients with SLE [21], patients with Sjögren's syndrome, including those with reversible blockage of expression of T_G Fc receptor, have normal concanavalin A-generated suppressor T cell activity in the pokeweed mitogen-induced antisheep erythrocyte assay [24] (Table 4). In preliminary studies of patients with Sjögren's syndrome in association with SLE, the immunoregulatory abnormalities resemble those in SLE, such as irreversible quantitative deficiency of T_G and defective suppressor cell function. These findings suggest that there is a spectrum of disorders of immunoregulation among diseases that resembles the murine models of autoimmunity. This ranges from the restricted hyperreactivity of B cell function and reversible abnormalities of immunoregulatory T cells seen in Sjögren's syndrome to the irreversible abnormalities of immunoregulatory T cells in SLE. The gradation of immunoregulatory aberrations seems to be directly reflected in the severity of expression of autoimmunity in these diseases.

Table 4. Effect of con-canavalin-A-generated suppressor cells from normal controls and patients on the pokeweed mitogen-induced plaque-forming cell responses of normal allogeneic lymphocytes

Patients	% Suppressor
SLE (n = 15)	5 ± 10
Sjögren's syndrome (n = 9)	76 ± 8
Normal controls (n = 10)	79 ± 10

References

1. Moutsopoulos HM (1980) Sjögren's syndrome (sicca syndrome): current issues. Ann Intern Med 92 (1):212—226
2. Moutsopoulos HM, Webber BL, Vlagopoulos TP, Chused TM and Decker JL (1979) Diferences in the clinical manifestations of sicca syndrome in the presence and absence of rheumatoid arthritis. Am J Med 66:733
3. Moutsopoulos HM, Mann DL, Johnson AH and Chused TM (1979) Genetic differences between primary and secondary sicca syndrome. N Engl J Med 301:761—763
4. Alspaugh MA, Tan EM (1975) Antibodies to cellular antigens in Sjögren's syndrome. J Clin Invest 55:1067—1073
5. Heaton JM (1959) Sjögren's syndrome and systemic lupus erythematosus. Br Med J 1:466—469
6. Alarcon-Segovia D, Ibnez G, Velazquez-Forero F, Hernadez-Ortiz J, Gonzalez-Jimenez Y (1974) Sjögren's syndrome in systemic lupus erythematosus: clinical and subclinical manifestations. Ann Intern Med 81:577—583
7. Moutsopoulos HM, Klippel JH, Pavlidis N, Wolf RO Sweet JB, Steinberg AD, Chu FC, Tarpley TM (1980) Correlative histologic and serologic findings of sicca syndrome in patients with systemic lupus erythematosus. Arthritis Rheum 23 (1):36—40
8. Morgan WS, Castleman B (1953) A clinicopathologic study of "Mikulicz's disease". Am J Pathol 29:471—503
9. Maddison PJ, Provost TT, Reichlin M (1981) Serological findings in patients with "ANA-negative" systemic lupus erythematosus. Medicine (Baltimore) 60:87—94
10. Sontheimer RD, Stasny P, Maddison PJ (1980) Immunological and HLA association in subacute lupus erythematosus (abstract). Clin Res 28:502
11. Alexander EL, Hirsch TJ, Arnett FC, Provost TT, Stevens MD (1982) Ro(SSA) and La(SSB) antibodies in the clinical spectrum of Sjögren's syndrome. J Rheumatol 9:239—246
12. Reinertsen JL, Klippel JH, Johnson AH, Steinberg AD, Decker JL, Mann DL (1979) B-lymphocyte alloantigens assocated with systemic lupus erythematosus. N Engl J Med 299:515—518
13. Cohen PL, Ziff M (1977) Abnormal polyclonal B-cell activation in NZB/NZW F_1 mice. J Immunol 119:1534—1537
14. Moutsopoulos HM, Boehm-Truitt M, Kassan SS, Chused TM (1977) Demonstration of activation of B-lymphocytes in New Zealand black mice at birth by an immunoradiometric assay for murine IgM. J Immunol 119:2213—2219
15. Theofilopoulos AN, Eisenberg RA, Bourdon M, Crowell JS Jr, Dixon FJ (1979) Distribution of lymphocytes identified by surface markers in murine strains with systemic lupus erythematosus-like syndromes. J Exp Med 149:516—524
16. Cantor H, McVay-Bourdeau L, Hugenberger J, Naidorf K, Shen FW, Gershon RK (1978) Immunoregulatory circuits among T-cell sets: II. Physiologic role of feedback inhibition in vivo: absence in NZB mice. J Exp Med 147:1116—1125
17. Fauci AS, Steinberg AD, Haynes BD, Whalen G (1978) Immunoregulatory aberrations in systemic lupus erythematosus. J Immunol 121:1473—1470
18. Budman DR, Merchant EB, Steinberg AD, et al. (1977) Increased spontaneous activity of antibody forming cells in the peripheral blood of patients with active systemic lupus erythematosus. Arthritis Rheum 20:829—833
19. Glinski W, Gershwin ME, Steinberg AD (1976) Fractionation of cells on a discontinuous Ficoll gradient: study of subpopulations of human T-cells using anti-T-cell antibodies from patients with systemic lupus erythematosus. J Clin Invest 57:604—614
20. Sakane T, Steinberg AD, Green I (1978) Studies of immune functions of patients with systemic lupus erythematosus: I. Dysfunction of suppressor T-cell activity related to impaired generation of rather than response to suppressor cells. Arthritis Rheum 21:657—664
21. Horowitz S, Borcherding W, Moorthy AV, et al. (1977) Induction of suppressor T-cells in systemic lupus erythematosus by thymosin and cultured thymic epithelium. Science 197:999—1001

22. Twomey JJ, Laughter AH, Steinberg AD (1978) A serum inhibitor of immune regulation in patients with systemic lupus erythematosus. J Clin Invest 62:713—715
23. Steinberg AD, Klassen LW, Budman DR, Williams GW (1979) Immunofluorescence studies of anti-T cells antibodies and T-cells in systemic lupus erythematosus. Arthritis Rheum 22:114—122
24. Moutsopoulos HM, Fauci AS (1980) Abnormalities of immunoregulatory T-cell subsets in Sjögren's syndrome: influence of serum factors. J Clin Invest 65:519—528
25. Fauci AS, Moutsopoulos HM (1981) Polyclonally triggered B-cells in the peripheral blood and bone marrow of normal individuals and in patients with systemic lupus erythematosus and primary Sjögren's syndrome. Arthritis Rheum 24 (4):577—584
26. Talal N, Asofsky R, Lightbody P (1970) Immunoglobulin synthesis by salivary gland lymphoid cells in Sjögren's syndrome. J Clin Invest 49:49
27. Lane HC, Callihan TR, Jaffe ES, Fauci AS, Moutsopoulos HM (1983) Presence of intracytoplasmic IgG in the lymphocyte infiltrates of the minor salivary glands of patients with primary Sjögren's syndrome. Clin Exper Rheum 1:237—239
28. Alarcon-Segovia D, Ruiz-Arguelles A (1978) Decreased circulating thymus-derived cells with receptors for the Fc portion of immunoglobulin G in systemic lupus erythematosus. J Clin Invest 62:1390—1394
29. Moretta L, Webb SR, Grossi CE, Lydyard PM, Cooper MD (1977) Functional analysis of two human T-cell subpopulations: help and suppression of B-cell responses by T-cells bearing receptors of IgM or IgG. J Exp Med 146:184—200
30. Moretta L, Mingri MC, Romanzi CA (1978) Loss of Fc receptors for IgG from human T-lymphocytes exposed to IgG immune complexes. Nature 272:618—620

Pathology

W. ULRICH and G. SYRÉ

Introduction

Patients with signs and symptoms of SLE produce antibodies which react with a variety of endogenous tissue components. Subsequent to the release of such tissue components, e.g., of intracellular autoantigens in physiologic or pathologic histolysis, circulating immune complexes may develop. The diversity of autoantigens and the heterogeneity of immune complexes cause a series of morphologic changes that are characteristic of SLE as a prototype of a multisystemic disease. Various organs can be affected to a varying extent; of these the kidneys, the skin, the joints, the heart, the lymph nodes, and the serous membranes are most commonly involved. The pathologic anatomy of SLE thus covers a wide range and its diversity manifest itself not only in the gross and clinical changes but also in the microscopic and ultrastructural findings. The latter are of extraordinary importance, particularly for the morphologic assessment of renal changes. Therefore they will be more closely reviewed in the following in the light of some of our own cases.

Renal Changes

From a clinical and pathologic point of view, the kidneys play a central part in SLE as they are involved in nearly 100% [23] of cases. The deposition of immune complexes is regarded as a pathogenetic principle of lupus mephritis and leads to a broad spectrum of renal lesions. These manifest themselves in various types of glomerulonephritis which may be associated with more or less marked tubulointerstitial or vascular processes. Although classification of lupus glomerulonephritis is primarily based on the light microscopic changes, immunomorphology and electron microscopy are indispensable for an adequate assessment of the renal involvement in patients with SLE. According to the location of the immune complexes deposited within the glomerulus and both their quantity and their quality, glomerulonephritis can be classified into three morphological categories (Table 1). We have chosen this simplified classification, which deviates from the WHO classification [10, Table 1], since the criteria in the latter were not clear-cut and as transitory and mixed types occurred. The present classification

Pathology 205

Table 1. Morphologic classification of lupus nephritis

Own classification	WHO classification (modified, Churg 1982)
I. Minimal glomerular change (predominantly mesangial deposits)	1. Normal glomeruli 2. Pure mesangial alterations
II. Proliferative glomerulonephritis (focal segmental, diffuse segmentally accentuated, or diffuse global subtypes with predominantly mesangial and subendothelial deposits)	3. Focal segmental glomerulonephritis 4. Diffuse glomerulonephritis (severe mesangial, endocapillary, or mesangiocapillary proliferation and/or extensive subendothelial deposits)
III. Membranous glomerulonephritis (predominantly subepithelial deposits)	5. Diffuse membranous glomerulonephritis

is based on the location of immune complexes in the glomerulus which determined the light microscope pattern. Active and sclerosing lesions must be distinguished in all forms of glomerulonephritis, because the activity of the inflammatory reaction (exudation, proliferation, or sclerosis) is decisive for the course and the prognosis of the disease [5, 6]. Thus, chronicity items like glomerulosclerosis, fibrous crescents, tubular atrophy, and interstitial fibrosis are considered to be highly predictive of renal failure outcome. The data on the incidence of the various types of glomerulonephritis differ greatly. In the following, the relative incidence [7] will be given in parentheses alongside the headings and contrasted with the results of our own investigations. Of 40 serologically established and biopsied cases of SLE with renal involvement, 34 were female patients (85%, mean age 35.4 years, age range 17–63 years) and 6 male patients (15%, mean age 27.8 years, age range 13–50 years).

Minimal Glomerular Change
(Incidence 12%–22%; in Our Material 12.5%)

In light microscopy, minimal glomerular change is characterized by slight insular widening of the mesangial fields. By means of immunofluorescence and electron microscopy, however, immune deposits can be demonstrated in the mesangium and sometimes also in small amounts on the peripheral basement membranes.

Minimal glomerular change is only rarely seen in biopsy material as it mostly takes its course without any major clinical manifestations and thus provides no indication for biopsy. Overall, five (12.5%) belonged in this category; four of them were female patients with a mean age of 26.5 years, and one was a male patient at the age of 40. Light microscopy shows largely nonspecific changes with slight widening of the mesangial fields due to proliferation of mesangial cells and/or an increase in the amount of mesangial matrix (Fig. 1a). By means of immunomorphology and electron microscopy immune deposits can be de-

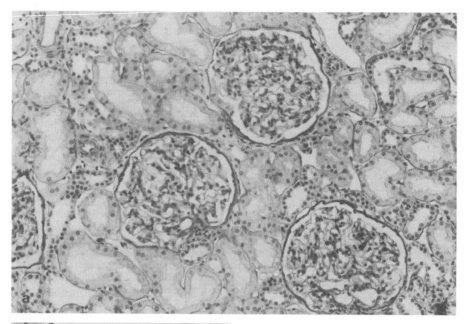

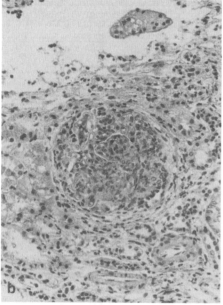

Fig. 1. a—e. a Minimal glomerular change in lupus erythematosus. The glomeruli show a slight widening of the mesangium as well as a proliferation of the mesangial cells (PAS, × 120). **b** Glomerulus in proliferative lupus glomerulonephritis. The glomerulus shows diffuse cell proliferation as well as segmental loop necroses and the beginning of a crescent formation. The periglomerular connective tissue contains mononuclear cells (H&E, × 120)

1. c, d. c So-called hematoxylin bodies *(arrows)* within a glomerular capillary loop (H&E, ×750). **d** Glomerulus in diffuse segmentally accentuated proliferative lupus glomerulonephritis. The peripheral basement membranes are thickened (so-called wire loops, *arrow*, H&E, ×360)

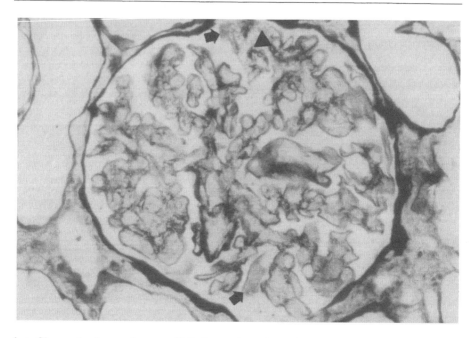

1. e. Glomerulus in membranous SLE glomerulonephritis. Besides a widening of the mesangium there is also a thickening of the peripheral capillary loop walls in several loop segments. Clear lacunae are recognizable in the thickened basement membrane *(arrow)*, and "spikes" *(arrowhead)* are seen on the outer aspect of the basement membrane (PASM, ×340)

tected even in histologically unremarkable sections of the glomeruli. Immunoglobulin and/or complement deposits are predominantly located in the mesangium; This is why Germuth chose the term "lupus mesangiopathy" [13, Fig. 2a]. Most of these deposits are IgM deposits. In two cases discrete segmental deposits of IgG, IgM, C3 and C1q were seen on the peripheral basement membranes. Electron microscopy mostly shows profuse electron dense deposits in the area of the mesangial fields (Fig. 3a). The peripheral basement membranes are either unremarkable or slightly widened, and only rarely are intramembranous, subendothelial, or subepithelial deposits found in the paramesangial zones. The only male patient proved to be immunomorphologically negative. Electron microscopy showed merely residues, i.e., dissolving subendothelial deposits, so this was likely to be a case of residual-stage glomerulonephritis or glomerulonephritis in remission.

Clinical Findings.
The findings are mostly negative or only minor (proteinuria) and nonspecific. Only in one of our own cases was hypertension found.

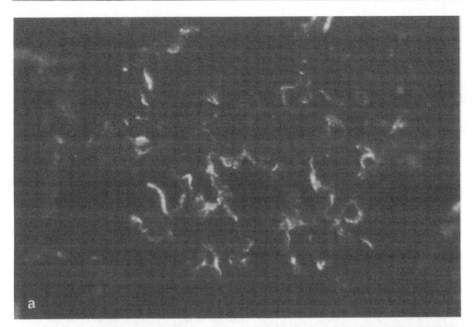
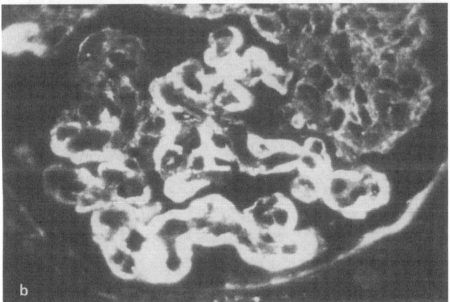

Fig. 2. a—d. a IgG deposits within the mesangium and only sparse deposits are seen on the peripheral capillary loop walls in minimal glomerular change (indirect immunofluorescence, anti-IgG, ×340). b Immunofluorescence microscopic appearance of a glomerulus in proliferative SLE glomerulonephritis. Granular and linear IgM deposits are recognizable within the mesangium and on the peripheral capillary loop walls (indirect immunofluorescence, anti-IgM, ×750)

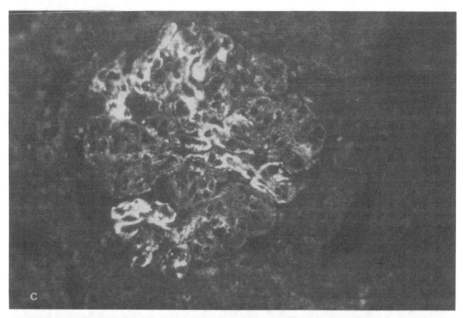

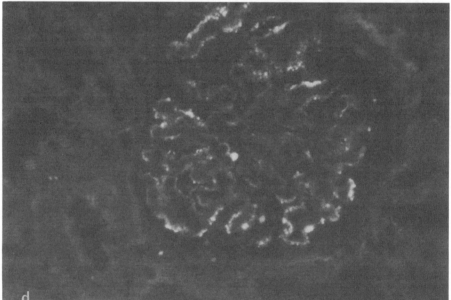

2. c, d. c Immunofluorescence microscopic appearance of a glomerulus in diffuse segmentally accentuated proliferative lupus glomerulonephritis. C3 deposits in segmental distribution within the mesangium and short linear deposits on the peripheral basement membranes are seen (indirect immunofluorescence, anti-C3, ×340). **d** Immunofluorescence microscopic appearance of a glomerulus in membranous SLE glomerulonephritis. Fine to coarsely granular deposits of C1q are predominantly seen on the peripheral basement membranes (indirect immunofluorescence, anti-C1q, ×340)

Proliferative Glomerulonephritis
(Incidence 22%—84%; in Our Material 77.5%)

Proliferative glomerulonephritis in SLE is characterized by a varying extent of segmental or global intraglomerular cell proliferation which may lead to a lobulation of the glomerular tuft. The peripheral basement membranes may be greatly thickened, (so-called wire loop glomeruli), and loop necrosis with capsular adhesions and crescent formations is commonly found. Immunofluorescence microscopy discloses granular deposits in the mesangium and short linear or granular deposits on the peripheral basement membranes with antibodies against IgG, IgM, IgA, C1q, and C3. Electronoptically, massive osmiophilic deposits are found in the mesangium and subendothelially, and to a lesser extent subepithelially or intramembranously. In this category, virus-like inclusion bodies are also quite commonly detected in the endothelial cells.

Thirty-one cases belonged in this group (77.5%); 4 were males with a mean age of 27.7 years and 27 were females with a mean age of 36.4 years. The light microscopic pattern of proliferative lupus nephritis varied greatly. According to the extent to which the glomerular loop segments were involved, segmental focal, diffuse segmentally accentuated, and diffuse global changes could be seen. In a total of ten cases, the segmental focal changes of a predominantly proliferative and partially sclerosing character prevailed. Part of the glomeruli showed segmental cell proliferation in the glomerular tuft, which was sometimes associated with segmental loop necrosis (Fig. 1b). Such cellular proliferation is partly caused by infiltration of mononuclear cells (lymphocytes, monocytes) and polymorphonuclear granulocytes, and partly by proliferation of local cells (mesangial cells). As a consequence of the exudation of fibrin into Bowman's capsule, capsular adhesions and crescents were commonly found due to proliferation of capsular epithelium (Fig. 1b). In one case (34 years, female) crescents were seen in more than 50% of the glomeruli, which suggests a course of extracapillary accentuation with a poor prognosis. Just once we found basophilic corpuscles, so-calles hematoxylin bodies, in necrotic loop segments. These were likely to precipitated complexes of nucleoprotein antibodies, which can be regarded as pathognomonic of SLE (Fig. 1c). Immunofluoresecence microscopy showed granular deposits of immunoglobulins and of complement in the mesangium, and short linear deposits in segmental distribution on the loop periphery. In three cases IgM, IgA, and C1q could be seen in diffuse global form despite marked segmental changes seen in light microscopy (Fig. 2b). Electron microscopic examination confirmed a mostly global deposition of electron dense immune deposits in the mesangium and segmental subendothelial deposits on the peripheral basement membranes of the affected glomeruli. In only three biopsies were deposits also found subepithelially — in addition to mesangial and subendothelial deposits — in the region of the lamina rara externa, and in one case at an intramembranous location.

In 16 cases the light microscopic diagnosis of "diffuse segmentally accentuated glomerulonephritis" was made. Proliferative glomerulonephritic changes were demonstrable in 100% of the glomeruli although the extent of such changes

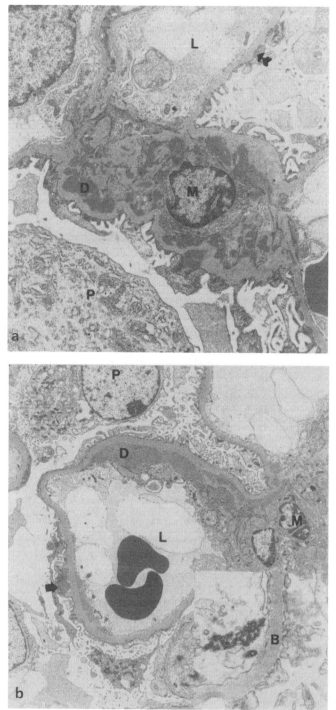

Fig. 3. a, b

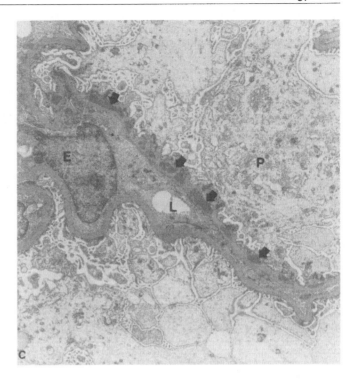

Fig. 3. c

Fig. 3. a—c. a Electron microscopy of a glomerulus in minimal glomerular change in SLE. The mesangium *(M)* is widened and contains a lot of electron-dense deposits *(D)*. Only sparse deposits are seen on the peripheral capillary loop wall *(arrow)*. L, lumen; P, podocyte (× 8400). b Electron microscopy of a glomerulus in proliferative SLE glomerulonephritis. Electron-dense deposits *(D)* are seen within the lamina rara interna. In addition there are also subepithelial deposits *(arrow)*, and the podocytic foot processes are fused. L, lumen; P, podocyte; M, mesangial cell (× 4000). *Inset:* Microtubular structures (virus-like particles) in the cytoplasm of an endothelial cell. B, basement membrane (× 13 500). c Electron microscopic appearance of a glomerulus in membranous lupus glomerulonephritis. A lot of electron-dense deposits are seen within the lamina rara externa *(arrows)*, and the podocytic foot processes are highly fused. L, lumen; P, podocyte; E, endothelial cell (× 5450)

varied within the individual loop segments. The morphologic changes essentially resemble those seen in segmental focally accentuated glomerulonephritis (see above). In three biopsies crescents were found in over 50% of the glomeruli. Numerous glomeruli showed a membranoproliferative component characterized by a lobulated tuft, double contours of the peripheral basement membrane, and interposition of the mesangial cells between the double lamellae of the basement membrane. The basement membrane was sometimes strikingly thickenes due to the deposition of hyaline material in the subendothelial space (so-called wire loops, Fig. 1d). In seven cases (17.5%) protein thrombi could be recognized within the lumina of the loops which predominantly appear, when cryoglobulinemia coexists. Immunofluorescence microscopy usually revealed a diffuse global pattern with granular or short linear deposits of IgG, IgM, IgA, C3, and C1q in the loop periphery (Fig. 2b). Only in four cases out of our own investigational material were segmental deposits seen in the mesangium and on the peripheral loop segments (Fig. 2c). The electron optical pattern was dominated by massive widening of the mesangial fields as well as thickening of the peripheral basement membranes with mesangial, subendothelial, and subepithelial electron-dense deposits of varying shape and distribution (Fig. 3b). In four cases intramembranous deposits were also detectable. In addition, double basement membranes were seen due to the neogenesis of mesangial matrix in the paramesangial zones of the glomerulus, as well as interposition of mesangial cells. The endothelial cells were mostly considerably hypertrophied and frequently contained microtubular cytoplasmatic inclusions ("virus-like structures," Fig. 3b, inset). Predominantly in the area of the most massive basement membrane deposits, the podocytic foot processes were fused or retracted over long stretches. The subepithelial deposits partly resembled those seen in genuine membranous glomerulonephritis. Occasionally, however, very large deposits occurred which were reminiscent of "humps" (see Fig. 2d in membranous glomerulonephritis). Contrary to the genuine humps in poststreptococcal glomerulonephritis, however, these were not located on the exterior of the basement membrane but within the lamina rara externa.

In 5 out of 31 cases the changes in the glomeruli were so evenly marked that they could be classified as diffuse global glomerulonephritides. The light microscopic pattern of one case correlated with an extracapillarily accentuated membranoproliferative glomerulonephritis with over 50% cresents. Mesangial cell proliferation with lobulation and hypersegmentation of the glomerular tuft were the predominant features. In addition, double contours of the peripheral basement membrane could be seen. The remaining four cases were classified as diffuse endocapillary glomerulitides; in these cases proliferation of mesangial and endothelial cells as well as an increase in the amount of mesangial matrix were the predominant features. In immunofluorescence microscopy, the diffuse mesangial deposition of IgG, IgM, IgA, and C1q prevailed. Although the light microscopic examination revealed diffuse lesions, the peripheral deposits of IgM and C1q were often limited to single loop segments only. The electron optical pattern corresponded to that of diffuse segmentally accentuated glomerulonephritis (see above). Electron-dense deposits of varying shape and size were found in the mesangium and in the lamine rara interna. In two cases, additional subepithelial deposits were recognizable which were associated with segmentally accentuated fusion of the podocytic foot processes. Sometimes virus-like inclusions were found in the hypertrophied endothelial cells. The mesangial matrix was globally increased.

Clinical Findings.

The clinical correlate of proliferative lupus nephritis was proteinuria in 95% of cases, in 47% of all cases associated with a nephrotic syndrome. In only two cases was proteinuria associated with macrohematuria. In 60% a distinctly raised creatinine level reflected the impairment of renal function. In one case the only sign was severe hypertension. Hypertension was associated with proteinuria in 45% and in 50% there was proteinuria with microhematuria.

Membranous Glomerulonephritis
(Incidence 7%—26%; in Our Material 10%)

Membranous glomerulonephritis is characterized by diffuse global thickening of the glomerular basement membranes. This is caused by the finely granular immune deposits visualized by immunofluorescence microscopy which mostly react with anti-IgG and anti-C1q. In most cases proliferation of mesangial cells is not very marked. The electron optical substrate consists in subepithelial electron-dense deposits in the lamina rara externa which are associated with retraction of the podocytic foot processes. Accordingly, the morphologic diagnosis of membranous glomerulonephritis is nearly exclusively based on the location of the immune deposits, which must be precisely determined by electron microscopy. In our material only four cases could be classified as membranous glomerulonephritides (10%); three were female patients (mean age 37 years) and one a 16-year old male. In only two cases did light microscopy suffice to make a diagnosis. In silver staining, the thickening of the basement membrane, the ostensible "perforation" of the basement, and the "spikes" on the exterior gave a characteristic pattern (Fig. 1e). In one case the glomeruli were unremarkable in light microscopy, like in stage 1 of membraneous glomerulonephritis, and in another case the segmental involvement of the glomerulus prevailed so that the primary diagnosis of segmental focal proliferative glomerulonephritis was made on the grounds of obvious segmental cell proliferation. Immunofluorescence microscopy also yielded a characteristic pattern with predominantly finely granular, but occasionally also coarse deposits of IgG, IgM, and C1q, either diffuse or segmentally accentuated to a varying extent on the peripheral loop segments (Fig. 2d). In addition to these peripheral deposits and unlike in genuine membranous glomerulonephritis, there was nearly always weak positive immunofluorescence in the mesangium which was associated with proliferation of mesangial cells. Electron microscopy confirmed the deposition of immune complexes in the peripheral basement membrane and in the mesangium; here, they were more irregularly arranged than in genuine membranous glomerulonephritis (Fig. 3c), and discreet subendothelial deposits were nearly always also present.

Clinical Findings.
The principal clinical sign of membranous glomerulonephritis is the nephrotic syndrome, which may be associated with hypertension and microhematuria.

Tubulointerstitial Nephritis in SLE
(Incidence in Our Material 27.5%)

Lupus glomerulonephritis is commonly associated with focal fibrosis of the interstitium, atrophy of the tubular system, and inflammatory interstitial cell infiltrates.

These infiltrates, which mainly consist of mononuclear cells, often lead to destruction or necrosis of the tubular epithelium. In our material, 29 (72.5%) lupus nephritides were associated with tubulointerstitial changes. These ranged from scanty periglomerular infiltrates (see Fig. 1b) to severe diffuse focally accentuated interstitial nephritis with desctuction of the tubules. Due to the fact that severe persisiting glomerular damage necessarily leads to tubular atrophy and interstitial fibrosis, it is often quite difficult to distinguish between primary interstitial nephritis in SLE and secondary changes due to glomerulonephritis. In our patients the most severe tubulointerstitial changes occured in the group of proliferative lupus nephritis and in particular in those taking an extracapillarily accentuated course. On the other hand, however, marked focal interstitial inflammatory signs with fibrosis of the interstitium were also detected in three of five cases of minimal change.

Thus it can be assumed that tubulointerstitial nephritis in SLE is caused by a primary pathomechanism which is independent of glomerular change [27]. Immunomorphologically, positive linear fluorescence was seen on the the tubular basement membranes in two cases (Fig. 4a), and in three cases tubular immune deposits were demonstrated by electron micrsocopy (Fig. 4b). As follows from the cases studied and from the literature, the amount of tubular or interstitial immune deposits does not correlate with the severity of interstitial nephritis [24].

Clinical Findings.
The degree of interstitial fibrosis and of tubular atrophy as well as the density of the cellular infiltrate are inversely proportional to renal function [our observations, 24]. Moreover, there are occasional disturbances of the urine-concentrating capacity, with polyuria. The severity of the tubular demage can be clinically assessed by measuring β^2-microglobulin secretion.

Vasculitis in Lupus Nephritis (Incidence in Our Material 5%)

Although a number of clinical manifestations in SLE are caused by vascular changes (Raynaud's disease) and although immune complexes are commonly deposited in vessels, vasculitis in the kidneys is a rare finding. Whereas immunofluorescence and electron microscopy demonstrated immune deposits in the vessel walls of 6 out of 40 cases of SLE (15%), the light microscopic diagnosis of arteritis could be made in merely two biopsies (5%). The changes were limited to fibroinoid necrosis with proliferation of local cellular elements in the interior parietal layers of the interlobular arteries and arterioles but without any appreciable inflammatory infiltration or thrombosis (Fig 5a). In all cases with detectable immune deposits in the vessel walls (Fig. 5b) there was coexisting severe diffuse or diffuse segmentally accentuated lupus glomerulonephritis with marked tubulointerstitial changes.

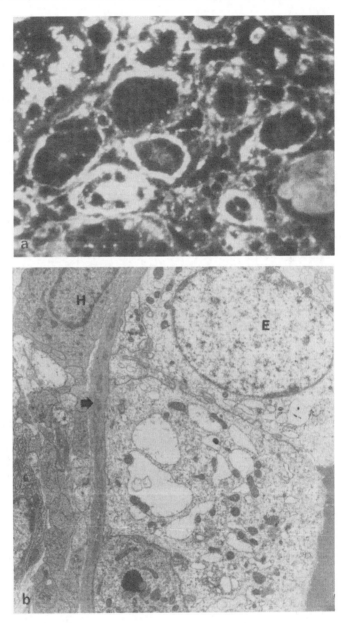

Fig. 4. a, b. a IgM deposits in the tubular basement membrane in intersitial lupus nephritis (indirect immunofluorescence, anti-IgM, × 180). b Electron-dense deposits in the tubular basement membrane *(arrow)*. E, tubular epithelial cell; H, histiocyte (× 9400)

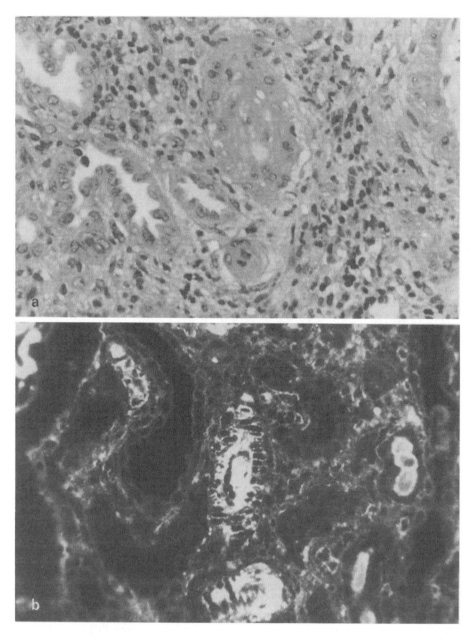

Fig. 5. a, b. a A small artery and an arteriole showing inflammatory changes of the vessel wall in SLE vasculitis (H&E, ×340). **b** Deposits of IgA within the vessel walls in SLE (indirect immunofluorescence, anti-IgA, ×180)

Clinical Findings.

Arteritis usually occurs only in combination with severe proliferative lupus nephritis and is commonly associated with malignant phase hypertension. The morphologic findings of vasculitis in renal biopsy therefore carries an unfavorable prognosis and terminal renal failure must be expected.

Morphologic Approaches to a Distinction Between Lupus Glomerulonephritis and Nonlupus Glomerulonephritis

In order to distinguish lupus glomerulonephritis from other types of glomerulonephritis for partical diagnostic purposes, the immunomorphologic findings in the 40 cases of lupus were contrasted with those in a group of 46 glomerulonephritides chosen at random. Statistical evaluation was carried of by means of the χ^2-test. The results were als follow:

1. Deposits of IgG both in the loop periphery and in the mesangium were significantly more common in lupus glomerulonephritis ($P < 0.05$).
2. Deposits of IgA in the loop periphery were significantly more common in lupus glomerulonephritis. After ruling out eight cases of IgA nephritis from the control group, IgA deposits in the mesangium were also significantly more commonly detected in lupus nephritis ($P < 0.05$).
3. Deposits of the complement component C1q were significantly more common in the lupus glomerulonephritis ($P < 0.05$).
4. No significant differences resulted with regard to deposits of IgM, C3, or fibrin.

In accordance with the literature [7, 18] the following criteria can therefore be applied in order to distinguish lupus nephritis from non-SLE nephritides for practical diagnostic purposes:

1. Heterogeneity of the immune deposits: The deposits vary in size, shape, and location from one glomerulus to the other, and even within the various loops of one glomerulus. Usually this finding can only by verified by electron microscopy.
2. Extraglomerular immune deposits.
3. Antinuclear antibodies seen on the tissue section in immunofluorescence microscopy.
4. Intraglomerular deposits of IgA and C1q besides IgG and IgM.
5. Microtubular virus-like inclusions in the endothelial cells.

In spite of being characteristic of SLE, the above criteria are nevertheless absolutely specific. Therefore particularly the combined occurrence of such findings suggests a high probability of the presence of SLE.

Pathogenesis of Lupus Nephritis

Both in proliferative and in membranous lupus glomerulonephritis, DNA molecules and/or DNA antibodies have been detected in the immune deposits [1—3]. Ribonucleoprotein, IgG (in combination with anti.idiotypic antibodies), and a cytoplasmic glycoprotein called Ro have been regarded as further antigens that might be involved in the development of immune deposits [7]. In addition, viral antigens (RNA viruses) are also being discussed as possible constituents of immune deposits [21]. The pathogenetic significance of viruses in the development of SLE is dealt with in another chapter. The various categories of lupus nephritis correspond to the varying location and amount of immune deposits in the glomerulus. For a long time it has generally been assumed that glomerulonephritis in SLE develops as a consequence of the deposition of preformed circulating immune complexes in the glomerulus after blockage of the mononuclear phagocytic system. This hypothesis plausibly accounts for the genesis of the mesangial and subendothelial deposits [13]. From animal experiments it is known that injected insoluble immune complexes do not penetrate the basement membrane but are primarily deposited in the mesangium and, after saturation of the mesangial clearance function, under the endothelium in the lamina rara interna. A more complex problem is the formation of the subepithelial deposits. Basically, four mechanisms can be taken into consideration which, however, have only partly been proved by experiments and are thus of a more or less hypothetical nature:

1. More than just one antigen—antibody system might be involved in the genesis of lupus nephritis. Besides insoluble large immune complexes, smaller soluble complexes might also be formed which penetrate the basement membrane and are deposited in the lamina rara externa [13].
2. Autoantibodies react with structural antigens of the glomerular basement membrane and so-called, in situ formation of immune complexes takes place [12].
3. Antigen and antibody penetrate the basement membrane separately and form an "in situ complex." This may happen either if there is particular affinity of the antigen molecule (DNA) for certain components of the basement membrane ("planted antigens", [17]) or — in the event of little avidity of the antibody — if there is a dissociation of preformed immune complexes in the subendothelial space and subsequent reassociation of the molecules after penetration of the basement membrane in the lamina rara externa [14]. Furthermore, it must be considered that preformed immune complexes may be altered by variation in the antibody titer or in the amount of antigens as well as by interaction with complement factors and other circulating plasma proteins.
4. Cationic proteins released from polymorphonuclear granulocytes, macrophages, or platelets as a consequence of the inflammatory processes are also being considered as further pathogenetic factors. These cationic molecules may lead to loss of the filtration function of the basement membrane by neu-

tralization of the glomerular polyanions [8]. The activation of the coagulation system with the development of fibrin thrombi leads to loop necrosis or obliteration.

Although extraglomerular immune deposits are repeatedly found in SLE, their amount does not correlate with the degree of interstitial nephritis and of impairment of renal function [24]. This suggests that deposition of tubular complexes does not constitute the only mechanism involved in the development of tubulointerstitial changes. In interstitial nephritides of different etiology it has been demonstrated that the majority of interstitial infiltrate consists of T-lymphocytes and macrophages; thus, cell-mediated immune reactions may play a crucial part in the pathogenesis of interstitial nephritis [16].

The genesis of vasculitis is likely to occur via similar mechanisms to glomerular changes. There is deposition of immune complexes in the subendothelial space and if these complexes are of extraordinary size or if they occur in great amounts, this may lead to proliferation of local cells and to necrosis of vessel walls. As recent studies have shown, the primary event seems to be damage to the endothelial cells by antiendothelial antibodies of the IgG class [11], which in turn renders the deposition of immune complexes in the vessel wall possible.

Thus it becomes clear that, overall, the pathogenesis of lupus nephritis is a complex process in which various immunologic and inflammatory reactions bring about glomerular, tubulointerstitial, and vascular changes which mutually influence each other.

Changes in Other Organs

Heart

Endocardium and myocardium are involved in about 50% of cases. Verrucous vegetations occur on the reverse side of the mitral and tricuspid valves, i.e., on that side which does not face the bloodstream. This change, known as "atypical verrucous endocardial Libmann-Sacks," must be distinguished from bacterial or rheumatic endocarditis. The deposits consist of fibrin, inflammatory cells, and fibroblasts which immigrate from the valve stroma. In the myocardium, perivascular round cell infiltrates may be found, and the intramural vessels sometimes show endovasculitic changes which in special cases may lead to necrosis of muscle fibers due to ischemia.

Serous Membranes

Inflammation on the serous membranes may be acute, subacute, or chronic. In the acute stage, the surface is covered with fibrinous exudate which later becomes organized; this leads to adhesions of the pleura, pericardium, or peritoneum.

Lungs

Apart from fibrinous pleuritis, marked changes occur in the lung parenchyma. Chronic interstitial pneumonia with interstitial lymphocytic infiltrates and mild interstitial fibrosis is commonly found. Acute lupus pneumonitis is rare but leads to severe clinical signs and symptoms. There is severe interstitial edema and inflammatory infiltrates are present with exudation into the alveoli and sometimes also hyaline membranes [19]. Intraalveolar hemorrhages reminiscent of Goodpasture's syndrome may occur. Immunomorphology and electron microscopy show immune deposits in the alveolar basement mambranes. Involvement of the pulmonary vessels in the form of vasculitis is rare. A more common finding is widening of the intima and periadvential fibrosis of the pulmonary arteries which may give rise to pulmonary hypertension.

Central Nervous System

The signs and symptoms with regard to the CNS can in most cases be attributed to acute vasculitis which may be associated with cerebral hemorrhage and infarctions. Immune complex deposits are sometimes detected in the basement membrane of the choroid plexus and in cerebral vessel walls [4, 9]. However, changes in SLE brains may not only be caused by primary vascular damage but also frequently be secondary complications like microemboli originating from SLE endocarditis or hypertensive vascular damage.

Muscles

The involvement of skeletal muscles in SLE manifests itself in myasthenia, myalgias, and signs of muscular atrophy. The incidence is about 50%, the proximal parts of the muscles being most severely affected [22]. The morphologic spectrum covers the following changes:

1. Inflammatory myopathy with predominantly perivascular lymphoplasmacellular infiltrates and segmental muscle fiber necrosis
2. Vasculitis with predominant involvement of the venous vessels
3. Perifascicular muscle fiber atrophy (= atrophy of muscle fibers in the periphery of the fascicles)
4. Vacuolar myopathy
5. Neurogenic damage of muscle fibers

Inflammatory myopathy and perifascicular atrophy are the changes most commonly observed. They correlate with the clinical diagnosis of polymyositis.

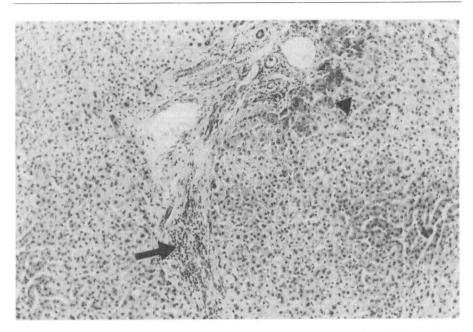

Fig. 6. Liver parenchyma in lupus hepatitis. The portal areas are widened and infiltrated with mononuclear cells *(arrow)*. In the periphery of the lobules focal liver cell necroses are seen *(arrowhead)* (H&E, × 100)

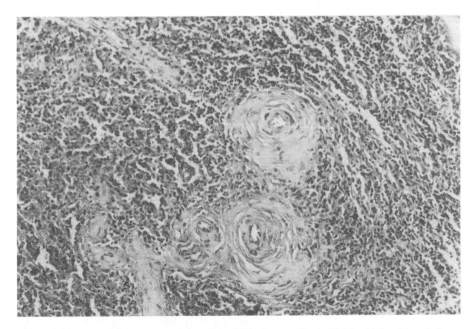

Fig. 7. Spleen in SLE. The vessel wall of the follicular arteries is highly thickened and shows perivascular onion-like fibrosis (H&E, × 100)

Joints

Arthritis is common in SLE and in the acute stage is characterized by synovitis with exsudation of neutrophil granulocytes and fibrin. The perivascular mononuclear cell infiltrates in the subsynovium and the hyperplasia of the synovial membrane are usually less pronounced than in rheumatoid arthritis [15]. So-calles LE cells (= neutrophil granulocytes which have phagocytized the nuclear debris of necrotic cells) may occasionally be found in the joint puncture fluid.

Liver

In lupus hepatitis there is nonspecific inflammation of the portal fields with lymphocytic infiltrates (Fig. 6) as well as the occasional presence of vasculitis of the rami of the hepatic artery. In addition, focal necroses of the parenchyma (Fig. 6) occur with predominantly plasma cellular infiltrates and proliferation of Kupffer's cells [26].

Lymphatic Tissue

Enlargement of the cervical or axillary lymph nodes is sometimes the first clinical sign of SLE. Involvement of the lymph nodes is quoted as occurring in 50%—66.7% [20, 25] of cases. The histological changes in the biopsy material are often nonspecific. At an early stage there is hyperplasia of the lymphatic follicles with florid germinal centers. Only rarely are focal fibrinoid necroses seen in whose surroundings irregularly shaped, structureless masses are found which appear lilac or bluish in the HE preparation. These masses correspond to confluent hematoxylin bodies arising from necrotic nuclei of lymphocytes which provide a characteristic but nonspecific criterion for SLE. They consist of DNA, alkaline proteins, and polysaccharides [20]. Part of the homogenized nuclear debris is phagocytized by leukocytes or histiocytes so that LE cells form in the tissue. In later stages, plasma cells come to the foreground which sometimes contain eosinophilic, PAS-positive inclusions (Russell's bodies). Diagnosing SLE through biopsy of lymph nodes is possible only in rare cases. Hematoxylin bodies and fibrinoid necroses are hardly seen except in autopsy material.

Moderate to severe splenomegaly can be observed in many cases. There is thickening of the spleen capsule as well as hyperplasia of the malpighian corpuscles. In the red pulp plasmacytosis is usually seen. Quite characteristic are the vascular changes in the spleen which primarily affect the follicular and penicillary arteries. The vessel walls are thickened and there are signs of perivascular onion-like fibrosis (Fig. 7).

Dermatological Changes

See chapter "Cutaneous Manifestations" (pp. 227—250).

References

1. Agnello V, Koffler D, Kunkel HG (1973) Immune complex systems in the nephritis of systemic lupus erythematosus. Kidney Int 3:90—97
2. Agnello V (1976) The immunopathogenesis of lupus nephritis. Adv Nephrol 6:119—136
3. Andres GA, Accinni L, Beiser SM, Christian CL, Cinotti GA, Erlanger BF, Hsu KC, Seegal BC (1970) Localization of fluorescein-labeled antinucleoside antibodies in glomeruli of patients with active lupus erythematosus nephritis. J Clin Invest 49:2106—2118
4. Atkins CHJ, Kondon JJ, Quismorio FP, Friou GJ (1972) The choroid plexus in systemic lupus erythematosus. Ann Intern Med 76:65—69
5. Austin HA, Muenz LR, Joyce KM, Antonovych TA, Kullick ME, Klippel JH, Decker JL, Balow JE (1983) Prognostic factors in lupus nephritis. Contribution of renal histologic data. Am J Med 75:382—391
6. Austin HA, Muenz LR, Joyce KM, Antonovych TT, Balow JE (1984) Diffuse proliferative lupus nephritis: identification of specific pathologic features affecting renal outcome. Kidney Int 25:689—695
7. Barba L, Pawlowski I, Brentjens JR, Andres GA (1983) Diagnostic immunopathology of the kidney biopsy in rheumatic diseases. Hum Pathol 14:290—304
8. Batsford SR, Takmiya H, Vogt A (1980) A model of in situ immune complex glomerulonephritis in the rat employing cationized ferritin. Clin. Nephrol 14:211—218
9. Budka H (1981) Brain pathology in the collagen vascular diseases. Angiology 32:365—372
10. Churg J (1982) Renal disease: Classification and atlas of glomerular diseases. Igaku-Shoin, Tokyo, p 128
11. Cines DB, Lyss AP, Reeber M, Bina M, DeHoratius RJ (1984) Presence of complement-fixing anti-endothelial cell antibodies in systemic lupus erythematosus. J Clin Invest 73:611—625
12. Couser WG, Salant DJ (1980) In situ immune complex formation and glomerular injury. Kidney Int 17:1—13
13. Germuth FG, Rodriguez E (1973) Immunopathology of the renal glomerulus. Little, Brown, Boston, pp 113—145
14. Germuth FG, Rodriguez E, Wise O (1982) Passive immune complex glomerulonephritis in mice. III. Clearance kinetics and properties of circulating complexes. Lab Invest 46:515—519
15. Goldberg D, Cohen AS (1978) Synovial membrane histology in the differential diagnosis of rheumatic diseases. Medicine 57:239—252
16. Husby E, Tung KSK, Williams RC jr (1981) Characterization of renal tissue lymphocytes in patients with interstitial nephritis. Am J Med 70:31—38
17. Izui S, Lambert PH, Miescher PA (1976) In vitro demonstration of a particular affinity of glomerular basement membrane and collagen for DNA: a possible basis of a local formation of DNA-anti-DNA complexes in systemic lupus erythematosus. J Exp Med 144:428—443
18. Jennette JC, Iskandar SS, Dalldorf FG (1983) Pathologic differentiation between lupus and non-lupus membranous glomerulopathy. Kidney Int 24:377—385
19. Katzenstein ALA, Askin FB (1982) Surgical pathology of non-neoplastic lung disease. Saunders, Philadelphia, pp 143—146

20. Lennert K (1961) Lymphknoten bei Lupus erythematodes. In: Lennert K (ed) Cytologie und Lymphadenitis. Springer, Berlin Heidelberg, p 371. (Handbuch der speziellen pathologischen Anatomie und Histologie, 1/3A)
21. Mellors RC, Mellors JW (1976) Antigen related to mammalian type C-RNA viral p30 proteins is located in renal glomeruli in human systemic lupus erythematosus. Proc Natl Acad Sci USA 73:233—237
22. Oxenhandler R, Hart MN, Bickel J, Scearce D, Durham J, Irvin W (1982) Pathologic features of muscle in systemic lupus erythematosus: a biopsy series with comparative clinical and immunopathologic observations. Hum Pathol 13:745—757
23. Robbins SL, Cotran RS (1984) Pathologic basis of disease, 3rd edn. Saunders, Philadelphia, p 184
24. Schwartz MM, Fennell JS, Lewis EJ (1982) Pathologic changes in the renal tubule in systemic lupus erythematosus. Hum Pathol 13:534—547
25. Symmers WStC (ed) (1978) Systemic pathology, 2nd edn. Churchill Livingstone, Edinburgh, pp 691—693
26. Thaler H (ed) (1982) Leberkrankheiten. Springer, Berlin Heidelberg New York, pp 123—133
27. Tron F, Ganeval D, Droz D (1979) Immunologically mediated acute renal failure of nonglomerular origin in the course of systemic lupus erythematosus (SLE). Am J Med 67:529—532

Cutaneous Manifestations

T. A. LUGER and D. BENESCH

Lupus erythematosus is an autoimmune disorder which defies any solitary explanation of its cause and pathogenesis. The term lupus was primarily used to characterize destructive ulcerations occurring mainly on the face. In 1828 for the first time Biett [136] described the clinical features of lupus erythematosus (LE), and in 1851 his student Cazanave appendes to them the name "lupus erythematosus" [15]. In 1872, over 100 years ago, Kaposi contended that systemic LE and chronic discoid lupus were one and the same disease [67]. Later, in 1934, O'Leary introduced a classification of LE similar to the one in use today. This included discoid LE (DLE), which was usually confined to the skin, acute disseminated LE (usually fatal), and subacute disseminated LE (usually benign).

Dermatological lesions are among the most important clinical manifestations of systemic LE, since the skin is easily accessible and extremely suitable for in depth clinical and immunohistopathologic studies, and since dermatologists have a unique opportunity of identifying LE subsets according to skin manifestations. Gilliam [42, 44] propsed a classification of cutaneous lupus erythematosus based strictly upon the clinical appearance of the skin lesions without consideration of the systemic aspect of the disease. The three major forms of skin disease specific for LE are as follows: chronic cutaneous LE (DLE), subacute cutaneous LE (SCLE), and acute cutaneous LE (Table 1).

Chronic Cutaneous Discoid Lupus Erythematosus

Discoid lupus erythematosus, the most common form of cutaneous LE, occurs predominantly in women between the ages of 20 and 60 with no particular racial incidence [107]. The lesions (Fig. 1) start as erythematous patches or are of papulosquamous character and usually are distributed on the light-exposed surfaces of the skin, such as the face, ears, upper chest, upper back and extensor aspect of the arms. Protected areas, including external ear canals as well as palmar and plantar surfaces, are also frequently affected. According to the distribution of the skin lesions two clinical types of DLE may be distinguished: a "localized form" confined to the head and neck, and a "generalized form," when lesions occur both above and below the neck. Depending on the thickness of the skin lesions, a third "hypertrophic form" can be distinguished. The primary erythematous or papulosquamous lesions develop into edematous plaques which are sharply circumscribed, covered with adherent scales, pink to violaceous, and have central scarring with borders of active inflammation. A magnifying glass will reveal follicular dilatation with keratin plugging of older plaques. These skin lesions can persist for months or years, but on healing they change into areas of atrophy and scarring with telangiectasia and hyper- and hypopigmentation (Fig. 2). Frequently extensive alopecia resulting from hair follicle damage occurs. A striking diagnostic feature is hyperesthesia, which can be proved by gently rubbing the fingertips over the skin lesions.

Early mucous membrane lesions occur as persistent erythema with a depressed or ulcerated center, whereas chronic lesions show a thickened epithelium with linear whitish scars. They are localized on the buccal mucosa, hard palate, tongue, lips, and nasal mucosa. Conjunctival, gingival, vaginal, and perianal lesions have also been described [30, 112, 144].

Most cases of DLE are not difficult to diagnose, but there are some skin disorders which occasionally may be confused with DLE, including chronic polymorphous light eruptions, actinic reticuloid, rosacea, tinea, poststeroid erythema, lymphocytic infiltration of the skin, seborrheic dermatitis, and psoriasis. Differential diagnoses from the mucous membrane LE lesions include oral leukoplakia, mucosal lichen planus, candidiasis, white sponge nevus, and morsicatio buccarum [4]. Usually the hiostologic and immunopathologic examination will allow a definite diagnosis.

The role of sunlight in the etiology of LE is well established. Repeated irradiation with high doses of UV light in the sunburn range can induce cutaneous LE and exacerbate systemic LE in most, though not all, patients [19, 31, 37]. The inducing wavelengths have been shown to be between 290 and 320 nm and can be blocked by window glass [144]. Recently antimalarials have also been shown to inhibit this effect of UV light [79]. In addition to sunlight, any form of trauma can provoke LE lesions. In general LE appears at sites of altered skin, such as tattoos, scars after thermal burns, and striae atrophicae [77, 89, 93, 128]. Koebner's phenomenon is suspected of being the underlying mechanism.

There is a low incidence of abnormal laboratory findings in patients with DLE. An elevated erythrocyte sedimentation rate which can be observed in 20% of the patients frequently correlates with the extent and activity of the skin lesions [107]. Occasionally the antinuclear antibody (ANA) test is positive at low titers and in these cases a particulate nuclear staining pattern may be observed [10]. A false reactive VDRL and leukopenia also may occur [12, 103]. Anti-double-stranded DNA antibodies are rarely present, but antibodies to single-stranded DNA can be found in 9%—25% of DLE patients [73]. Anticytoplasmatic antibodies are usually not present, and low levels of complement components and total hemolytic complement do not occur [107, 119]. Some studies also show an increased frequency of the HLA-B7 phenotype [87]. Taken together, the yield of conclusive laboratory tests in patients with DLE is low, and to date there is no test which will reliably select those patients who will eventually develop systemic manifestations.

The histologic pattern of DLE skin lesions shows epidermal hyperkeratosis with follicular plugging (Fig. 3), loss of the normal orientation, and organization of basal cells and hydropic degeneration of the basal cell layer. Acanthosis and

Table 1. Classification of cutaneous lupus erythematosus

1. Chronic cutaneous (discoid) lupus erythematosus (DLE)
   a) Localized DLE
   b) Generalized DLE
   c) Hypertrophic DLE (verrucous DLE)
   d) LE profundus (LE panniculitis)
2. Subacute cutaneous lupus erythematosus (SCLE)
   a) Papulosquamous (psoriasiform) SCLE
   b) Annular — polycyclic SCLE
3. Acute cutaneous lupus erythematosus (ACLE)
   a) Malar erythema ("butterfly rash")
   b) Widespread erythema
4. Neonatal lupus erythematosus
5. Overlap syndrome

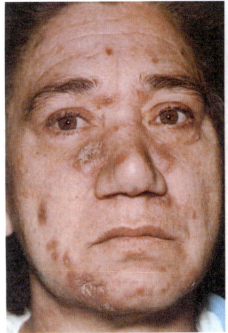

Fig. 1. Chronic cutaneous (discoid) lupus erythematosus

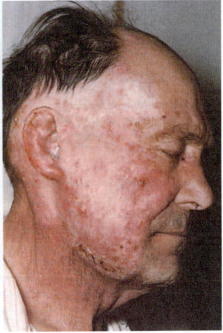

Fig. 2. Chronic cutaneous lupus erythematosus with scarring, depigmentation, and hyperpigmentation

focal atrophy of the malpighian cell layer may also be seen. Moreover there is evidence of increased production of melanin and accumulation of pigment in the upper dermis. In older lesions thickening of the PAS-positive basement membrane is typical. The most striking pathologic feature is a dense infiltration of mononuclear cells in the upper dermis around the blood vessels and hair

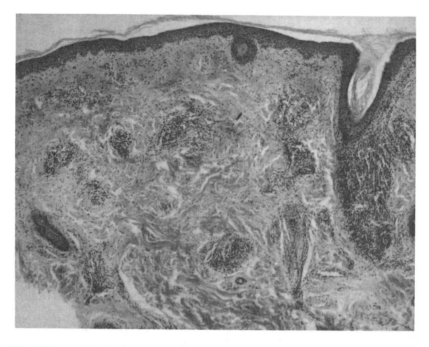

Fig. 3. Histopathologic features of DLE, showing hyperkeratosis, keratotic plugging, and a patchy perivascular and periappendageal mononuclear cell infiltrate (H&E, ×63)

follicles, extending into the deep dermis. The mononuclear cells consit primarily of lymphocytes, plasma cells, and monocytes. The density and depth of the dermal mononuclear cell infiltration are greatest in DLE and diminish increasingly in SCLE and ACLE [3, 107]; they thus provide additional support in distinguishing the different cutaneous manifestations of LE.

In diagnostic problems the lupus band test is widely regarded as a specific and sensitive test for DLE [149]. In DLE lesions a positive lupus band test is only present in clinically involved skin. Deposits of IgG, IgM, IgA, fibrin, and complement in a homogeneous, granular or thready pattern are found in the dermal—epidermal junction. In DLE the immunoglobulin deposits are usually homogeneous, and may become thick in older lesions. In contrast in patients with SLE the lupus band test of uninvolved skin is positive in 82% and may have some predictive value by identifying a subset of SLE patients with more aggressive renal disease and decreased long-term survival [22].

Since laboratory evaluation in patients with DLE will usually be normal, a careful history and physical examination but no extensive laboratory investigation is recommended. Only 5%—10% of DLE patients will subsequently develop systemic symptoms [12, 89], which frequently are milder than those of patients with SLE without discoid lesions [104]. At present, local treatment of choice for DLE is intralesional injection of triamcinolone acetonide. Topical steroids, especially fluorinated steroid ointments, are usually successful when the lesions are small, but for resistant lesions, occlusive dressings and steroid-impregnated tapes may be needed. Local application of CO_2 snow or trichloracetic acid may on occasion be quite effective and worth a try [114].

In systemic treatment of DLE, antimalarial therapy maintains a prominent place despite its possible side-effects. The mode of action of antimalarials in LE is unknown at present. Chloroquine sulfate is the first drug of choice: the usual dosage is two tablets of 250 mg daily for 10 days, followed by one tablet daily. More than 15 g per treatment should not be given. Hydroxychloroquine, 200 mg daily, is particularly useful in patients with widespread DLE. Toxic effects are proportional to the accumulated dose; the most important is retinal damage, which is usually seen after prolonged chloroquine therapy. Other side-effects include corneal deposits, pigmentation of the palate, nails, and legs, bleaching of the hair and moustache, exfoliative dermatitis, lichenoid rashes, myasthenia, myopathy, extrapyramidal, involuntary movements, neuropathy and mental disturbances, nausea, and dizziness. Although quinacrine may be added when hydroxychloroquine is ineffective [13], combinations of antimalarials should be avoided [114].

In resistant cases low dose prednisone 5—10 mg per day may help. Among other drugs shown to be effective in some patients are cyclophosphamide 50—200 mg per day [121], thalidomide [71], β-carotine [94] and clofazimine [83]. These drugs should preferably only be used if systemic disease has developed. Since sunlight exacerbates lesions in about 60% of patients, sun exposure should be avoided and a sunscreen prescribed [114]. Some patients may discontinue drug therapy during the winter months [72].

Variants of DLE

Lupus erythematosus panniculitis (LEP) ist a rare clinical variety of DLE, first described by Kaposi in 1883 [66]. LEP, or less accurately „lupus erythematosus profundus," appears as a manifestation of DLE but is also seen in approximately 50% of patients with SLE [24, 152]. It develops as firm, sharply defined, freely movable, subcutaneous nodules several centimeters in diameter [2, 34, 57, 141]. The inflammatory infiltrate occurs primarily in the deeper areas of the dermis and subcutis; the overlying skin often is unaffected but may be drawn inward and attached to the underlying nodule. Occasionally ulcerations can be observed [57]. The nodules, which may or may not be painful, occur most commonly on the forehead, cheeks, chin, back, buttocks, and thighs. Sun exposure does not seem to provoke the lesions, but trauma may precede their appearance [141]. When the nodules resolve, they leave depressed, scarred areas with subcutaneous atrophy.

Histologically these lesions are characterized by lobular panniculitis, fat necrosis, hyaline degeneration of the fat, hyaline papillary bodies, and patchy lymphohistiocytic infiltrations (Fig. 4). Calcification and mucinosis may also be seen [57, 116]. Often epidermal and dermal manifestations of DLE are seen, and the immunopathologic features of LE may be present. Frequently immunoglobulin and complement deposits in the vessel walls of the deep dermis and subcutis are

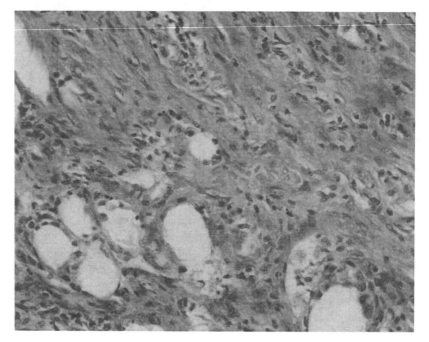

Fig. 4. LE panniculitis showing lymphocytic panniculitis (H&E, ×250)

noted [142, 145]. Essential for the diagnosis are the response to antimalarial therapy, the presence of a positive linear basement membrane zone stain of involved skin by direct immunofluorescence microscopy, and any signs of lupus, either cutaneous or systemic. This helps to differentiate LEP from other pathologic types of panniculitis, such as Weber-Christian disease associated with pancreatitis or pancreatic neoplasm, erythema nodosum, erythema induratum, subcutaneous sarcoidosis, nodular vasculitis, and connective tissue diseases.

Lupus erythematosus hypertrophicus is a relatively rare variant of DLE with severe lymphocytic infiltration [62, 146]. The lesions are commonly located on the face, the lower lips, and the chin, and resemble the clinical picture of warts. They vary from violaceous to red, consist of sharply outlined, elevated plaques with indurated borders, and are covered with thick, verrucous, hyperkeratotic scales. The differential diagnosis consists of lymphadenosis cutis benigna and nodular sarcoidosis.

Chilblain lupus: These lesions resemble chilblains in the early stages. Erythematosus patches develop on cold-exposed areas of the skin, such as the face (especially the nose and ears), hands, and feet, subsequently changing to blue—red infiltrated plaques with sparse adherent scales and hyperesthesia. The typical lesions are chronic and aggravated by cold weather [144].

Bullous Lesions: The coexistence of SLE with dermatitis herpetiformis (DH) and bullous pemphigoid (BP) has been reported previously [20, 50, 63, 92, 96, 133, 138, 139]. Bullous lesions in patients with SLE clinically are indistinguishable from those of BP or DH. Transient vesicles are common whereas giant bullae occur relatively rarely [97]. The bullous eruption may be generalized but is usually limited to the face, neck, shoulders, and proximal upper extremities. Although the clinical, histopathologic, and immunologic features in these immune complex-mediated autoimmune diseases closely resemble each other, there are several diagnostic criteria suggesting that the bullous lesions are a specific manifestation of SLE and not a coexistent bullous disease [96, 138, 139]. Patients with BP usually have demonstrable circulating BP antibodies, whereas SLE patients with BP-like lesions failed to have anti-basement membrane zone (BMZ) antibodies [38, 96, 134]. The pattern of immunofluorescence, showing linear deposition of IgG on C3 at the BMZ, is indistinguishable from that characteristic for BP. However, immune electronmicroscopy reveals that immune deposits are predominantly located immediately subadjacent to the basal lamina and in the superficial layer of the dermis. These features are characteristic for SLE [120, 153] since in BP the deposits are confined to the lamina lucida [54]. In typical DH lesions IgA deposits are in close association with dermal microfilar bundles [133, 154] and in linear IgA dermatoses the presence of other immunoglobulins in rarely observed [68]. The absence of HLA B8 and subtotal villous atrophy of the small bowel provides additional evidence against DH [50]. These findings support the hypothesis that blisters are a specific manifestation of SLE and not a coexistent bullous disease.

Treatment of bullous lesions of LE includes local as well as systemic corticosteroids. Sulfones also appears to be very useful, particularly in cases where the bullous lesions are not controlled by relatively high doses of corticoseroids [50].

Erythema Multiforme: Erythema multiforme-like lesions have been described in association with DLE and SLE ("Rowell syndrome") [59, 75, 113]. The early erythema multiforme-like lesions begin as erythematous papules and progress to ring shapes with a vesicular edge. Since bullae and necrosis may also occur, the possibility of other bullons diseases has to be excluded by histologic and immunologic findings. Usually these patients have speckled ANA deposits upon indirect immunofluorescence.

Neoplastic Changes: Squamous cell as well as basal cell carcinoma may rarely develop in chronic lesions od DLE [56, 100], particularly in the scalp, ears, and nose. The occurrence of keratoacanthoma in a DLE lesion has also been reported [88].

Complement deficiency, including C1q, C1s, C1r, C2, C4, C5, C6, C7, C8, and C9, has been reported in patients with DLE and SLE [26, 70, 84, 95, 132]. The characteristic clinical picture involves high sensitivity to sunlight and cold, associated with Raynaud's phenomenon. Skin lesions are found predominantly in locations typical for SCLE and on the palms and soles [70]. Systemic features, including rheumatoid arthritis, may occur, but renal involvement is unusual.

Subacute Cutaneous Lupus Erythematosus

In 1977 a clinically distinct subset, "subacute cutaneous LE," was added to the spectrum of cutaneous LE by Gilliam [42]. SCLE lesions are clinically different from the typical, well circumscribed DLE lesions. These patients have a symmetrical, widespread, superficial, nonscarring form of cutaneous LE. The involvement includes areas of skin exposed to sunlight, such as the upper trunk (Fig. 5), face, shoulders, neck, and extensor surface of the upper extremities. SCLE lesions are rarely seen below the waist, on the lateral part of the trunk, on the axillae, or on the inner aspect of the arms and knuckles. The incidence is approximately 10% and the patients are mostly (70%) white [45]. SCLE may be divided into two subtypes according to clinical features: a "papulosquamous or psoriasis-like variety" appearing as erythematous papillary lesions with a scaly surface and an "annular—polycylic variety" with peripherally expanding annular or polycyclic lesions. Sometimes both patterns are seen in the same patient but one is usually predominant.

In contrast to DLE lesions, which remain separate and well circumscribed, the SCLE lesions have a tendency to coalescence and to build large areas of involvement. Annular lesions are bordered by erythema and a superficial scale, while the center shows grayisch hypopigmentation and telangiectasia (Fig. 6). Because of epidermal separation due to basal layer injury, occasionally vesiculae may

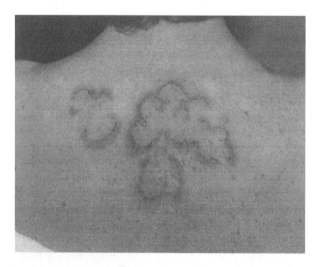

Fig. 5. Subacute cutaneous lupus erythematosus, annular polycyclic variety

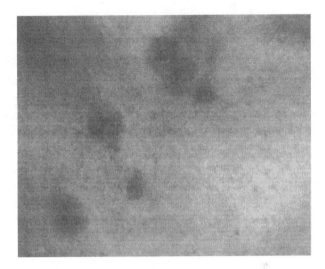

Fig. 6. Early erythema multiforme like lesion of SCLE

appear in the margin of these lesions [82]. Following the resolution of SCLE lesions, pigmentary changes and teleangiectasia may remain but eventually disappear after months. More than half of the patients with SCLE have diffuse nonscarring alopecia. Compared with DLE, follicular plugging and adherent hyperkeratosis are not prominent features, and scarring areas with dermal atrophy are rarely seen. SCLE is somewhat less persistent than DLE and more widespread in distribution, and clinically significant photosensitivity is more common.

Mucous membrane lesions are present in 40% of patients. Livedo reticularis and periungual telangiectatic changes occur in 20% [45]. Twenty percent of SCLE patients additionally have localized scarring DLE lesions, which mostly appear on the scalp, often many years before the onset of SCLE. In contrast to DLE, most patients with SCLE have mild systemic involvement, marked by musculoskeletal symptoms, fever, and malaise, whereas severe central nervous system or renal disease is unusual [128]. Often the SCLE patient will satisfy four or more criteria established by the "American Rheumatism Association Criteria Laboratory."

The histological picture of biopsies from SCLE lesions (Fig. 7) is similar to that of DLE lesions. Follicular plugging, hyperkeratosis, and the density as well as the depth of the cellular infiltrate are significantly less in SCLE. Marked hydropic changes along the epidermal basal cell layer with a loss of the normal organization and orientation of the basal cells, edema, and vacuolar degeneration which may lead to subepidermal bullae formation are usually present [48, 82]. The mononuclear cell infiltration is not as heavy as in DLE, and is usually restricted to the perivascular and periappendageal areas of the upper dermis [3]. Whereas in over 90% of skin biopsies taken from DLE lesions immune deposits can be detected in the dermal—epidermal junction [65], at least 40% of SCLE lesions fail to reveal immunoglobulin deposition upon direct immunofluores-

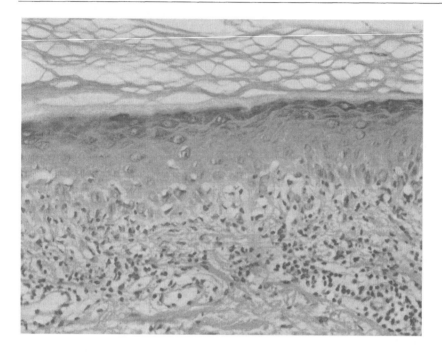

Fig. 7. Histopathologic features of SCLE, showing vacuolar degeneration of the epidermal basal cell layer and mononuclear cell infiltration confined to the superficial dermis (H&E, ×250)

cence [128]. Therefore negative direct immunofluorescence cannot be used to exclude SCLE. However, 23% of SCLE patients have immune deposits at the dermal−epidermal junction in biopsies taken from clinically normal sun-protected skin, whereas no DLE patients without systemic involvement [105] and 55% of unselected SLE patients [40] show this finding.

The histopathologic pattern of SCLE appears very similar to that seen in lichenoid skin lesions of graft versus host (GVH) disease [78, 131]. Skin lesions of some patients with GVH resemble those of patients with SCLE [55] or DLE [49], and in the case of GVH disease are probably T-lymphocyte-mediated, suggesting a similar mechanism of cutaneous injury may occur in LE [45]. This is further supported by the presence of HLA-DR antigens on T-lymphocytes and keratinocytes in skin lesions of patients with LE [8, 151] or GVH disease [47], which may represent activated CD8 T cells with cytotoxic activity against basal keratinocytes.

The most common laboratory features of SCLE are leukopenia, an elevated erythrocyte sedimentation rate, positive LE cell preparation, and positive ANA test. Using the "fluorescence antinuclear antibody test" (FANA) with human cells (Hep-2) as the nuclear substrate [106], 81% of patients with SCLE but only 29% of patients with DLE were positive, whereas over 90% of SLE patients have a positive FANA test. Patients with SCLE frequently have antibodies to the cellular antigens Ro/SSA and LA/SSB [23], and low serum concentrations of antibody to double-stranded DNA are present in approximately 30%. HLA typing of patients with SCLE yielded a significant association with HLA B8 and DR3 [129]. In all patients with the annular form of SCLE, HLA DR3 has been found. In addition, a striking concordance of anti-Ro and the HLA DR3 phenotype in SLE [6] as well as SCLE patients [130] has been reported, suggesting that a specific immune response gene for Ro antigen may be closely linked to the HLA DR3 locus and possibly may be responsible for the development of LE.

Patientes with SCLE are a subgroup of patients with LE who have an illness which appears to be intermediate in severity between DLE and SLE. Thus complete laboratory studies and a thorough physical examination must be performed. Since serious systemic disease such as CNS or renal involvement is uncommon, treatment of patients with SCLE will usually be similar so that of patients with DLE, including topical corticosteroids, systemic corticosteroids, or antimalarial agents either alone or in combination [5, 128]. When corticosteroids fail to control skin disease an immunosuppressive therapy using cyclophosphamide may be tried [128]. Thalidomide [148] and etretinate [80] also have been used successfully in some cases.

Acute Cutaneous Lupus Erythematosus

Skin involvement is one of the most obvious clinical features of SLE, being present in 60%—72% of patients [29, 140]. The acute cutaneous lupus erythematosus (ACLE) lesions frequently coincide with exacerbation of systemic disease and are present in 30%—52% of SLE patients [33, 111]. They often arise after sun exposure and are abrupt in onset, appearing as an inflammatory rash marked by edema and erythema, lasting for hours to days. The typical cutaneous finding is the classic malar "butterfly rash," also termed the "localized, indurate erythematous form" of ACLE. The lesions are located on both cheeks and the nose. Sometimes the patient's entire face may be involved, sparing only the eyelids and periorbital regions. Occasionally the eyelids may similarly be involved, as in dermatomyositis. Facial swelling sometimes resembles granuloma faciale, contact dermatitis, seborrheic dermatitis, rosacea, and cellulitis. The second most common form of ACLE is a widespread, indurated erythema with papulous, vesiculous changes, sometimes accompanied by adherent scales or atrophy. These maculopapular lesions are often pruritic and may be located anywhere on the body above the waistline (Fig. 8). This clinical type may resemble a drug eruption, erythema multiforme, or toxic epidermal necrolysis.

The development of ACLE skin lesions is unpredictable. The skin changes can obstinately persist for hours to days as previously described, or suddenly vanish, leaving atrophy and postinflammatory hyperpigmentation. Other cutaneous manifestations of SLE include a necrotizing vasculitis which may lead to digital nodules, cutaneous infarcts, leg ulcers, and digital gangrene [28]. Ryanaud's phenomenon is found in about 20% of SLE patients [25, 143]. Livedo reticularis is often an early sign of SLE [143], and erythromelalgia has also been reported

[109]. Acral lesions with diffuse patchy erythema on plantar and palmar areas, extending to the distal part of fingers and toes, also may be seen. Telangiectatic changes on the fingertips and subungual bleeding are common. Diffuse or patchy alopecia, usually healing without scarring, and fractured frontal hairs may be noted [29].

Oral and anal mucous membrane lesions are associated with a greater tendency toward ulceration and bleeding as compared with DLE. The lesions are usually found on the oral mucosa, with predilection for the buccal mucosa and the hard palate. They appear as erythematous or white patches or plaques with telangiectasia, atrophy, erosion, or ulceration [112]. When they become older, they show atrophy and a white keratotic border. Rarely the tongue is involved, with erythema, fissuring, and atrophy of the papillae; more frequently the lips show the picture of an exudative, encrusting cheilitis with a tendency to atrophy. Conjunctival and gingival lesions have also been observed in SLE. Urticaria and erythema multiforme may occur, and these patients often have an increased prevalence of glomerulonephritis and frequently anti-DNA, anti-Sm, and anti-Ro antibodies [135].

The laboratory abnormalities in patients with ACLE show much variability but generally reflect the presence of active systemic disease and therefore will not be discussed in detail in this chapter. In 60%—80% of the patients high concentrations of anti-dsDNA antibodies are present and often they are also found to be positive for ANA. Anemia, leukopenia, hypergammaglobulinemia, proteinuria, hematuria, pyuria, cylindruria, and hypocomplementemia are common.

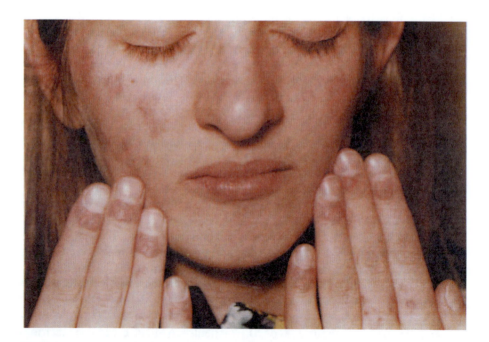

Fig. 8. Acute systemic lupus erythematosus, maculopapular lesions

High titers of anti-DNA antibodies have been considered to be pathognomonic of an active state of disease [122]. Patients with antibodies to an extractable nuclear antigen (Sm) usually have a prominent skin eruption and necrotizing vasculitis but less severe renal and CNS dysfunction [137]. Anti ribonuclein (RNP) antibodies are characteristic for overlap diseases or mixed connective tissue diseases [53, 126], and the cytoplasmatic antigens anti-Ro and anti-La usually occur in patients with mild disease [16, 85, 101, 102].

Direct immunofluorescence demonstrates immunoglobulin and complement deposits in normal (75%—80%) as well as lesional (95%) skin (Fig. 9) [35, 149]. These deposits in normal skin appear to be a result of circulating antibodies to DNA and have provided us with a useful diagnostic test for SLE (LE band test). The lupus band test (LBT) of normal skin is usually netative in patients with DLE or SCLE. Biopsies from the deltoid area of the shoulder apparently most frequently yield a positive test (88%) [64].

The histopathology of ACLE may not be characterisctic in the early stages. However, usually many of the features seen in DLE or SCLE skin lesions can also be observed in ACLE lesions, including hydropic changes along the epidermal basal layer, a sparse mononuclear cell infiltrate, and upper dermal edema. In general the only histologic difference between DLE, SCLE, and ACLE skin lesions is the intensity of the inflammatory process. In some cases of ACLE the upper dermal edema can be so intensive that subepidermal blisters develop which subsequently rupture and leave small erosions.

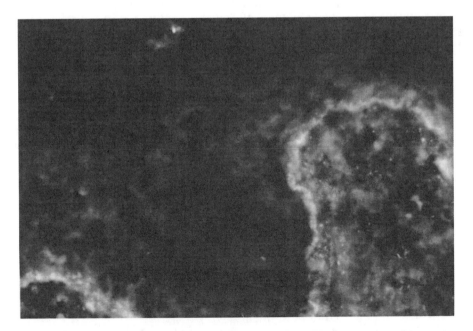

Fig. 9. SLE; direct immunofluorescence of lesional skin demonstrating IgG deposition at the dermal – epidermal junction (× 400)

Usually SLE patients with dermatologic involvement have a better than expected 5-year survival when compared with patients without such lesions. The local therapy for SLE lesions is the same as in DLE lesions, but normally the rash vanishes with systemic treatment, which is discussed in detail in another chapter of this book. Protection against sun and avoidance of stress should be recommended.

Neonatal Lupus Erythematosus

Neonatal LE (NLE) is a rare, recently described, but well recognized syndrome, characterized by transient LE skin lesions, cardiac or hematologic disorders, and organomegaly, either singly or in a multiorgan fashion [9, 76, 86]. The disease occurs more commonly in female infants [27] and is usually but not always self-limited. Mothers of these affected infants have diagnosable LE (SLE), an underlying connective tissue disorder, or symptoms of Sjögren's syndrome [36, 39]. However, 25% of the mothers are apparently asymptomatic [150].

The most common skin changes are a transient nonscarring form of cutaneous LE, which generaly appears in light-exposed areas such as the face, chest, upper trunk, arms, legs, and back. The facial lesions mostly appear as erythematous scaling patches of the midfacial of periorbital areas, associated with prominent telangiectasia. The skin lesions of the other sun-exposed parts of the trunk are often annular scaling erythematous patches with hypopigmented atrophic centers, resembling the annular form of SCLE in adults. Follicular plugging has been noted in some patients. The rash may be present at birth but is usually seen at 1—2 months and disappears within 6 months without scarring [115].

It is presumed that the manifestations in the neonate result from transplacental passage of maternal antibodies directed against the cytoplasmic antigens Ro/SSA and La/SSB. By the age of approximately 6 months maternal immunoglobulins have been cleared, the infant has begun production of its own antibodies, and the skin lesions usually disappear, suggesting that maternal anti-Ro or anti-La antibodies in some way trigger the expression of LE in affected infants [39, 69, 76, 150].

Although other hematologic abnormalities may be present, affected infants rarely fulfill the criteria for SLE. The most serious complication of NLE is the development if cardiac conduction abnormalities as infalmmation leads to fibrosis and different types of heart block [32, 51]. Anti-Ro antibody was present in every child with cardiac conduction defects. Although other organs may be involved and some cases of hepatic dysfunction, hepatomegaly, thrombocytopenia, anemia, and leukopenia have been noted, multisystem disease is unusual [36]. Remembering the association of anti-Ro antibodies and photosensitivity in adults with LE [101], it is of interest to observe that cutaneous discoid skin lesions were sun-induced in most infants [39].

The histological and immunofluorescent picture reveals similar findings to adult lupus, such as keratotic plugging, alternate areas of atrophy and acanthosis, vacuolar degeneration of the basal cell layer, pigment incontinence, lymphocytic perivascular and periappendageal infiltration, and immunoglobulin deposits at the dermal—epidermal junction.

As NLE disease is self-limited, no treatment is necessary in most cases. The eruptions clear at the latest by 10—12 months of age, but may leave mild residua of atrophy, scarring, hypopigmentations, and telangiectasia. However, there have been reports of children with NLE who developed multisystem connective tissue disease in later life [32, 60]. Therefore long-term follow-up laboratory investigations should be performed. Moreover, every pregnant woman with a history of connective tissue disorder should be screened for anti-Ro and anti-La antibodies and monitored during pregnancy for fetal bradycardia. It seems that the fetus is less likely to be affected when the LE appears in the last trimester of pregnancy. Earlier in pregnancy the incidence of miscarriage or stillbirths seems higher [86]. There is no known risk for women who have circulating anti-Ro antibodies in giving birth to a child which eventually may develop NLE. On the other hand, the sera of all infants with the symptoms of congenital heart block and discoid skin lesions should be tested for cytoplasmic antibodies.

Overlap Syndromes

Mixed Connective Tissue Disease

The term mixed connective tissue disease (MCTD) was first described by Sharp and co-workers in 1972 [124] as a syndrome with overlapping features of systemic sclerosis, polymyositis, rheumatoid arthritis, and LE. Over 50% of patients with MCTD develop chronic, subacute, or acute cutaeous LE. Usually the course of LE in patients with MCTD is more benign with less serious renal involvement. The characteristic features of MCTD are the association of the overlapping syndromes with circulating antibodies to the RNP component of extractable nuclear antigen, a low incidence of renal disease, and a good prognosis [125, 126]. Except for cutaneous LE lesions, the most suggestive cutaneous features of MCTD are Raynaud's phenomenon, pigmentary changes, swollen hands and fingers, and diffuse alopecia. In many cases Raynaud's phenomenon is the earliest symptom and only after months to years is the onset of MCTD recognized. However, approximately 75% of patients with Raynaud's phenomenon have or will develop scleroderma, and only the remaining 25% will develop SLE. The diffuse intermittent swelling of hands and fingers is a typical symptom of MCTD and leads to the digits having a "sausage-like" appearance.

Chronic alopecia is often seen (65%), usually being diffuse, nonscarring, and persistent in character. The pigmentary disturbances include telangiectasia, both diffuse and focal, hyperpigmentation, and depigmentation with follicular retention of pigment as seen in scleroderma or repigmenting vitiligo [46]. Other prominent features are joint pain, fever, weight loss, generalized lymphadenopathy, inflammatory polymyositis involving proximal muscles, serositis, and evidence of myocardial involvement. Most patients have high levels of antibodies to the RNP component of extractable nuclear antigen [64], a thymic extract consisting of two different components, a ribonuclease (RNAse), and a trypsin-resistant molecular antigen Sm [101]. Both of these antibody systems to mRNP and Sm yield speckled nuclear patterns by indirect immunofluorescence. An interesting direct immunofluoerescence pattern is seen in skin biopsies of these patients: in addition to immunoglobulin deposition at the dermal—epidermal junction, speckled immunofluorescence is apparent within nuclei in the epidermis [7, 41, 58, 127]. This positive nuclear staining only occures in those patients with high levels of antibodies to RNP, but not to other nuclear antigens such as Sm ans nDNA [41, 58]. Although this pattern seems to be an artifact which is seen only in patients with extremely high anti-RNP antibodies [41, 64], it is a useful marker for those patients with an overlapping syndrome.

In spite of the relatively good prognosis of MCTD it is not a totally benign process and may delay recognition of a more serious disease. Thus, patients with this syndrome should be observed closely for the appearance of antinuclear or anticytoplasmic antibodies other than anti-RNP, which may indicate a progression to a more serious disease process.

Lupus Erythematosus and Lichen Planus

The lupus erythematosus, lichen planus overlap syndrome refers to a group of patients who demonstrate clinical, histologic, and immunopathologic characteristics of two diseases with unknown etiology. Lichen planus (LP) may appear in patients with DLE as well as those with SLE [1, 17, 61, 98, 117, 147]. Skin lesions clinically resembling DLE or ACLE are usually present in these patients. These may be accompanied by typical LP skin lesions existing of tiny flat-topped red to violaceous polygonal glisterning papules with thin adherent scales. Mild itching is common [147]. Sometimes they may be more verrucous, with marked hyperkeratosis and acanthosis, or "lichenoid," with an edematous mononuclear infiltrate in the upper dermis, epidermal exocytosis, and coloid ("Civatte") bodies. Most of the lesions affect the volar aspects of arms and legs, palms, soles, and oral mucous membranes [14, 17]. Alopecia and nail changes may be observed [1]. Mucosal changes consist of whitish or erythematous, occasionally erosive patches in a reticulated, linear, or speckled pattern.

Although LE and LP are different entities, they overlap in such a way that definite diagnosis is sometimes not easy; thus it has to be supported by immunofluoresecence and histopathology in nearly all patients. The lupus band test is positive in most cases of SLE and is negative in LP, which is extremely helpful in distinguishing the two diseases if they occur simultaneously [1]. Indirect immunofluorescence using patients serum and autologous lesional skin as substrates shows consistent staining of the stratum granulosum in LP lesions and may provide a useful tool for separation of LP from LE lesions [14]. The criterion for LP is the presence of fibrin in the basement membrane region in a "fibrillar, rainshower pattern," with or without combination with cytoid bodies and C_3.

Histopathologic features are hyperkeratosis, vacuolar degeneration of the basal cell layer with the presence if intraepidermal or subepidermal colloid bodies, and a papillary dermal band-like lymphocytic infiltrate. Based on histopathology two types are proposed: the "papillary dermal cell-rich" variant (LP type) and the "cell-poor" variant (LE type) [110].

Local therapy is difficult, as verrucous and DLE-like lesions run a very chronic course and are rather resistant to therapy. Intralesional steroids seem the most effective treatment of the verrucous lesions. In severe cases systemic steroids may also be used [147].

The similarities in the clinical pictures and histopathology of LE and LP could be regarded as the result of common pathophysiologic pathways [21], and a viral, genetic, autoimmune, or drug etiology has been suggested in both diseases [35, 108]. In addition, the lichenoid tissue reaction, consisting of a specific form of inflammatory cell infiltrate at the dermal—epidermal junction and cytolysis of keratinocytes [99], may occur in numerous dermatoses besides LE and LP, including GVH disease and drug eruptions [118]. Thus the immunogenetic predisposition of the patient may be responsible for the final clinical picture.

Lupus Erythematosus and Psoriasis

Systemic and discoid LE have both been described in association with psoriasis [52, 81, 90, 91]. The diagnosis of LE has usually relied on clinical findings and limited immunologic studies. Recently an increased frequency of cytoplasmic anti-Ro antibodies in SLE patients with coexisting psoriasis has been reported [74].

Moreover, since anti-Ro correlates with photosensitivity, LE/psoriasis patients may have an increased risk of photosensitivity. High titer of ANAs and negative anti-Ro have also been decribed [52]. As patients with psoriasis are often treated with ultraviolet phototherapy, they may develop severe systemic disease following the treatment. Thus SLE/psoriasis patients may present therapeutic problems: ultraviolet B light, the therapy for psoriasis, exacerbates LE, and antimalarials, the therapy for LE, exacerbates psoriasis. Therefore it would be advisable to screen those psoriatic patients with a positive history of photosensitivity for anti-Ro antibodies.

Lupus Erythematosus and Porphyria Cutanea Tarda

Several cases of lupus erythematosus and coexisting porphyria cutanea tarda (PCT) have been reported [11, 18]. Although the mechanism of association is unclear, urine and serum analysis for porphyrins should be done in LE patients with bullous lesions in light-exposed areas. Sometimes ANA or anti-Ro determination may also be a helpful diagnostic criterion in patients with PCT. Treatment of these patients may be challenging, as phlebotomy can exacerbate LE and antimalarials may provoke PCT.

244 T. A. Luger and D. Benesch

Relationship Between Cutaneous and Systemic Lupus Erythematosus

Some type of cutaneous involvement may be present in about 70% of patients with SLE [12, 29, 89]. However, chronic discoid lesions have been reported by Tuffanelli [140] as the initial manifestation in approximately 10% of patients with systemic LE. During the course of disease discoid lesions occurred in 30% of the patients. Fifty patients having systemic LE with discoid skin lesions have recently been studied by Prystowsky and Gilliam [107]. This clinical subset of SLE patients with discoid lesions usually have a more benign form and survival is increased as compared with LE patients without discoid LE lesions [123, 144]. Lupus nephritis and progressive renal insufficiency are rarely noted in this group of patients. Serological abnormalities such as a positive ANA test and mild depression of serum complement are not uncommon. Elevations of Anti-DNA are infrequent. Persistence of ANA, leukopenia, and thrombocytopenia may be associated with progression of the disease. Sometimes central nervous system disease and systemic vasculitis occur [107].

Gilliam [43] has proposed a relationship between the different types of cutaneous LE and their position in the clinical spectrum of LE. Thus the cutaneous injury in DLE may be predominantly cell mediated with little autoantibody production and little evidence of immune complex disease. In contrast, SLE with renal and CNS involvement appears to be immune complex mediated with little evidence of cell-mediated cutaneous injury. Patients with SCLE occupy an intermediate position.

Acknowledgments. We wish to thank Mrs. Monika Bednar for her expert secretarial assistance.

References

1. Ahmed AR, Schreiber P, Abramovits W, Ostreicher M, Lowe NJ (1982) Coexistence of lichen planus and systemic lupus erythematosus. J Am Acad Dermatol 7:478—483
2. Arnold HL jr (1956) Lupus erythemaosus profundus: commentary and report of four more cases. Arch Dermatol 73:15—33
3. Bangert JL, Freeman RG, Sontheimer RD, Gilliam JN (1984) Subacute cutaneous lupus erythematosus and discoid lupus erythematosus. Arch Dermatol 120:332—337
4. Banoczy J (1983) Oral leukoplakia and other white lesions of the oral mucosa related to dermatological disorders. J. Cutan Pathol 10:238—256
5. Bardach H (1982) ANF-negativer subackuter kutaner Lupus erythematosus mit Anti-Ro Antikörpern. Hautarzt 33:537—541
6. Bell DA, Maddison PJ (1980) Serologic subsets in systemic lupus erythematosus. An examination of autoantibodies in relationship to clinical features of disease and HLA antigens. Arch Rheum 23:1268—1273
7. Bentles-Philips CP, Geake TMS (1980) Mixed connective tissue disease characterized by speckled epidermal nuclear IgG deposition in normal skin. Br J Dermatol 102:529—533

8. Bjerke JR, Matre R (1983) Demonstration of Ia-like antigens of T lymphocytes in lesions of psoriasis, lichen planus and discoid lupus erythematosus. Acta Derm Venerol (Stockh) 63:103—107
9. Bremers H, Golitz LE, Westen WL, Hays WG (1979) Neonatal lupus erythematosus. Cutis 24:287—290
10. Burnham TK (1975) Antinuclear antibodies II. The prognostic significance of nuclear immunofluorescent patterns in lupus erythematosus. Arch Dematol 111:203—207
11. Callen JP, Ross L (1981) Subacute cutaneous lupus erythematosus and porphyria cutanea tarda. J Am Acad Dermatol 5:269—273
12. Callen JP (1982) Chronic cutaneous lupus erythematosus. Arch Dermatol 118:412—416
13. Callen JP (1982) Therapy of cutaneous lupus erythematosus. Med Clin North Am 66:795—805
14. Camisa C, Neff JC, Olsen RG (1984) Use of indirect immunofluorescence in the lupus erythematosus/lichen planus overlap syndrome: an additional diagnostic clue. J Am Acad Dermatol 11:1050—1059
15. Cazenave PLA (1851) Lupus erythemateux (erytheme centrifuge). Ann Malad Peau Syph 3:297—299
16. Clark G, Reichlin M, Tomasi TB Jr (1969) Characterization of a soluble cytoplasmic antigen reactive with sera from patients with systemic lupus erythematosus. J Immunol 102:117—122
17. Copeman PW, Schroeter AL, Kierland RR (1970) An unusual variant of lupus erythematosus or lichen planus. Br H Dermatol 83:269—272
18. Cram DL, Epstein JH, Tuffanelli DL (1973) Lupus erythematosus and porphyria: coexistence in seven patients. Arch Dermatol 108:779—784
19. Cripps DJ, Rankin J (1973) Action spectra of lupus erythematosus and experimental immunofluorescence. Arch Dermatol 107:563—567
20. Davies MG, Marks R, Waddington E (1976) Simultaneous systemic lupus erythematosus and dermatitis herpetiformis. Arch Dermatol 112:1292—1294
21. Davies MG, Gorkiewicz A, Knight A, Marks R (1977) Is there a relationship between lupus erythematosus and lichen planus? Br J Dermatol 96:145—154
22. Davis BM, Gilliam JN (1984) Prognostic significance of subepidermal immune deposits in uninvolved skin of patients with systemic lupus erythematosus: a 10-year longitudinal study. J Invest Dermatol 84:242—247
23. Deng JS, Sontheimer RD, Gilliam JN (1984) Relationships between antinuclear and anti-Ro/SS-A antibodies in subacute cutaneous lupus erythematosus. J Am Acad Dermatol 11:494—499
24. Diaz-Jovanen E, DeHoratius RJ, Alarcon-Segovia D, Messner RP (1975) Systemic lupus erythematosus presenting as panniculitis (lupus profundus). Ann Intern Med 82:376—379
25. Dinant J, Ginzler E, Schlesinger M (1979) The clinical significance of Raynaud's phenomenon in systemic lupus erythematosus. Arthritis Rheum 22:815—819
26. Douglass M, Lamberg SI, Lorincz AL, Good RA, Noorbibi KD (1976) Lupus erythematosus-like syndrome with a familial deficiency of C2. Arch Dermatol 122:671—674
27. Draznin TH, Esterly NB, Furey NL, Debofsky H (1979) Neonatal lupus erythematosus. J Am Acad Dermatol 1:437
28. Dubois EL, Arterberry JD (1962) Gangrene as a manifestation of systemic lupus erythematosus. JAMA 181:366—373
29. Dubois EL, Tuffanelli DI (1964) Clinical manifestations of systemic lupus erythematosus. JAMA 190:104—111
30. Dubois EL (1976) Lupus erythematosus: a review of the current status of discoid and systemic lupus erythematosus and their variants, 2nd edn. University of Southern California Press, Los Angeles, pp 213—293
31. Epstein JH, Tuffanelli DL, Dubois EL (1965) Light sensitivity and lupus erythematosus. Arch Dermatol 91:483—495
32. Esscher E, Scott JS (1979) Congenital heart block and maternal systemic lupus erythematosus. Br Med J 2:1234—1238
33. Estes D, Christian CL (1971) The natural history of systemic lupus erythematosus studied by prospective analysis. Medicine 50:85—95

34. Fellner MJ (1980) Lichen planus. Int J Derm 19:71—75
35. Fountain RB (1968) Lupus erythematosus profundus. Br J Dermatol 80:571—579
36. Franco HI, Weston WL, Peebles C, Forstot SL, Phanuphak P (1981) Autoantibodies directed against sicca syndrome antigens in the neonatal lupus syndrome. J Am Acad Dermatol 4:67—72
37. Freeman RG, Knox JM, Owens DW (1965) Cutaneous lesions of lupus erythematosus induced by monochromatic light. Arch Dermatol 100:677—682
38. Gammon WR, Briggaman RA, Inman AO. Merrit CC, Wheeler C (1983) Evidence supporting a role for immune complex-mediated inflammation in the pathogenesis of bullous lesions of systemic lupus erythematosus. J Invest Dermatol 81:320—325
39. Gawkrodger DJ, Beveridge GW (1984) Neonatal lupus erythematosus in four successive siblings born to a mother with discoid lupus erythematosus. Br J Dermatol 111:683—687
40. Gilliam JN, Cheatum DE, Hurd ER, Stastny P, Ziff M (1974) Immunoglobin in clinically uninvolved skin in systemic lupus erythematosus: association with renal disease. J Clin Invest 53:1434—1440
41. Gilliam JN, Prystowsky SD (1977) Mixed connective tissue disease syndrome. Cutaneous manifestations of patients with epidermal nuclear staining and high titer serum antititer in clinical diagnosis of cutaneous disease. Ann Intern Med 71:753—762
42. Gilliam JN (1977) The cutaneous signs of lupus erythematosus. Contin Educ Fam Rhys 6:34—40
43. Gilliam JN (1981) Immunopathology and pathogenesis of cutaneous lupus erythematosus. In: Good AD, Day SB (eds) Comprehensive immunology. Plenum, New York, pp 323—343
44. Gilliam JN, Sontheimer RD (1981) Distinctive cutaneous subset in the spectrum of lupus erythematosus. J Am Acad Dermatol 4:471—475
45. Gilliam JN, Sontheimer RD (1982) Subacute cutaneous lupus erythematosus. In: Callen JP (ed) Clinics in rheumatic disease, vol 8. Saunders, Philadelphia, pp 343—352
46. Gilliam JN, Sontheimer RD (1982) Clinically and immunologically defined subsets of LE. Rheum Dis 2:165.
47. Gomes MA, Schmitt DS, Souteyrand P (1982) Lichen planus and chronic graft-versus-host reaction. In situ identification of immunocompetent cell phenotypes. J Cutan Pathol 9:249—257
48. Grant JM (1981) Annular vesicular lupus erythematosus. Cutis 28:90—912
49. Gratwohl AA, Moutsopoulos HM, Chused TM (1977) Sjögren's-type syndrome after allogeneic bone marrow transplantation. Ann Intern Med 87:703—706
50. Hall RP, Lawley TJ, Smith HR, Katz SI (1982) Bullous eruption of systemic lupus erythematosus: dramatic response to dapsone therapy. Ann Intern Med 97:165—170
51. Hardy JD, Solomon S, Banwell GS, Beach R, Wright V, Howard FM (1979) Congenital complete heart block in the newborn associated with maternal systemic lupus erythematosus and other connective tissue disorders. Arch Dis Child 54:7
52. Hays SB, Camisa Ch, Luzar MJ (1984) The coesistence of systemic lupus erythematosus and psoriasis. J Am Acad Dermatol 10:619—622
53. Holman AR (1965) Partial purification and characterization of an extractable nuclear antigen which reacts with SLE sera. Ann NY Acad Sci 124:800—806
54. Holubar K, Wolff K, Konrad K, Beutner EH (1975) Ultrastructural localization of immunoglobulins in bullous pemphigoid skin: employment of a new peroxidase-antiperoxidase multistep method. J Invest Dermatol 64:220—227
55. Hood AF, Soter NA, Rapperport J, Gigli I (1977) Graft-versus-host reaction: cutaneous manifestations following bone marrow transplantation. Arch Dermatol 113:1087—1091
56. Ingber A, Sterry W, Grünwald MH, Feuermann EJ (1983) Plattenepithelkarzinome in discoiden Lupus erythematodes-Herden. Z Hautkr 58:1289—1297
57. Izumi AK, Takiguchi P (1983) Lupus erythematosus panniculitis. Arch Dermatol 119:61—64
58. Izuno GT (1978) Observations on the in vivo reaction of antinuclear antibodies with epidermal cells. Br J Dermatol 98:391—398
59. Jablonska S, Blaszczyk M, Chorzelski T (1972) Syndrome de Rowell: lupus erythemateux avec des lesions co-existantes de type erytheme polymorphe bulleux. Med Hyg 30:1390

Cutaneous Manifestations 247

60. Jackson R, Gulliver M (1979) Neonatal lupus erythematosus progressing into systemic lupus erythematosus. Br J Dermatol 101:81—86
61. Jamison TH, Cooper NM, Epstein WV (1978) Lichen planus and discoid lupus erythematosus. Arch Dermatol 114:1039—1042
62. John MD, Gruber GG, Turner JE, Callen JP (1981) Lupus erythematosus hypertrophicus: two case reports and a review of the literature. Cutis 28:290—292
63. Jordon RE, Muller SA, Hale WL (1969) Bullous pemphigoid associated with systemic lupus erythematosus. Arch Dermatol 99:17—25
64. Jordon RE (1982) Cutaneous immunofluorescence. In: Callen JP (ed) Clinics and rheumatic disease, vol 8. Saunders, Philadelphia, pp 479—491
65. Kay DM, Tuffanelli DL (1969) Immunofluorescent techniques in clinical diagnosis of cutaneous disease. Ann Intern Med 71:753—762
66. Kaposi M (ed) (1883) Pathologie und Therapie der Hautkrankheiten. Urban and Schwarzenberg, Wien, 642
67. Kaposi M (ed) (1895) Pathology and treatment of disease of the skin for practitioners and students. William Wood, New York, pp 505—510
68. Katz SI, Hall RP, Lawley TJ (1980) Dermatitis herpetiformis: the skin and the gut. Ann Intern Med 93:857—874
69. Kephart DC, Hood AF, Provost TT (1981) Neonatal lupus erythematosus: new serologic findings. J Invest Dermatol 77:331—333
70. Klein G, Tappeiner G, Hintner H, Scholz S, Wolff K (1984) Systemischer Lupus erythematodes bei hereditärer Defizienz der vierten Komplementkomponente. Hautarzt 35:27—32
71. Knop J, Bonsmann G, Vakilzadeh F, Happle R (1980) Behandlung des discoiden Lupus erythematodes mit Thalidomid. Zentralbl Haut- u Geschlechtskrankh 144:1—20
72. Koranda FC (1981) Antimalarials. J Am Acad Dermatol 4:650—655
73. Kulick KB, Provost TT, Reichlin M (1981) Antibodies to SS-DNA in patients with discoid lupus erythematosus. J Invest Dermatol 77:309
74. Kulick KB, Mogavero H, Provost TT, Reichlin M (1983) Serological studies in patients with lupus erythematosus and psoriasis. J Am Acad Dermatol 8:631—634
75. Lawrence CM, Marshall TL, Byrne JPH (1982) Lupus erythematosus associated with erythema multiforme-like lesions in identical twins. Br J Dermatol 107:349—356
76. Lee LA, Lillis PJ, Fritz KA, Huff JC, Norris DA, Weston WL (1983) Neonatal lupus syndrome in successive pregnancies. J Am Acad Dermatol 9:401—406
77. Lerchin E, Sturman S, Lockwood M (1975) Discoid lupus erythematosus occuring in red pigment of tattoos. J Assoc Milit Dermatol 1:18
78. Lerner KG, Kao GF, Strob R, Buckner CD, Cliff RA, Thomas ED (1974) Histopathology of graft-versus-host reaction (GHVR) in human recipients of bone marrow from HLA-matched sibling donors. Transplant Proc 6:367—371
79. Lester RS et al (1967) Immunologic concepts of light reactions in lupus erythematosus and polymorphous light eruption. Arch Dermatol 96:1—10
80. Lubach D, Wagner G (1984) Erfolgreiche Behandlung eines subakuten Lupus erythematodes mit Etretinat. Aktuel Dermatol 10:142—144
81. Lynch WA, Roenigk HH Jr (1978) Lupus erythematosus and psoriasis vulgaris. Cutis 21:511—525
82. Maciejewski W (1980) Annular erythema as an unusual manifestation of chronic disseminated lupus erythematosus. Arch Dermatol 116:450—453
83. Mackey JP, Barnes J (1974) Clofazimine in the treatment of discoid lupus erythematosus. Br J Dermatol 91:93—96
84. Massa MD, Connolly SM (1982) An association between C1 esterase inhibitor deficiency and lupus erythematosus: report of two cases and review of the literature. J Am Acad Dermatol 7:255—264
85. Mattioli M, Reichlin M (1974) Heterogeneity of RNA protein antigens reactive with sera of patients with systemic lupus erythematosus. Arthritis Rheum 17:421—429
86. McCuishion CH, Schoch EP (1983) Possible discoid lupus erythematosus in newborn infant. Arch Dermatol 119:615—618
87. Millard LG, Rowell NR, Rajah SM (1977) Histocompatibility antigens in discoid and systemic lupus erythematosus. Br J Dermatol 96:139—144

88. Millard LG, Barker DJ (1977) Development of squamous cell carcinoma in chronic discoid lupus erythematosus. Clin Exp Dermatol 3:161
89. Millard LG, Rowell NR (1979) Abnormal laboratory test results and their relationship to prognosis in discoid lupus erythematosus: a long-term follow-up study of 92 patients. Arch Dermatol 115:1055—1058
90. Millns JL, McDuffic FC, Muller SA, Jordon RE (1978) Development of photosensitivity and an SLE-like syndrome in a patient with psoriasis. Arch Dermatol 114:1177—1181
91. Millns JR, Muller SA (1980) The coexistence of psoriasis and lupus erythematosus. Arch Dermatol 116:658—663
92. Moncada B (1974) Dermatitis herpetiformis: an association with systemic lupus erythematosus. Arch Dermatol 109:723—725
93. Moskowitz R, Freundlich B, Petrozzi J (1983) Lupus erythematosus arising in striae distensae. Cutis 31:503—505
94. Newbold PCH (1976) Beta-carotene in the treatment of discoid lupus erythematosus. Br. J Dermatol 95:100—101
95. Nishino H, Shibuya K, Nishida Y, Mushimoto M (1981) Lupus erythematosus-like syndrome with selective complete deficiency of C1q. Ann Intern Med 95:322—324
96. Olansky AJ, Briggaman RA, Gammon WR, Kelly TF, Mitchell Sams W (1982) Bullous systemic lupus erythematosus. J Am Acad Dermatol 7:511—520
97. Penneys NS, Wiley HE III (1979) Herpetiform blisters in systemic lupus erythematosus. Arch Dermatol 115:1427—1428
98. Piamphongsant T, Sawarrapreecha S, Gritiyacangson P, Sawchome Y, Kullavanijaya P (1978) Mixed lichen planus lupus erythematosus disease. J Cutan Pathol 5:209—215
99. Pinkus H (1973) Lichenoid tissue reactions. A speculative review of the clinical spectrum of epidermal basal cell damage with special reference to erythema dyschromicum perstans. Arch Dermatol 107:840—946
100. Presser SE, Tylor JR (1981) Squamous cell carcinoma in blacks with discoid lupus erythematosus. J Am Acad Dermatol 4:667—669
101. Provost TT (1979) Subsets in systemic lupus erythematosus. J Invest Dermatol 72:110—113
102. Provost TT, Reichlin M (1981) Antinuclear antibody-negative systemic lupus erythematosus. J Am Acad Dermatol 4:84—89
103. Prystoxsky SD, Herndon JH, Gilliam JN (1975) Chronic cutaneous lupus erythematosus (DLE). Medicine 55:183—191
104. Prystowsky SD, Gilliam JN (1975) Discoid lupus erythematosus as part of a larger disease spectrum: correlation of clinical features with laboratory findings in lupus erythematosus. Arch Dermatol 111:1448—1452
105. Prystowsky SD, Gilliam JN (1976) Chronic cutaneous lupus erythematosus (DLE): a clinical and laboratory investigation of 80 patients. Medicine 55:183—191
106. Prystowsky SD, Gilliam JN (1977) Antinuclear antibody studies in chronic cutaneous discoid lupus erythematosus. Arch Dermatol 113:183—186
107. Prystowsky SD, Gilliam JN (1983) Cutaneous subsets of lupus erythematosus. Dermatol Clin 4:449—460
108. Quimby FW, Schwartz RS (1978) The etiopathogenesis of systemic lupus erythematosus. Pathobiol Annu 8:35—39
109. Ratz JL, Bergfeld WF, Steck WD (1979) Erythermalgia with vasculitis: a review. J Am Acad Dermatol 1:443—450
110. Romero RW, Nesbitt LT, Rees RJ (1977) Unusual variant of lupus erythematosus or lichen planus. Arch Dermatol 113:741—748
111. Rothfield NF (1979) Lupus erythematosus. In: Fitzpatrick TB, Eisen AZ, Wolff K, Freedberg IM, Austen KF (eds) Dermatology in general medicine, 2nd McGraw Hill, New York, pp 1273—1298
112. Roundtree J, Weigand D, Burgdorf W (1982) Lupus erythematosus with oral and perianal mucous membrane involvement. Arch Dermatol 118:55—56
113. Rowell NR, Beck JS, Anderson JR (1963) Lupus erythematosus and erythema multiforme-like lesions. Arch Dermatol 88:176

114. Rowell NR (1982) The management of lupus erythematosus, scleroderma, lichen sclerosus and dermatomyositis. Clin Exp Dermatol 7:407—414
115. Rowell NR (1984) The natural history of lupus erythematosus. Clin Exp Dermatol 9:217—231
116. Sanchez NP, Peters MS, Winkelmann RK (1981) The histopathology of lupus erythematosus panniculitis. J Am Acad Dermatol 5:673—680
117. Santa Cruz DJ, Uitto J, Eisen AZ, Prioleau P (1983) Verrucous lupus erythematosus: ultrastructural studies on a distinct variant of chronic discoid lupus erythematosus. J Am Acad Dermatol 9:82—90
118. Scholtz M (1922) Lupus erythematosus acutus disseminatus haemorrhagicus. Arch Dermatol Syph 6:466
119. Schrager MA, Rothfield NF (1977) Pathways of complement activation in chronic discoid lupus: serologic and immunofluorescence studies. Arthritis Rheum 20:637—647
120. Schreiner E, Wolff K (1970) Systemic lupus erythematosus: Electron microscopic localization of in vivo bound globulins at the dermal—epidermal junction. J Invest Dermatol 55:325—328
121. Schulz EJ, Menter MA (1971) Treatment of discoid and subacute lupus erythematosus with cyclophosphamide. Br J Dermatol 85 [Suppl 7]:60—65
122. Schur PH, Sandson J (1968) Immunologic factors and chemical activity in lupus erythematosus. N Engl J Med 278:533—538
123. Scott A, Rees EG (1969) The relationship of systemic lupus erythematosus and discoid lupus erythematosus. Arch Dermatol 79:422—435
124. Sharp GC, Irwin WS, Tan EM, Gould RG, Holman HR (1972) Mixed connective tissue disease — an apparently distinct rheumatic disease syndrome associated with a specific antibody to an extractable nuclear antigen (ENA). Am J Med 52:148—159
125. Sharp GC, Irvon WS, May CM (1976) Association of antibodies to ribonucleoprotein and Sm antigens with mixed connective tissue diseases. N Engl J Med 295:1149—1154
126. Sharp GC, Anderson PC (1980) Current concepts in the classification of connective tissue diseases. J Am Acad Dermatol 2:269—279
127. Shu S, Provost T, Croxdale MD, Reichlin M, Beutner EH (1977) Nuclear depostis of immunoglobulin in skin of patients with systemic lupus erythematosus. Clin Exp Immunol 27:238—244
128. Sontheimer RD, Thomas JR, Gilliam JN (1979) Subacute cutaneous lupus erythematosus: a cutaneous marker for a distinct lupus erythematosus subset. Arch Dermatol 115:1409—1415
129. Sonntheimer RD, Stastny P, Gilliam JN (1981) HLA associations in subacute cutaneous lupus erythematosus. J Clin Invest 67:312—316
130. Sontheimer RD, Maddison PJ, Reichlin M, Jordon RE, Stastny P, Gilliam JN (1982) Serologic and HLA associations in subacute cutaneous lupus erythematosus, a clinical subset of lupus erythematosus. Ann Intern Med 97:664—666
131. Stanstny P, Stembridge VA, Ziff M (1963) Homologous disease in the adult rat, a model for autoimmune disease. J Exp Med 118:635—648
132. Stern R, Fu SM, Fotine M, Agnello V, Kunkel HG (1976) Hereditary C2 deficiency. Arthr Rheum 19:517—522
133. Stingl G, Hönigsmann H, Holubar K, Wolff K (1976) Ultrastructural localization of immunoglobulins in skin of patients with dermatitis herpetiformis. J Invest Dermatol 67:507—512
134. Stoll DM, King LE (1984) Association of bullous pemphigoid with systemic lupus erythematosus. Arch Dermatol 120:362—366
135. Synkowski D, Dore N, Provost TT (1982) Urticaria and urticaria-like lesions. In: Callen JP (ed) Clinics in rheumatic disease, vol 8. Saunders, Philadelphia, pp. 383—395
136. Talbot JH (1974) Historical background of discoid and systemic lupus erythematosus. In: Dubois EL (ed) Lupus erythematosus, 2nd edn. University of Southern California Press, Los Angeles, pp 1—9
137. Tan EM, Kunel HE (1966) Characteristics of a soluble antigen precipitating with sera of patients with systemic lupus erythematosus. J Immunol 96:464—471

138. Tani M, Shimizu R, Ban M, Murata Y, Tamaki A (1984) Systemic lupus erythematosus with vesiculobullous lesions. Arch Dermatol 120:1497—1501
139. Thomas JR, Daniel Su WP (1983) Concurrence of lupus erythematosus and dermatitis herpetiformis. Arch Dermatol 119:740—745
140. Tuffanelli DL, Dubois EL (1964) Cutaneous manifestations of systemic lupus erythematosus. Arch Dermatol 90:377—386
141. Tuffanelli DL (1971) Lupus erythematosus panniculitis (profundus): clinical and immunologic studies. Arch Dermatol 103:231—242
142. Tuffanelli DL (1972) Lupus erythematosus. Arch Dermatol 106:553—566
143. Tuffanelli DL (1981) Lupus erythematosus. J Am Acad Dermatol 4:127—142
144. Tuffanelli DL (1982) Discoid lupus erythematosus. In: Callen JP (ed) Clinics in theumatic diseases, vol 8., Saunders, Philadelphia, pp 327—341
145. Tuffanelli DL (1982) Lupus erythematosus (panniculitis) profundus. Hawaii Med J 41:394—395
146. Uitto J, Santa-Cruz DJ, Eisen AZ (1978) Verrucous lesions in patients with discoid lupus erythematosus. Clinical, histological and immunofluorescence studies. Br J Dermatol 98:507—520
147. Van der Horst JC, Cirkel PKS, Nieboer CN (1983) Mixed lichen planus-lupus erythematosus disease: a distinct entity? Clinical, histopathological and immunopathological studies in six patients. Clin Exp Dermatol 8:631—640
148. Volc-Platzer B, Wolff K (1983) Behandlung eines subakutkutanen Lupus erythematosus mit Thalidomid. Hautarzt 34:175—178
149. Weigand DA (1984) The lupus band test: a re-evaluation. J Am Acad Dermatol 11:230—234
150. Weston WL, Harmon C, Peebles C, Manchester D, Franco HL, Hugo JC, Norris DA (1982) A serological marker for neonatal lupus erythematosus. Br J Dermatol 107:377—386
151. Willemze R, Vermeer BJ, Meijer CJLM (1984) Immunohistochemical studies in lymphocytic infiltration of the skin (Jessner) and discoid lupus erythematosus. J Am Acad Dermatol 11:832—840
152. Winkelmann RK (1970) Panniculitis and systmic lupus erythematosus. JAMA 211:472—475
153. Wolff-Schreiner E, Wolff K (1973) Immunoglobulins at the dermal—epidermal junction in lupus erythematosus: ultrastructural investigations. Arch Dermatol Res 246:193—210
154. Yaoita H, Katz SI (1976) Immunoelectronmicroscopic localization of IgA in skin of patients with dermatitis herpetiformis. J Invest Dermatol 67:502—506

Neurological Manifestations

E. MAIDA and E. HORVATITS

Introduction

Neurological manifestations are common features of systemic lupus erythematosus (SLE). They concern all levels of the central nervous system as well as peripheral nerves and muscles [1]. Depending on the type and extent of the lesions and on different combinations located throughout the nervous system, they present a great variety of neurological symptoms and syndromes. This led Dubois [28] to state that nervous system SLE has replaced neurosyphilis to be the "big imitator". Indeed, the diversity of clinical findings may pose diagnostic problems, especially in cases of first manifestations of SLE in the nervous system, and in cases with non-focal, non-specific symptoms of multiple possible origins like depression and headache. The diagnostic difficulties are sustained by the fact that there exists no relevant examination by which nervous system SLE can be indentified with certainty. However, early diagnosis of nervous system involvement in SLE is not a medical problem alone. Because the manifestations may lead to incapacitation, predominantly in young people, they are also of important social relevance.

Neuropathology and Pathophysiology

There is no neurological symptom which may not occur in nervous system SLE. This is due to the widespread involvement of nervous system structures, in which no preferential affinity to special levels or functional entities is seen. However, pathophysiological mechanisms of nervous system manifestations in SLE are not completely clear. Predominantly small parenchymal and meningeal vessels show fibrinoid and hyalin degeneration and endothelial proliferation with micro-occlusions, perivascular lymphocytic infiltrations, micro-haemorrhages or — more rarely — a typical vasculitis with inflammatory infiltrates within the vessel walls [20, 29, 38, 39, 45, 57, 67]. These alterations are obviously responsible for infarctions and haemorrhages and may explain particular focal symptoms. But it is an interesting and poorly understood fact that there is a remarkably weak correlation between clinical and neuropathological findings [29, 38, 81]. Nearly half of the patients with clinically evident neurological symptoms do not show pathological nervous system alterations. On the other hand, about half of the patients without neurological complaints demonstrate nervous system manifestations by neuropathological examinations [29, 57, 81].Moreover, infarctions and the other findings mentioned above may not account sufficiently for non-focal neurological symptoms. This suggests that changes other than vascular ones may affect the nervous system. Autoimmune phenomena with formation of different autoantibodies are typical features of SLE [52, 64]. The nervous system is an immunologically active organ, which is capable of local immune responses and which often becomes the target of autoimmune reactions, e.g. in multiple sclerosis or postinfectious acute encephalomyelitis. Therefore, it was supposed that local autoimmune mechanisms may be directed against nervous system constituents. They may damage the nervous system alone or in combination with vascular alterations [10, 17, 52, 62, 74]. The important findings which first pointed to the existence of local immune mechanisms were the detection of immune complex deposits within the choroid plexus [3, 32, 47, 65], and of cerebrospinal fluid (CSF) alterations of immunoglobulin and complement levels [44, 69, 70, 72, 73, 83, 84, 93, 96], and the occurrence of anti-DNA antibodies and immune complexes in the CSF of SLE patients [46, 58, 74, 90]. Later on, autoantibodies against the nervous system were demonstrated, i.e. IgM and IgG anti-neuronal antibodies, brain-reactive lymphocytotoxic antibodies and antiglycolipid antibodies [9—13, 16, 18, 50, 53, 86, 92]. CSF or serum autoantibody titres correlate well with the clinical activity of nervous system SLE [9, 16, 50, 106, 110, 111]. Experimental studies support the assumption that local autoimmunity is responsible at least for non-focal neurological signs, and possibly for a part of the focal lesions. Antineuronal antibodies placed into the CSF of experimental animals produce cerebral oedema, meningeal inflammation and epileptic seizures [95], and antibodies against synaptosomal membranes cause significant memory impairment [60]. These animal models may help to elucidate the pathogenetic mechanisms of nervous system SLE in humans and encourage the search for further target antigens for autoimmunity within the nervous system.

At present, no definite explanation exists of the pathomechanisms in nervous system SLE, especially of the role and mode of action of autoimmune phenomena. Current hypotheses postulate a disturbance of the blood-brain-barrier (BBB) due to immune complex deposits in the choroid plexus, or else SLE-related vascular alterations, by which the transudation of autoantibodies against nervous tissue and lymphocytes is facilitated [10, 62]. However, there are still unresolved problems, such as the nature and role of thecally produced immunoglobulins, the effect of immune regulatory dysfunctions on the lymphoid tissue of the nervous system (which is known to react autochthonously and independently from the peripheral blood) and the role of immune mediators in the extent of the lesions. Further questions are whether there are one or more primary targets of autoimmunity within the nervous tissue, or also secondary autoantigens, which are set free during a first immunologic attack on the nervous tissue, and whether reactions against different nervous tissue antigens produce different clinical symptoms.

Peripheral nerves and muscles are less frequently involved than the central nervous system, but there are similar discrepancies between frequency and intensity of clinical symptoms and of pathological findings [52, 54]. Histological examinations in cases of polyneuritis show axonal or occasionally demyelinating lesions which are caused by alterations of nerve vessels. In addition, the nervous tissue may be damaged directly by immunoglobulin deposits within the nerve fascicles, like in paraproteinaemic neuropathies [99], and by local immune complex formations at the site of the complement receptors within the peripheral nerves [80]. The latter pathomechanisms might be responsible for the development of Guillain-Barré syndrome in SLE patients, but action of cross-reacting antineuronal antibodies against peripheral nervous tissue constituents cannot be ruled out in these cases.

Muscles show either a true polymyositits, with inflammatory alterations of vessels and perivascular and interstitial infiltrations with lymphocytes and macrophages, or a myopathy with fibre atrophies, which follows steroid medication [63]. A direct action of autoantibodies against muscles is unlikely. The rare occurrence of acetylcholine-receptor autoantibodies and of myasthenic symptoms [104] is an accidental coincidence of multiple autoimmune diseases rather than an SLE-related phenomenon, which is possibly associated with a special pattern of HLA-antigens.

Clinical Features

Neurological symptoms in SLE may be focal or diffuse, and they refer to either localization within the nervous system — such as brain cortex, basal ganglia, brain stem, cerebrellum, spinal cord, nerve roots, peripheral nerves and muscles. The manifestations either appear during a single episode of active disease, or are relapsing-remitting, presenting with symptoms which may be different or identical during individual bouts, or they are chronically existent [28, 39, 52].

While involvement of the nervous system — especially of the central nervous system — used to be viewed as a rather rare condition of poor or even fatal prognosis, these manifestations are now seen much more frequently, due to the generally better prognosis and prolonged survival of SLE patients, and they are no longer considered to be more life-shortening than other organ mifestations [31, 32, 42, 48, 91, 107]. A recent multicentre study of 1103 SLE patients showed that central nervous system involvement had no influence on survival rates, and that it was the cause of death in only 10% of the patients who died from SLE during an observation period of 10 years, i.e. 2% of the total number of patients [40, 89].

About 60% of SLE patients show central nervous system manifestations at any time during the course of the disease, fewer than 10% present with clinical symptoms of peripheral nerve lesions and nearly 50% suffer from muscle involvement [1, 8, 31, 32, 34, 39, 52, 54, 62, 81, 94]. A survey of the different neurological manifestations, including psychiatric symptoms, is given below:

Headache (migraine)
Psychiatric disorders
  Organic mental syndrome
  Depression
  Psychosis
Epileptic seizures
Stroke
Haemorrhages
Cerebral venous thrombosis
Brainstem dysfunctions
Cranial nerve lesions
Cerebellar symptoms
Chorea
Meningitis
Myelitis
Polyneuritis
Muscle disorders

About two—thirds of the central nervous system manifestations consist of non-focal signs like headache and psychiatric symptoms. The frequency of headache undoubtedly attributable to SLE is difficult to determine, because headache is such a non-specific symptom of multifactorial origin, having a high incidence in the normal population. It can be associated with central nervous system SLE with some certainty if it appears during a relapse with serologically evident alterations, and if it is sensitive to steroid treatment. In most instances the headache is of migraine-type with scotoma and hemicrania; sometimes it is complicated by transient focal neurological deficits [15, 55]. The pathomechanism of migraine in SLE is not clear. It might be attributable to SLE-specific vascular dysfunctions and perivascular inflammations (which enhande the action of vasoactive substances) [15], or to autoimmune phenomena.

The estimations in the literature of frequency of psychiatric symptoms in SLE are contradictory; between 10% and 50% have been described [5, 6, 8, 28, 31, 32, 52, 81]. The reasons for this are general difficulties of diagnosing psychiatric disorders, especially in mild cases, and the frequency of psychiatric examinations, i.e. whether the patients were seen at regular intervals during the course of the disease and in all relapses, or only when psychiatric symptoms became evident. Organic mental syndromes and depressions are found most frequently, often in association with other neurological symptoms like migraine or epileptic seizures [5, 6, 52, 81].

Epilepsy is another frequently occurring sign of central nervous system SLE. About 20—30% of patients suffer from seizures at one or more times during the course of the disease. Focal seizures are seen as well as primarily generalized seizures, the latter dominating markedly [28, 31, 32, 39, 52, 62, 81].

Stroke is a serious but rare event in central nervous system SLE, occurring in only about 10% of cases [1, 28, 29, 31, 48, 52, 62, 91]. Complete stroke is mostly caused by occlusions of medium-sized arteries like posterior cerebral artery and the branches of carotid, basilar and middle cerebral arteries. Massive haemorrhages are seen exceptionally [109]; the same is true for occlusions of the carotid, basilar, vertebral and subclavian arteries [33, 52] and for venous occlusions due to cerebral thrombophlebitis [77]. Cerebrovascular infarctions are often preceded by migraine and by transitory neurologcal deficits, because large areas of cerebral vessels are usually involved. For that reason cases of transitory ischaemic attacks may be difficult to distinguish from migraine with focal neurological symptoms. Although stroke is a potentially fatal complication of central nervous system SLE, Rosner et al. [89] found it to be the cause of death in only 5% of patients who died from SLE.

Other central nervous system manifestations are seen occasionally. Most reports concern only a single or a few cases, as is the case with descriptions of myelitis and myelopathy [59, 108], brain stem and cranial nerve involvement [25, 66, 78, 98], aseptic meningitis [31, 36], cerebellar symptoms [103] and chorea [2, 19, 27, 76]. For the development of chorea, Bruyn and Padberg [19] postulated an immunological pathomechanism by which neurotransmission within the extrapyramidal system is disturbed.

Peripheral nervous system involvement is only seen in less than 10% of SLE patients [1, 28, 52]. It manifests with typical paraesthesias or hypaesthesia of stocking- or glove-like distribution and diminished tendon reflexes, and exceptionally with true Guillain-Barré syndrome [41, 94]. As has already been mentioned, axons or myelin sheaths are directly damaged by SLE-specific vascular changes and/or immunologically mediated alterations. Sweet et al. [100] mentioned the appearance of amyloidosis in SLE patients. This might be caused by SLE-related amyloid deposits; but it might just as well be an occasional coincidence of two unrelated diseases.

The clinical features of muscle involvement are predominantly proximal muscle weakness and pains. These symptoms occur in about 50% of SLE patients [52, 54]. Like peripheral nerve lesions, they do not leave major incapacities. Sometimes it may be difficult to distinguish pains due to muscle or peripheral nerve involvement from those af adjacent joints [54, 79].

For practical reasons, e.g. for therapeutic considerations, it may be important to differentiate between symptoms due to primary or direct SLE-related lesions

Table 1. Indirect nervous system involvement in systemic lupus erythematosus

Symptom	Causes
Headache	Uraemia, hypertension, hypoxia (anaemia, cardiac insufficiency)
Psychiatric disturbance	Uraemia, hypoxia, steroid treatment
Epileptic seizures	Uraemia, hypoxia
Stroke	Hypertension, embolism (endocarditis), hypoxia, steroid treatment
Haemorrhage	Hypertension, thrombopenia
Meningitis	Infection (leucopenia, immunosuppressive treatment)
Polyneuropathy	Uraemia, cytostatic/antimalarial drugs
Myopathy	Steroid/antimalarial treatment

and those due to secondary or indirect alterations, which result from other organ manifestations or treatments. The different possibilities of secondary nervous system alterations in SLE are displayed in table 1.

The most important symptoms are the sequelae of renal failure, i.e. headache, psychiatric symptoms, epileptic seizures and polyneuropathy due to uraemia, as also headache, stroke and haemorrhages resulting from hypertension. Hypoxia due to anaemia or cardiac insufficiency may induce non-focal neurological symptoms such as headache and psychiatric symptoms, or cerebrovascular insufficiency. Immunosuppressive treatments, as well as leucopenia, markedly increase the risk of infections in SLE patients, including meningitis [1, 31, 68, 87, 89, 97]. Other neurological complications following treatments of SLE are often seen, especially the side-effects of steroid administration, such as myopathy, which may occur after only a few weeks of therapy [63]. Ayoub et al. [4] reported central nervous system manifestations in 3 out of 18 patients who had received steroid pulse therapy for active SLE without evidence of nervous system involvement. The patients developed seizures, hemiplegia and psychosis respectively, which resolved after a few days. The high incidence of neurological symptoms in these patients, compared to the lack of such complications in multiple sclerosis patients treated by pulse therapy by us and several others, and also the rapid remission of the symptoms, suggest that they were not caused by pulse therapy but by manifestation in the course of relapse, or by activation of a pre-existing latent involvement of the central nervous system. Possibly, pulse therapy of three days' duration was too short for these patients to suppress an as yet unapparent central nervous system involvement. When using 3-day pulse therapy for multiple sclerosis relapses, we saw a rapid remission but a recurrence of the same or even enhanced symptoms after a few days in some patients, whereas this was never observed with 5- or 7-day treatments [unpublished data]. Other neurological complications of SLE therapies refer to polyneuropathy or myopathy following administration of cytotoxic and antimalarial drugs. Induction of aseptic meningitis by ibuprofen has been described [101], but the association is difficult to appraise, as aseptic meningitis is a known manifestation of SLE.

Another rare indirect nervous system lesion, carpal tunnel syndrome due to fasciitis [112], should be mentioned, because it is a frequently diagnosed syndrome among neurologically affected patients. The neurologist should bear SLE in mind for aetiology of the syndrome, if the presence of SLE or cutaneous LE is already known. Even in the absence of such knowledge, and, in particular, if there is no evident mechanical influence or other reason to explain its occurrence in a young, often female patient, and if the patient suffers from arthralgias or an elevated blood sedimentation rate, the syndrome might be an early sign of as yet undiagnosed SLE.

In about 25% of SLE patients, the disease first appears with neurological manifestations, predominantly of the central nervous system [1, 23, 32, 39, 52, 56, 61, 78, 113, 114]. Neurological symptoms sometimes occur as the only signs of SLE and may precede evident systemic disease for many months or years [2, 71, 78]. Recurrent episodes of neurological deficits and of aseptic meningitis have been reported [22, 30, 36, 43]. Cendrowski and Stepien [22] described a clinical variant of SLE resembling multiple sclerosis with relapsing, disseminated neurological deficits. Devos and Destee [26] observed a patient with clinically evident multiple sclerosis, who developed signs of typical SLE 42 years after the onset of the neurological disorder, but it semed to them more likely that the patient suffered from two unrelated autoimmune diseases. As has been mentioned, a certain pattern of histocompatibility antigens might be responsible for such rare associations of autoimmune diseases like SLE and myasthenia gravis or multiple sclerosis.

Table 2a. Neurological symptoms in 26 patients[a] with nervous system and muscle involvement during the course of systemic lupus erythematosus (39 relapses)

Symptom	No. of patients	%
Headache	9	34.6
Transitory ischaemic attack	2	7.7
Epileptic seizures	6	23.1
Organic mental syndrome	5	19.2
Depression	2	7.7
Stroke	2	7.7
Brain stem dysfunction	8	30.8
Cerebellar syndrome	2	7.7
Cranial nerve lesion	1	3.8
Polyneuritis	2	7.7
Myalgia	5	19.2
Muscle weakness	3	11.5
Myasthenic syndrome	1	3.8

[a] Group 1, taken from 50 patients registered at the Second Department of Medicine of the University Clinic of Vienna

Table 2b. Neurological symptoms in 27 patients[a] with acute nervous system involvement in systemic lupus erythematosus

Symptom	No. of patients	%
Headache	3[b]	11.1
Transitory ischaemic attack	6[b]	22.2
Epileptic seizures	5[b]	18.5
Organic mental syndrome	4	14.8
Depression	1	3.7
Stroke	4	14.8
Brain stem dysfunction	8[c]	29.6
Chorea	2	7.4
Aseptic meningitis	1	3.7
Cranial nerve lesion	1	3.7
Polyneuritis	1	3.7
Muscle weakness	1	3.7
Myalgia	3	11.1

[a] Group 2 patients of different neurological, medical and children's hospitals, whose cerebrospinal fluid was examined at the Vienna University Neurological Clinic
[b] One patient belonged to group 1
[c] Two patients belonged to group 1

First manifestations of SLE mostly present with migraine, psychiatric symptoms, especially depressions, epileptic seizures and stroke or transient ischaemic attacks [23, 61, 62, 81].

The authors' own observations refer to 50 SLE patients registered at the Second Department of Medicine of the University Clinic of Vienna (group 1) and 27 patients whose CSF was examined at the Vienna University Neurological Clinic at the time of active nervous system SLE (group 2). Five patients of group 2 belonged to group 1, the others were patients of different internal, neurological and children's hospitals. A summary of the neurological manifestations of SLE in the two groups is presented in Tables 2a, b.

Twenty-six (52%) of the 50 patients of group 1 presented with nervous system manifestations during the course of SLE. The observation period was between 1 and 32 years (mean, 10.2 years). In 10 patients (20%) SLE started with nervous system affections. The frequency of neurological symptoms which occurred throughout the course of the disease was nearly the same as was described in the literature, except regarding brain stem and cranial nerve lesions, which were found with greater and less frequency respectively. This might be explained by the discrepancies in clinical diagnosis of lesions of these locations, which are sometimes difficult to discriminate.

Group 2 (Table 2b) showed a higher rate of cerebrovascular accidents and a lower one of headache and muscle involvement, because CSF examinations tend to be performed in severely affected patients. Among the 22 patients were three children. Five patients (27.3%, including two of the three children) suffered from onset of SLE with neurological symptoms.

Twenty of the 26 patients in group 1 showed in isolated involvement of either central or peripheral nervous system or muscles; the remaining six patients presented with combined manifestations. The 26 patients had experienced 39 relapses during the course of SLE, the majority of which remitted. Only four patients had chronic symptoms, which predominantly concerned muscles (Table 3). Most patients had suffered one realpse in the past, and they showed signs of

Table 3. Frequency and type of neurological manifestations in 50 patients with systemic lupus erythematosus (group 1)

Type	No. of patients	Course		No. of relapses
		Remitting	Non-remitting	
CNS	14	13	1	20
CNS + PNS	3	3	—	7
CNS + muscles	2	2	—	4
PNS	1	1	—	1
PNS + muscles	1	1	—	1
Muscles	5[a]	2	3[a]	6[a]
Total	26	22	4	39

CNS, Central nervous system; PNS, peripheral nervous system

[a] Including one patient with myasthenic syndrome

lesion in only one location more frequently than in more than one location. The more relapses had occurred in a patient, the more locations were affected (Table 4).

Table 4. Distribution of disseminated nervous system involvement in relation to relapses with neurological symptoms in 26 patients with nervous system manifestations in systemic lupus erythematosus (group 1)

No. of relapses	No. of patients	No. of localizations	
		1	>1
1	18	11	7
2	4	2	2
3	3	—	3
4	1	—	1

Table 5. Distribution of relapses with focal and non-focal neurological symptoms in 19 patients with central nervous system manifestations in systemic lupus erythematosus (group 1)

CNS symptoms	No. of relapses	%
Focal	8	28.6
Non-focal	16	57.1
Both	4	14.3
Total	28	

Central nervous system manifestations occurred more frequently with non-focal than with focal signs, as was described in the literature. In a few patients both focal and non-focal lesions appeared during individual relapses (Table 5).

Altogether, group 2 showed a similar distribution of total relapse number and relapse rate in individual patients and of dissemination of lesions throughout the nervous system, and this is therefore not shown in additional tables. The only difference to group 1 was a higher incidence of central nervous system manifestations and a lower one of muscle involvement, which obviously can be attributed to a greater selection within that group of patients.

Laboratory Examinations

Different technical examinations are performed with the aim of proving the existence of nervous system involvement in SLE, estimating its extent and distinguishing between a primary or a secondary manifestation. No specific test is available to serve that purpose, nor, probably, will be in the future, because of the diversity of SLE-related alterations already mentioned, and because different pathomechanisms are responsible for the neurological symptoms, (e.g. hypoxia due to local vessel changes and autoimmune reactions which directly damage the nervous tissue).

As has been demonstrated with neuropathological examinations, laboratory findings do not correlate well with the clinical picture, either [28, 39, 52, 96]. They are therefore neither suitable to prove a nervous system involvement during an acute relapse nor to affirm the diagnosis in cases of first manifestations of SLE with neurological symptoms, without searching for typical serological alterations or other organ manifestations. Except with muscle biopsies, most of the examinations ascertain a nervous system affection only indirectly and do not allow of an exact causative differentiation.

Muscle biopsies are the most appropriate means to demonstrate muscle involvement in SLE. Inflammatory infiltrations are seen in cases of polymyositis. By contrast, a secondary alteration of muscles due to steroid therapy is accompanied by type II fibre atrophies. For therapeutic reasons it may be important to distinguish between these two causes of muscle symptoms, because polymyositis demands an increased dosage of steroids, something which in cases of steroid myopathy should be avoided unless really necessary. Nevertheless, in many patients electromyography (EMG) is sufficient for routine differential diagnosis. In cases of myopathy as well as myositis, amplitude and spontaneous activity are decreased and positive sharp waves are seen, which in myositis occur much more frequently and are accompanied by big potentials. EMG is also useful to distinguish between pain caused by myositis or resulting from neuritis or arthritis of adjacent joints [1, 52, 79]. EMG was performed in 20 of the 50 of our own group 1 SLE patients (Table 6), among whom were six of the eight patients with clinical signs of muscle involvement. Four of these six patients showed a pathological pattern consistent with myositis, which was confirmed by biopsy. One patient displayed the typical EMG and clinical features of myasthenic syn-

Table 6. Findings of pathological laboratory examinations in relation to clinical symptoms of neurological manifestations in 50 patients with systemic lupus erythematosus (group 1)

Examinations	No. of patients	Pathological			Normal		
		Total	sy+[a]	sy−[b]	Total	sy+[a]	sy−[b]
EEG	17	13	12	1	4	2	2
CT	7	1	1	—	6	5	1
Brain scan	10	2	2	—	8	8	—
Xenon clearance	5	4	4	—	1	1	—
Angiography	1	1	1	—	—	—	—
EMG	20	12	5	7	8	1	7
Muscle biopsy	4	4	4	—	—	—	—
Electroneurography	15	11	3	8	4	1	3
CSF	5	4	4	—	1	1	—
Neuropsychological test	4	4	3	1	—	—	—

[a] Relevant symptoms present
[b] Relevant symptoms not present

drome. EMG was normal in one patient with muscle weakness which was clinically attributed to myositis. Seven of the remaining 14 patients without clinically evident muscle involvement demonstrated pathological EMG alterations, namely that of myopathy in six patients and of myositis in one patient. Altogether, the observations give evidence of the importance of EMG examinations in SLE patients, particularly in the absence of clinical symptoms, in early recognition of the development of steroid myopathy.

Electroneurographic (ENG) alterations are found in peripheral nervous system manifestations in SLE. These are signs of axonal degeneration with diminished nerve conduction velocity, which is associated with SLE-related vessel alterations, and also by toxic effects of drugs or by uraemia. Occasionally, they are of the demyelinating type with prolonged distal latency, which is predominantly observed in cases of polyneuritis or Guillain-Barré-syndrome in SLE [41]. Altogether, ENG is of minor diagnostic value in SLE, because it is difficult to distinguish primary SLE-specific alterations from polyneuropathy due to a secondary manifestation or even due to an unrelated cause, as polyneuropathy is a frequently observed disorder of multifactorial origin. Fifteen of our 50 patients were examined for ENG alterations, of whom a remarkably high number (11) showed pathological findings. These were three with and eight without clinical symptoms of polyneuropathy. The three patients developed signs of peripheral nerve lesions during an acute relapse. This was also the case in one patient whose ENG reading was normal. Since in that patient the symptoms responded quickly to treatment, ENG might have been already normal at the time of its performance. One of the eight patients without clinical signs of polyneuropathy and positive ENG findings had received vincristine therapy, in the other patients renal dysfunction was assumed to be the cause auf polyneuropathy.

Electroencephalography (EEG) is another non-specific examination by which focal or non-focal cerebral dysfunctions or — more rarely — an increased cortical excitability (i.e. a tendency for seizures) can be demonstrated. EEG abnormalities are found in a large proportion of patients with different central nervous system disorders, and even in about one quarter of healthy individuals. One should keep this in mind when interpreting EEG findings in SLE patients. A very high proportion, up to two—thirds, of SLE patients show pathological EEG alterations, mostly of the diffuse type with increased occurrence of slow waves, sometimes with signs of a functional lateralization, seldom with paroxysms [15, 32, 52, 67, 81, 96]. Our own observations refer to 17 of the 50 SLE patients in group 1, on whom EEG was performed. Among these 17 patients were 14 of the 19 patients with central nervous system manifestations. Of these 14 patients, 12 showed abnormalities (signs of a diffuse brain dysfunction in 11 patients and paroxysms in one patient); the other two gave normal readings. We cannot reach a conclusion about the value of EEG examinations in recognizing latent cerebral involvement, becaue we have too little data concerning EEG findings in SLE patients without central nervous system affections.

Neuropsychological tests were also performed in too few patients for an estimation to be formed of its diagnostic usefulness. Signs of organic mental syndrome were present in three patients with corresponding clinical findings and in one patient without evident mental disturbance. Neuropsychological tests should routinely be done in all patients, because psychiatric disorders occur frequently in SLE and slight disturbances are often difficult to recognize by clinical examinations.

Brain scan abnormalities are seen in association with dysfunctions of the BBB. Previous reports of brain scan findings in central nervous system SLE have described their poor correlation with clinical features [32, 39, 96]. This agrees with our own observations. Ten of the 19 group 1 patients with cerebral involvement underwent static brain scan, but only two demonstrated pathological radionuclide accumulation. Both suffered from acute stroke. The six other patients with focal and two with non-focal neurological deficits had normal static brain scans. Taken together, this examination is of no diagnostic importance in SLE.

Dynamic brain scans using xenon-133 are more practicable in cerebral SLE, because they are sensitive to diffuse as well as focal reductions of the cerebral blood flow. The findings correlate well with the clinical picture and with the activity of central nervous system SLE [7, 85]. Our own observations refer only to five patients with cerebral manifestations, of whom four demonstrated pathological findings (Table 6).

Examination of cerebral blood flow and metabolism by positron emission tomography has recently been introduced, and it promises well for use in cerebral SLE [49]. Besides its diagnostic value, this technique offers the possibility of sensitive monitoring of therapeutic effects in acute cerebral SLE. Nuclear magnetic resonance is another new technique, which is appropriate to detection of small focal or scattered central nervous system manifestations in SLE [105]. It is superior to computerized tomography (CT) because of its higher resolution. CT can reveal hypodense foci due to ischaemia, sometimes of multifocal distribution, and severe haemorrhages may be demonstrable in acute relapses [88], as well as cerebral atrophy or other late sequelae of central nervous system SLE [14, 82]. In a large proportion of patients, however, the vascular alterations of cerebral SLE are too small to be detected by CT. Our own observations refer to seven patients, of whom six suffered from acute central nervous system involvement. Only one of these patients showed CT alteration (Table 6).

Angiography also is of minor importance in SLE, because it does not show the typical small vessel alterations [102, 115]. Moreover, it is associated with an increased risk because of the frequent allergies in SLE patients and its performance might therefore do more harm than good.

Examination of the CSF seems to be more valuable, because it is the only way to prove nervous system inflammations and the most sensitive one to determine a disturbance of the BBB. The CSF cell count is normal or — especially in acute relapses — slightly elevated, usually to less than 150 cells/mm^3 [21, 32, 52, 67, 70, 72, 96], except in the rare instances of aseptic meningitis, which may present between a few hundred and a thousand cells/mm^3. Activated lymphocytes and plasma cells are found by cytological examinations. If there is pronounced tissue damage or haemorrhage, additional macrophages with vacuoles and haematophages are seen. The occurrence of LE cells within the CSF has been described [37]. Our own material showed slight pleocytosis, below 150 cells/mm^3, in 12 out of 27 patients (group 2), all of whom presented with central nervous system manifestations. The cytological picture showed up to 85% lymphocytes and 5% plasma cells in all instances and thus was indistinguishable from findings in multiple sclerosis or other chronic inflammations.

A disturbance of the BBB is indicated by an increase of CSF total protein concentration and — for a more accurate estimation — by an elevated CSF/serum-albumin ratio. Slightly elevated total protein levels, below 70 mg/dl, are seen in about half of the patients with central nervous system SLE, mostly in active phases of the disease [32, 52, 67, 96]. CSF alterations are not usually associated with peripheral nervous system and muscle involvement. Albuminocytologic dissociation may be observed in cases of Guillain-Barré syndrome [41].

Our own observations of 27 patients who were all in realpse showed a dysfunction of the BBB with increased total protein content, up to 88 mg/dl in 16 cases, and an elevated CSF/serum-albumin ratio of up to 0.012 in 21 patients. In 8 cases the disturbance of the BBB was so pronounced that high molecular weight protein — like α2-macroglobulin — was allowed to enter the CSF.

CSF immunoglobulins have been reported to be increased, but occasionally also to be decreased [22, 32, 47, 52, 67, 69, 70, 72, 73, 96]. The latter finding might be attributed to local consumption with formation of immune complexes [65, 90]. Immunoglobulin levels within the CSF are elevated either because of an increased transudation rate, due to a disturbance of the BBB or increased serum immunoglobulin levels, or else — more importantly — because of thecal antibody production. Elevated immunoglobulin and autoantibody concentrations in the serum have been described in conjuction with neuropsychiatric disorders in SLE [11, 16, 35]. Increased passage of anti-nervous tissue autoantibodies into the nervous system, due to a disturbance of the BBB, has been suggested for an immune-mediated pathomechanism in nervous system SLE [17, 18, 47, 62, 86]. Anti-DNA antibodies, which have been demonstrated in the CSF, probably reach the central nervous system across the BBB [46, 58, 74]. However, disturbance of the BBB might not be the only mechanism by which the nervous system becomes the target of autoimmunity. According to Krankenhagen and Cohen

Table 7. Frequency of pathological cerebrospinal fluid alterations in 27 patients with nervous system manifestations during acute relapses of systemic lupus erythematosus

CSF alteration	No. of patients	%
Pleocytosis	12	44.4
Total protein elevation	16	59.3
Elevated CSF/serum-albumin ratio	21	77.8
Thecally produced IgG	20	74.1
IgA	22	81.4
IgM	4	14.8
Thecally decreased C4, C3	18	66.7
C1 inactivator	4[a]	57.1
increased C4, C3	1	31.7
C1 inactivator	1[a]	14.3

[a] C1 inactivator was only determined in seven of the 27 patients

[61], and Small et al. [96], immunoglobulins may be produced within the central nervous system. This opinion was confirmed by our own observations in group 2 SLE patients. Local synthesis was estimated for IgG in 20 patients, for IgM in four patients, and for IgA in 22 patients (Table 7), using radial immunodiffusion technique and a formula which has been described elsewhere [75]. Thecal IgA synthesis has been found more frequently in connective tissue diseases than in any other inflammatory disease of comparable symptomatology [73]. Obviously the pathomechanism is similar to that of IgA production in synovial fluid in rheumatoid arthritis [51]. We do not know the antibody specifity of thecally produced immunoglobulins. The local synthesis might be caused by thecal activation of B lymphocytes, due to a disturbance of local suppressor cell activity by lymphocytotoxic antibodies which have passed the BBB. That way, autoantibodies might be synthesized within the nervous tissue. Bluestein [10, 13] was able to demonstrate markedly higher titres of antineuronal antibodies in the CSF than in the serum during an acute SLE relapse in patients who suffered from neurological symptoms.

Complement decrease in the CSF of SLE patients with neurological manifestations also suggests local immune phenomena [44, 72, 83, 84]. The method of estimating the ratio of CSF and serum complement concentrations in relation to the CSF/serum-albumin ratio (that means regarding the actual function of the BBB) allows an accurate determination of local activation or consumption of complement factors [73]. In this way we found a local decrease of complement C3 and C4 in 18 out of 27 patients, and a local activation in one case. C1 inactivator was examined in seven patients, four of whom showed locally decreased and one thecally increased levels.

Altogether, the combined occurrence of slight pleocytosis or normal cell count, minor disturbance of the BBB, thecal production of immunoglobulins, especially IgA and IgG, and local consumption of complement seems to be the pathognomonic CSF syndrome for active central nervous system involvement in SLE. Occasionally, an elevation of myelin basic protein can be observed in the CSF [24], which indicates acute demyelination. In cases of first manifestations of SLE with neurological symptoms, this finding may aggravate the difficulties in distinguishing nervous system SLE from multiple sclerosis. Like SLE, the latter is associated with local IgG production and slight pleocytosis, but thecal IgA production and complement decrease are usually not present [73].

Conclusion

Neurological manifestations are observed with increasing frequency due to the better prognosis of SLE and longer survival of patients. They are no longer seen as a major cause of death from the disease, bute are instead often the first signs of SLE; in these cases they may pose diagnostic difficulties because they occur with such a great variety of neurological symptoms. At present no specific tests are available for diagnosis of nervous system SLE. The demonstration of autoan-

Neurological Manifestations **265**

tibodies against nervous tissue in the CSF is a promising finding. Specific alterations are to be expected from CSF analysis rather than from other technical investigations. However, as long as the pathomechanisms of nervous system involvement remain unknown, it is doubtful whether the diagnosis can ever be made by a single specific test. In all probability, different mechanisms are responsible for different neurological symptoms. Above all, SLE is a clinical diagnosis of which neurologists should be aware, so that they may recognize, as early as possible, neurological manifestations of that serious disease.

References

1. Aita JA (1975) Neurologic manifestations of general diseases. Thomas, Springfield
2. Arisaka O, Obinata K, Sasaki H, Arisaka M, Kaneko K (1984) Chorea as an initial manifestation of systemic lupus erythematosus: a case report of an 10-year-old girl. Clin Peditr 23(5):298—300
3. Atkins CJ, Kondon JJ, Quismorio FP, Friou GJ (1972) The choroid plexus in systemic lupus erythematosus. Ann Intern Med 75:65—73
4. Ayoub WT, Torretti D, Harrington TM (1983) Central nervous system manifestations after pulse therapy for systemic lupus erythematosus. Arthritis Rheum 26(6):809—810
5. Baker M (1973) Psychopathology in systemic lupus erythematosus: I. Psychiatric observations. Semin Arthritis Rheum 2:95—10
6. Baker M (1973) Psychopathology in systemic lupus erythematosus: II. Relation to clinical observations, corticosteroid administration and cerebrospinal fluid C4. Semin Arthritis Rheum 2:111—126
7. Bennahum DA, Messner RP, Shoop JD (1974) Brain scan findings in central nervous system involvement by lupus erythematosus. Ann Intern Med 81:763—765
8. Bennett R, Hughes GRV, Bywaters EGL, Holt PHL (1972) Neuropsychiatric problems in systemic lupus erythematosus. Br Med J 4:342—345
9. Bluestein HG, Zvaifler NJ (1976) Brain reactive lymphocytotoxic antibodies in the serum of patients with systemic lupus erythematosus. J Clin Invest 57:509—516
10. Bluestein HG (1978) Neurocytotoxic antibodies in serum of patients with systemic lupus erythematosus. Proc Natl Acad Sci USA 75:3965—3969
11. Bluestein HG, Williams GW, Steinberg AD (1981) Cerebrospinal fluid antibodies to neuronal cells: association with neuropsychiatric manifestations of systemic lupus erythematosus. Am J Med 70:240—246
12. Bluestein HG, Woods VL (1982) Antineuronal antibodies in systemic lupus erythematosus. Arthritis Rheum 25(7):773—778
13. Bluestein HG (1984) Antineuronal antibodies in the pathogenesis of neuropsychiatric manifestations of systemic lupus erythematosus. In: Behan PO, Spreafico F (eds) Neuroimmunology. Raven, New York
14. Borenstein DG, Jacobs RP (1982) Aqueductal stenosis — a possible late sequela of central nervous system inflammation in systemic lupus erythematosus. Southern Med J 75(4):475—477
15. Brandt KD, Lessell S (1978) Migrainous phenomena in systemic lupus erythematosus. Arthritis Rheum 1:7—16
16. Bresnihan B, Oliver M, Grigor G, Hughes GRV (1977) Brain reactivity of lymphocytotoxic antibodies in systemic lupus erythematosus with and without cerebral involvement. Clin Exp Immunol 30:333—337
17. Bresnihan B, Oliver M, Williams B, Hughes GRV (1979) An antineuronal antibody cross-reactivity with erythrocytes and lymphocytes in systemic lupus erythematosus. Arthritis Rheum 22:313—320

18. Bresnihan B, Hohmeister R, Cutting J, Travers RL, Waldburger M, Black C, Hones T, Hughes GRV (1979) The neuropsychiatric disorder in systemic lupus erythematosus: evidence for both vascular and immune mechanisms. Ann Rheum Dis 38:301—306

19. Bruyn GW, Padberg G (1984) Chorea and systemic lupus erythematosus: a critical review. Eur Neurol 23(4):278—290

20. Burning RD, Laureno R, Barth WF (1982) Florid central nervous system vasculitis in a fatal case of SLE. J Rheumatol: 9(5):735—738

21. Canoso JJ, Cohen AS (1975) Aseptic meningitis in systemic lupus erythematosus: report on three cases. Arthritis Rheum 4:369—374

22. Cendrowsi W, Stepien M (1974) Clinical variant of lupus erythematosus resembling multiple sclerosis. Eur Neurol 11:373—376

23. Chin D, Zilko P (1983) Stroke as an early manifestation of systemic lupus erythematosus. J Neurol Neurosurg Psychiatry 46(7):688

24. Daras M, Tuchman AJ, Chengot MT (1982) Myelin basic protein elevation in myelopathy due to systemic lupus erythematosus. NY State J Med 82(3):357—358

25. Davalos A, Matiasguin J, Codina A (1984) Painful ophthalmoplegia in systemic lupus erythematosus. J Neurol Neurosurg Psychiatry 47(3):323—324

26. Devos P, Destee A (1984) MS and systemic lupus erythematosus. Rev Neurol (Paris) 140:513—515

27. Donaldson IM, Espiner EA (1971) Disseminated lupus erythematosus presenting as chorea gravidarum. Arch Neurol 25:240—244

28. Dubois EL (1974) Lupus erythematosus. University of Southern California Press, Los Angeles

29. Ellis SG, Verity MA (1979) Central nervous system involvement in systemic lupus erythematosus: a review of neuropathologic findings in 57 cases 1955—1977. Semin Arthritis Rheum 3:212—221

30. Estebanez C, Alonso JM, Viano J, Quereda C, Losada M, Ortuno J (1982) Focal, relapsing neurological manifestations as the main signs of systemic lupus erythematosus. Med Clin (Barc) 79(1):39—42

31. Estes D, Christian CL (1971) The natural history of systemic lupus erythematosus by prospective analysis. Medicine (Baltimore) 2:85—95

32. Feinglass EJ, Arnett FC, Dorsch CA, Zizic TM, Stevens MB (1976) Neuropsychiatric manifestations of systemic lupus erythematosus: diagnosis, clinical spectrum and relationship to other features of the disease. Medicine (Baltimore) 4:323—337

33. Ferrante FM, Myerson GE, Goldman JA (1982) Subclavian artery thrombosis mimicking the tortic arch syndrome in systemic lupus erythematosus. Arthritis Rheum 25(12):1501—1504

34. Fessel WJ (1961) Disturbed serum proteins in chronic psychosis. Arch Gen Psychiatry 68:154—159

35. Fessel WJ, Solomon G (1960) Psychosis and systemic lupus erythematosus — review of the literature and case reports. California Med 92:266—270

36. Finelli PF, Yockey CC, Herbert AJ (1976) Recurrent aseptic meningitis in an elderly man: unusual prodrome of systemic lupus erythematosus. JAMA 235(11):1142—1143

37. Fulford KWM, Catterall RD, Delhany JJ, Doniach D, Kremer M (1972) A collagen disorder of the nervous system presenting as multiple sclerosis. Brain 95:373—386

38. Funata N (1979) Cerebral vascular changes in systemic lupus erythematosus. Bull Tokyo Med Dent Univ 2:91—112

39. Ginzler EM, Diamond HS, Weiner M (1982) A multicenter study of outcome in systemic lupus erythematosus: I. Entry variables as predictors of prognosis. Arthritis Rheum 25(6):601—611

40. Goldberg M, Chitanon DH (1959) Polyneuritis with albuminocytologic dissociation in the spinal fluid in systemic lupus erythematosus. Am J Med 17:342—350

41. Gibson T, Myers AR (1976) Nervous system involvement in systemic lupus erythematosus. Ann Rheum Dis 35:398—406

42. Grigor R, Edmonds J, Lewkonia R, Bresnihan B, Hughes GRV (1978) Systemic lupus erythematosus — a prospective analysis. Ann Rheum Dis 37:121—128

43. Haas LF (1982) Stroke as an early manifestation of systemic lupus erythematosus. J Neurol Neurosurg Psychiatry 45(6):554—556
44. Hadler NM, Gerwin RD, Frank MM, Whitaker JN, Decker JL, Baker M (1973) The fourth component of complement in the cerebrospinal fluid in systemic lupus erythematosus. Arthritis Rheum 4:507—521
45. Harada K (1960) Histopathology of central nervous system in patients with systemic lupus. Folia Psychiatr Neurol Jpn 62:490—497
46. Harbeck RJ, Hoffman AA, Carr RI, Bardana EJ (1973) DNA antibodies and DNA: anti DNA complexes in the cerebrospinal fluid (CSF) of patients with SLE. Arthritis Rheum 4:552
47. Harbeck RJ, Hoffman AA, Hofmann SA, Shucard DW (1979) Cerebrospinal fluid and the choroid plexus during acute immune complex disease. Clin Immunol Immunopathol 13:413—425
48. Hashimoto H, Maekawa S, Nasu H, Okada T, Shiokawa Y, Fukuda Y (1984) Systemic vascular lesions and prognosis in systemic lupus erythematosus. Scand J Rheumatol 13(1):45—55
49. Hiraiwa M, Nonaka C, Abe T, Iio M (1983) Positron emission tomography in systemic lupus erythematosus — relation of cerebral vasculitis to PET findings. Am J Neuroradiol 4(3):541—543
50. Hirano T, Hashimoto H, Shiokawa Y (1980) Antiglycolipid autoantibody detected in the sera from systemic lupus erythematosus patients. J Clin Invest 66:1437—1440
51. Hrnčiř Z, Tichy J (1978) Subclasses IgA_1, and IgA_2 in serum and synovial fluid in rheumatoid arthritis and reactive synovitis of local origin. Ann Rheum Dis 37:518—521
52. Hughes GRV (1977) Connective tissue disease. Blackwell, Oxford
53. Inoup T (1982) Antineuronal antibodies in brain tissue of patients with systemic lupus erythematosus. Lancet I:852
54. Isenberg DA, Snaith ML (1981) Muscle disease in SLE: a study of its nature, frequency and cause. J Rheumatol 8(6):917—924
55. Isenberg DA, Meyrickthomas D, Snaith ML, McKeran RO, Royston JP (1982) A study of migraine in systemic lupus erythematosus. Ann Rheum Dis 41(1):30—32
56. Jentsch HJ, Haas H, Haffner B, Berger H (1971) Fokale Anfälle und Hemiplegie als Erstmanifestation eines systemischen lupus erythematosus. Therapiewoche 29:1187—1194
57. Johnson RT, Richardson EP (1968) The neurological manifestations of systemic lupus erythematosus. Medicine (Baltimore) 4:337—369
58. Keeffe EB, Bardana EJ, Harbeck RJ, Pilowsky B, Carr R (1974) Lupus meningitis — antibody to deoxyribonucleic acid (DNA) and DNA: anti-DNA complexes in cerebrospinal fluid. Ann Intern Med 80:58—60
59. Kewalramani LS, Orth MS, Salem S, Bertrand D (1978) Myelopathy associated with systemic lupus erythematosus (erythema nodosum). Paraplegia 16:282—294
60. Kobiler D, Fuchs S, Samuel D (1976) The effect of antisynaptosomal plasma membrane antibodies on memory. Brain Res 115:129—138
61. Krankenhagen B, Cohen G (1975) Frühmanifestation des Lupes erythematodes im Zentralnervensystem. Dtsch Med Wochenschr 100:2328—2337
62. Krüger KW (1984) Lupus erythematodes und Zentralnervensystem. Nervenarzt 55:165—172
63. Kruse K (1984) Myopathien bei endokrinen Störungen. Monatsschr Kinderheilkd 132:581—586
64. Lachmann PJ, Peters DK (1982) Clinical aspects of immunology, Vol 2. Backwell, Oxford
65. Lampert PW, Oldstone MBA (1973) Host immunoglobulin G and complement deposits in the choroid plexus during spontaneous immune complex disease. Science 180:408—413
66. Lanham JG, Elkon KB, Hughes GRV (1982) Ptosis in systemic lupus erythematosus. Postgrad Med J 58(685):688—698
67. Lapresle J (1962) Neurospychiatric manifestations of disseminated lupus. Sem Hop Paris 38:35—39
68. Lehman TJA, Bernstein B, Hanson V, Kornreich H, King K (1981) Meningococcal infection complicating systemic lupus erythematosus. J Pediatr 99(1):94—96

69. Levin AS, Fudenberg HH, Petz LD, Sharp GC (1972) IgG levels in cerebrospinal fluid of patients with central nervous system manifestations of systemic lupus erythematosus. Clin Immunol Immunopathol 1:1—5
70. Lindström FD, Sjöholm AG (1975) Cerebrospinal fluid changes in systemic lupus erythematosus with and without central nervous system involvement. Arthritis Rheum 18:413—414
71. Locotura Ruperez J, Mijan de la Torre A (1983) Systemic lupus erythematosus manifesting with neurologic involvement as a single sign. Med Clin (Barc) 81(14):646—647
72. Maida EM (1980) Zur Differentialdiagnose der Liquorveränderungen bei entzündlichen Hirngefäßerkrankungen. In: Reisner H, Schnaberth G (eds) Fortschritte der technischen Medizin in der neurologischen Diagnostik und Therapie. Selbstverlag Neurologische Universitätsklinik Wien, Vienna
73. Maida EM (1983) Liquorproteinprofile bei entzündlichen Erkrankungen des Nervensystems. Maudrich, Vienna
74. Maida E, Kristoferitsch W (1982) Central nervous participation in systemic lupus erythematosus. Wien Klin Wochenschr 94(16):439
75. Maida EM, Horvatits E (1986) Cerebrospinal fluid alterations in bacterial meningitis. Eur Neurol 25:110—116
76. Martin P, Bedoucha P (1981) Acute chorea and disseminated lupus erythematosus. Rev Neurol (Paris) 137(11):671—676
77. Molle D, Guillevin L, Herreman G, Godeau P (1982) Thrombophlebitis of the superior sagittal sinus in a patient with systemic lupus erythematosus. Sem Hop Paris 58(20):1215—1219
78. Moster MM, Kennerdell JS (1983) Isolated sixth nerve palsy as initial manifestation of systemic lupus erythematosus: a case report. J Clin Neuro Ophthalmol 3(2):109—111
79. Nassonova KA, Alekverova ZS, Folomeyev MY, Mylov NM (1984) Sacroiliitis in men with SLE. Scand J Rheumatol [Suppl] 52:172—174
80. Nyland H, Matre R, Tönder O (1979) Complement receptors in human peripheral nerve tissue. Acta Pathol Microbiol Immunol Scand [C] 87:7—10
81. O'Connor JF, Musher DM (1966) Central nervous system involvement in systemic lupus erythematosus. Arch Neurol 14:157—164
82. Ostrov SG, Quencer RM, Gaylis NB, Altman RD (1982) Cerebral atrophy in systemic lupus erythematosus: steroid- or disease-induced phenomenon? Am J Neuroradiol 3(1):21—24
83. Petz LD, Sharp GS, Cooper NR, Irvin WS (1971) Serum and cerebrospinal fluid complement and serum autoantibodies in systemic lupus erythematosus. Medicine 4:259—275
84. Petz LD (1978) Measurement of spinal fluid complement in immunological mediated neurologic disorders. In: Opferkuch W, Rother K, Schultz RD (eds) Clinical aspects of the complement system. Thieme, Stuttgart
85. Piching AJ, Travers RL, Hughes GRV (1978) Detection of cerebral involvement in systemic lupus erythematosus using 15-oxygen brain scanning. Lancet I:898—901
86. Quismorio FP, Friou GJ (1972) Antibodies reactive with neurons in SLE patients with neuropsychiatric manifestations. Int Arch Allergy Appl Immunol 43:740—748
87. Reinitz E, Hubbard D, Grayze L (1982) Central nervous system systemic lupus erythematosus versus central nervous system infection — low cerebrospinal fluid glucose and pleocytosis in a patient with a prolonged course. Arthritis Rheum 25(5):583—587
88. Reinitz E, Hubbard D, Zimmermann RD (1984) Central nervous system sdisease in systemic lupus erythematosus — axial tomographic scan as an aid to differential diagnosis. J Rheumatol 11(2):252—254
89. Rosner S, Ginzler EM, Diamond HS (1982) A multicenter study of outcome in systemic lupus erythematosus: II. Causes of death. Arthritis Rheum 25(6):612—617
90. Schmidt RE, Ryan PFJ, Hughes GRV, Stroehmann J (1981) Antineuronal antibodies in patients with systemic lupus erythematosus. Med Welt 32(32—3):1216—1222
91. Schur PH (1982) Complement and lupus erythematosus. Arthritis Rheum 25(7):793—798
92. Seibold RJ, Buckingham RB, Medsger TA, Kelly RH (1982) Cerebrospinal fluid immune complexes in systemic lupus erythematosus involving the central nervous system. Semin Arthritis Rheum 12(1):68—74

Neurological Manifestations 269

93. Sergent JS, Lockshin MD, Klempner MS, Lipsky BA (1975) Central nervous system disease in systemic lupus erythematosus — therapy and prognosis. Am J Med 58:644—654
94. Sheinberg L (1956) Polyneuritis in systemic lupus erythematosus. N Engl J Med 255:416—421
95. Simon J, Simon O (1975) Effect of passive transfer of antibrain antibodies to a normal recipient. Exp Neurol 47:523—34
96. Small P, Mass MF, Kohler PF, Harbeck RJ (1977) Central nervous system involvement in SLE — diagnostic profile and clinical features. Arthritis Rheum 3:869—878
97. Staples PJ, Gerding DN, Decker JL, Gordon RS Jr (1974) Incidence of infection in systemic lupus erythematosus. Arthritis Rheum 1:1—10
98. Stoudemire A, Stork M, Simel D, Houpt JL (1982) Neuroophthalmic systemic lupus erythematosus misdiagnosed as hysterical blindness. Am J Psychiatry 139(9):1194—1196
99. Swash M, Perrin J, Schwartz S (1979) Significance of immunoglobulin deposition in peripheral nerve in neuropathies associated with paraproteinaemia. J Neurol Neurosurg Psychiatry 42:179—183
100. Sweet J, Bear RA, Lang AP (1981) Amyloidosis and systemic lupus erythematosus. Hum Pathol 12(9):853—856
101. Treves R, Gastine H, Richard A (1983) Aseptic meningitis and acute renal failure induced by ibuprofen during the treatment of systemic lupus erythematosus. Rev Rheum Mal Osteoartic 50(1):75—76
102. Trevor RP, Sontheiner FK, Fessel WJ, Wolpert SM (1972) Angiographic demonstration of major cerebral vessel occlusion in systemic lupus erythematosus. Neuroradiology 4:202—207
103. Tuchmann AJ, Daras M, David S (1983) Cerebellar ataxia in systemic lupus erythematosus. NY State J Med 83(7):983—984
104. Valesini G (1983) Appearance of anti-acetylcholine receptor antibodies coincident with onset of myasthenic weakness in patient with systemic lupus erythematosus. Lancet I:831
105. Vermess M, Bernstein RM, Byoder GM, Steiner RE, Young IR, Hughes GRV (1983) Nuclear magnetic resonance (NMR) Tomography of the central nervous system: comparison of two imaging sequences. J Comput Assist Tomogr 7(3):461—467
106. Von Wicman MD, Tarres MV (1983) Clinical value of antineuronal antibodies in systemic lupus erythematosus. Medicina Clinica 80(4):229—230
107. Wallace DJ, Podell T, Weiner J, Klingenberg J, Forouzesh S, Dubois EL (1981) Systemic lupus erythematosus—survival patterns. JAMA 9:934—938
108. Warren RM, Kredich DW (1984) Transverse myelitis and acute central nervous system manifestation of systemic lupus erythematosus. Arthritis Rheum 27(9):1058—1061
109. Weil MH (1955) Disseminated lupus and massive hemorrhagic manifestations and paraplegia. Lancet I:358—360
110. Williams GW, Bluestein HG, Steinberg AD (1981) Brain-reactive lymphocytotoxic antibodies in the cerebrospinal fluid of patients with systemic lupus erythematosus: correlation with central nervous system involvement. Clin Immunol Immunopathol 1:126—132
111. Wilson HA, Winfield JB, Lahita RG, Koffler D (1979) Assosiation of IgG antibrain-antibodies with central nervous system dysfunction in systemic lupus erythematosus. Arthritis Rheum 22:458—467
112. Winkelman RK, Connolly SM, Doyle JA (1982) Carpal tunnel syndrome in cutaneous connective tissue disease—generalized morphea, lichen sclrosus, fasciitis, discoid lupus erythematosus and lupus pannivulitis. J Am Acad Dermatol 7(1):94—99
113. Wong K, Ai E, Jones DV, Young D (1981) Visual loss as the initial symptoms of systemic lupus erythematosus. Am J Ophthalmol 92(2):238—244
114. Yancey CL, Doughty RA, Athreya BH (1981) Central nervous system involvement in childhood systemic lupus erythematosus. Arthritis Rheum 24(11):1389—1395
115. Zeiler K, Brunner G, Schnaberth G (1979) Das zerebrale Angiogramm bei Kollagenosen und Arteriitiden anderer Genese. Fortschr Neurol Psychiatr 47:490—497

Radiographic Features

G. Seidl

Radiographic changes in systemic lupus erythematosus (SLE) represent sequelae of mechanisms which lead to tissue destruction. Although there are no radiologic abnormalities pathognomonic of SLE, the radiologist can be helpful to the clinician in establishing certain patterns of organ involvement and in the differential diagnosis. In this respect, X-rays of the chest and joints are of particular importance. With regard to abnormalities of the heart, liver, lymph nodes, kidney, and exocrine glands, sonography and isotope scanning techniques can often be helpful, whereas computerized tomography or angiography will only rarely be indicated for these organs.

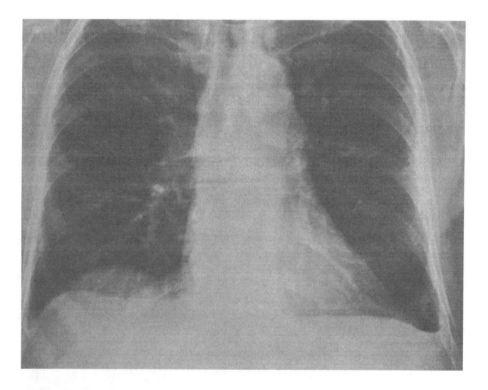

Fig. 1. Chest film showing small pleural effusions in both costophrenic angles tending to obliterate

Intrathoracic Manifestations

Pleural Abnormalities

In SLE, chest X-rays often reveal uni- or bilateral effusions which tend to recur and to obliterate (Fig. 1) [11, 28]. They are often accompanied by pleurisy which, however, can also be present without any evidence of effusions [28]. Being detected in 20%—30% of all patients, effusions represent the most common intrathoracic roentgenographic symptom of SLE [14, 23].

Intrapulmonary Abnormalities

Acute pneumonitis may be reflected by variable homogeneous opacities which are usually located in the bases of the lungs and are situated in the periphery (Fig. 2). These changes often occur bilaterally with or without concomitant pleu-

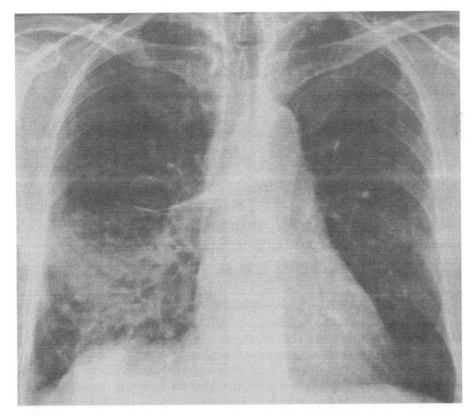

Fig. 2. Opacification of the right lower lobe with recognizable air bronchogram in a patient with acute SLE pneumonitis. Small pleural marking of the interlobar fissure

ral effusions [11, 28]. Such opacities, which may be due to parenchymal infiltration with lymphocytes and plasma cells, are observed in less than 10% of patients with SLE [14, 16]. In therapeutic follow-up studies there was no response to antibiotic therapy, but rapid remission was observed after the institution of corticosteroid treatment. With respect to this differential diagnosis must take into account infectious and thrombembolic parenchymal consolidations.

Occasionally, wide-spread acinar shadows sometimes confluent, can be found in the perihilar regions in both lungs; these changes may represent extensive immune complex pneumonitis with alveolar hemorrhage. This is, however, a rare condition in SLE [12].

Reticulonodular interstitial structures, predominantly in the bases of the lungs, reflect the chronic stage of interstitial lung disease (fibrosis, Fig. 3) [11, 14, 22, 28]. The pattern is indistinguishable from interstitial changes of other connective tissue diseases, e.g., scleroderma, dermatomyositis, or rheumatoid arthritis.

Linear, often bilateral and migratory shadows, which are most commonly located in the lung bases, are attributable to platelike atelectases (Fig. 4) [11, 22, 28] and may develop in association with diaphragm dysfunction [28]. In some instances, however, they may represent incomplete lung infarction caused by pulmonary vasculitis.

Nodular manifestations occur occasionally in patients with SLE [5, 31]. These may represent areas of ischemic necrosis caused by vasculitis. The majority of cavitary nodules in SLE are found to be bacterial or fungal abscesses and occur as a consequence of immunosuppressive therapy [31] — in fact, approximately 50% of radiologic pulmonary abnormalities in patients with SLE are caused by infectious processes. Steroid therapy and prolonged immunosuppression lead in many of these patients to acquisition of opportunistic and fulminant pulmonary infections with variable opacifications on chest X-ray [11, 27]. Furthermore, pulmonary embolism may be responsible for several abnormalities. This occurs mainly in patients with circulating anticoagulant. There may be occasional evidence of pulmonary hypertension [25, 28] as a consequence of the changes mentioned above. Sarcoid reaction with bilaterial hilar adenopathy may, rarely constitute an additional complication [28].

Enlargement of the Cardiac Silhouette

Cardiomegaly in SLE has generally to be regarded as the result of pericardial effusion (Fig. 5) [28]. The liquid nature can be proved by sonography, which also gives an impression of the amount of the effusion. However, lateral chest X-ray may also detect pericardial effusion, through a thickening of the anterior pericardial stripe.

Lupus myocarditis is a rare cause of cardiomegaly. When pleural effusions are present, the possibility of an underlying left heart failure with vascular signs of redistribution must also be borne in mind, whereas in pure lupus pericarditis the pulmonary vascular structures remain unchanged.

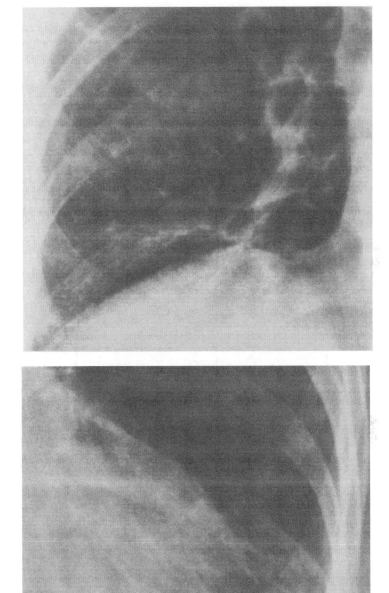

Fig. 3. Detailed enlargement of both lung bases showing a subtle reticular, nodular interstitial pattern

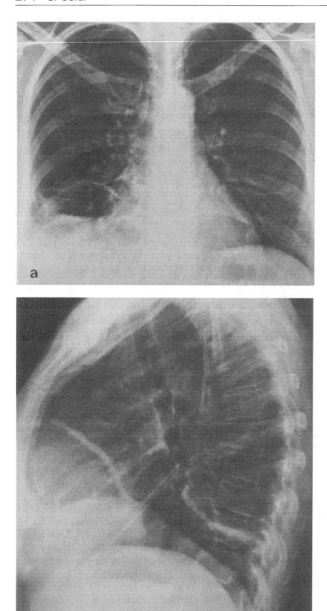

Fig. 4a,b. a Posteroanterior (PA) and **b** lateral chest film demonstrating linear shadows in the right lung base due to platelike atelectases. Note also the diaphragm elevation and the small pleural effusion

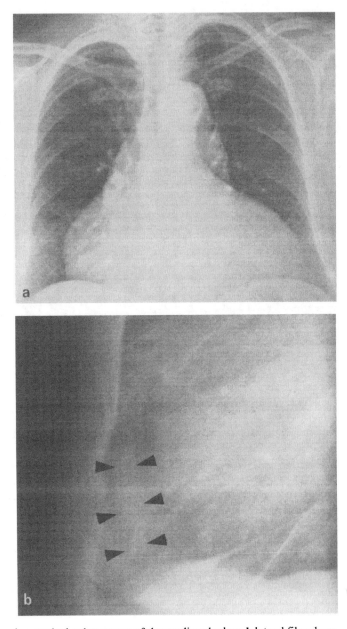

Fig. 5a-c. a PA film showing marked enlargement of the cardiac shadow. **b** lateral film showing a widening of the anterior pericardial stripe *(arrows)*, reflecting pericardial effusion

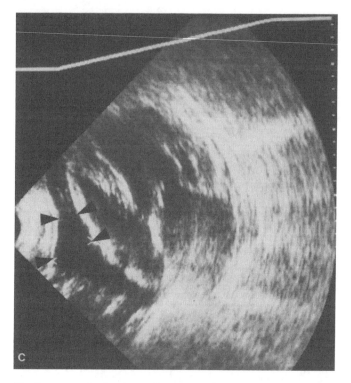

Fig. 5a-c. c sagittal echocardiogram outlining the fluid accumulation in the anterior and epiphrenic part of the pericardium *(arrows)*

Elevation of the Diaphragm

Bilateral elevation of the diaphragm is a characteristic appearance on the chest Y-ray of SLE patients, and is in fact often the only roentgenographic abnormality. Diaphragm involvement can be accompanied by linear shadows in the lung bases, by pleural effusions, or by obliteration of the costophrenic angles. The cause of this abnormality appears to be a weakness of the diaphragm rather than pulmonary restriction [28].

Joints

Episodes of polyarthralgia constitute the most common clinical feature in SLE and are present in 75% to 90% of patients [15, 19], in whom the pattern of joint involvement is usually bilateral and symmetrical. The interphalangeal joints of the hands, wrists, knees, and shoulders are those most frequently affected. Although the occurence of arthralgia and joint tenderness is common, radiographic changes are generally slight. These radiographic findings and their frequency have been defined on hand X-rays in several studies [2, 15, 21, 24, 32, 33].

Swelling of the Soft Tissue

Lupus synovitis (Fig. 6) is characterized by fusiform soft tissue swelling in about 20% of the patients [24, 32]. The percentage of soft tissue swelling appears to be significantly higher in late onset SLE: in a group of SLE patients aged over 50 years, 60% were reported to suffer from soft tissue swellings [3]. This corresponds with the observation of a somewhat higher incidence of SLE-associated arthritis in the elderly [10].

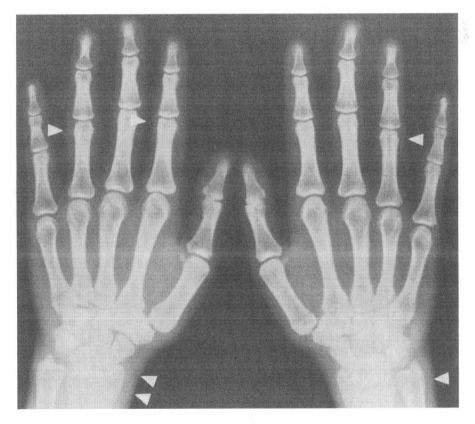

Fig. 6. Radiograph of the hands showing several joints with soft tissue swelling *(arrows)*

Osteoporosis

On X-rays, osteoporosis is the most common abnormality and is observed in 40%—60% of patients with SLE [24, 32]. Juxta-articular osteoporosis, in particular, can be observed at both the proximal interphalangeal and metacarpophalangeal joints and is consistent with uncomplicated synovitis (Fig. 7); this abnormality simulates early rheumatoid arthritis. In contrast to the latter, cartilagineous and osseous destructions are rare or absent in SLE-associated joint changes. Differential diagnosis of osteoporosis must take into account immobilisation and — in cases of more generalized osteoporosis — the consequences of prolonged therapy with corticosteroids.

Alignment Abnormalities

Abnormalities of joint alignment which resemble Jaccound-arthropathy are a characteristic feature of SLE (Fig. 8); they are observed in 10%—40% of the patients and are related to inflammatory changes in the periarticular structures,

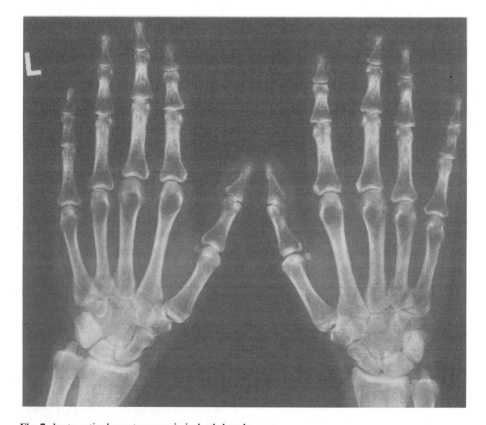

Fig. 7. Juxta-articular osteoporosis in both hands

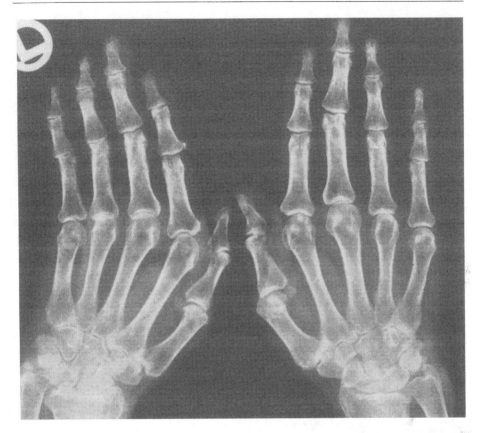

Fig. 8. Nonerosive arthropathy. Swan neck deformities (flexion at the distal interphalangeal joints and extension at the proximal interphalangeal joints, more pronounced on the left). Ulnar deviation of the metacarpophalangeal joints. Note also a small periarticular calcification in the left second digit

especially of the capsule and the ligaments [2, 15, 21, 24, 32]. The usual involvement of the interphalangeal joints leads to bilateral symmetric hyperextensions of the proximal and hyperflexions of the distal interphalangeal joints ("swan neck deformities"). Boutonnière deformities and ulnar deviations may also be observed. Since the deformities are mobile and voluntarily correctable, they may disappear when the hand is firmly placed onto the cassette during exposure. An X-ray of the hands taken in a lateral oblique position may provoke the appearance of these deformities. Fixed deformities can also sometimes be observed [8, 21]. The appearance of alignment abnormalities without associated erosions (the nonerosive, deforming arthropathy) is the most important radiographic clue for the diagnosis of SLE in a differentiation against rheumatoid arthritis.

Atlantoaxial subluxation should also be mentioned in this context. This can occur in SLE and is due to ligamentous laxity [17].

Acro-osteosclerosis

Sclerosis of the terminal phalanges is a nonspecific finding in SLE, present in 10%—30% of all patients (Fig. 9) [24, 32], and often occurs associated with Raynaud's phenomenon; similar findings have been reported in scleroderma, dermatomyositis, rheumatoid arthritis, and sarcoidosis, but occasionally even in healthy women [7, 32].

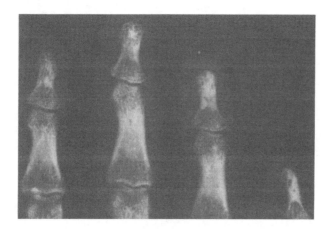

Fig. 9. Acral osteosclerosis. Localized areas of increased densities in the tufts

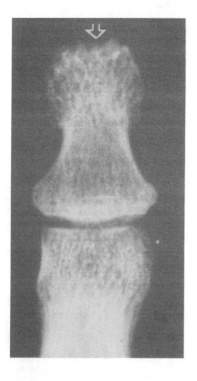

Fig. 10. Small tuftal resorption *(arrow)*

Tuftal resorptions

Localized bony defects of the tufts of the terminal phalanges occur in about 5% of SLE patients (Fig. 10) [24, 32]. These can be associated, although not necessarily so, with Raynaud's phenomenon. Such lesions are more characteristic, however, of scleroderma and can be also found in psoriasis, hyperparathyroidism, and after thermal injuries [18]. In particular, they can be present in SLE patients with endstage kidney disease and secondary hyperparathyroidism.

Soft Tissue Calcification

Calcinosis of the joint capsule or surrounding structures has been reported with a frequency of 8%—40% [4, 24, 32]. Diagnostic accuracy is increased by the routine use of magnification radiography, leading to the detection of calcium deposits which are usually very small [24]. The incidence of calcinosis increases with the duration of the disease (Fig. 11). Calcinoses may reflect regressive changes in the joint capsule or periarticular tissue, and a connection with Raynaud's phenomenon is evident. Degenerative changes as a consequence of alignment abnormalities may also be of pathogenetic significance. Occasional calcifications of subcutaneous soft tissue can be observed in the finger tips of SLE patients [24], although amorphous periarticular and subcutaneous calcifications are more characteristic of scleroderma. Similar calcifications can be seen in hyperparathyroidism, other collagen vascular diseases, hypervitaminosis D, and fat necrosis [18].

Joint Space Narrowing

Since destruction of cartilage is not a typical feature of SLE, joint space narrowing is seen only rarely. When present, it relates rather to atrophy or pressure from subluxated articular bones [19] than to cartilage destruction.

Articular Erosions

Destruction of articular bones is said to be absent in SLE [2, 15, 21]. However, occasional erosive defects can be seen in SLE patients (Fig. 12) [19, 24]. If they occur, they do not resemble the polyarticular, marginal osseous lesions of rheumatoid arthritis, but affect only a few joints and are asymmetrical. A detailed analysis of X-rays of the hands of our patient population revealed erosions of this kind in as many as 20%, despite the exclusion of cases with overlap disorders of SLE with rheumatoid arthritis, other connective tissue disorders, and patients with azotemia. The majority of the erosions were found in the metacarpophalangeal joints and were radially located. Such lesions have been termed "hook-erosions." They probably result from mechanical damage of the subluxated, ulnarly drifted joints [19]. Rarely locations of erosions are found at the proximal interphalangeal joints.

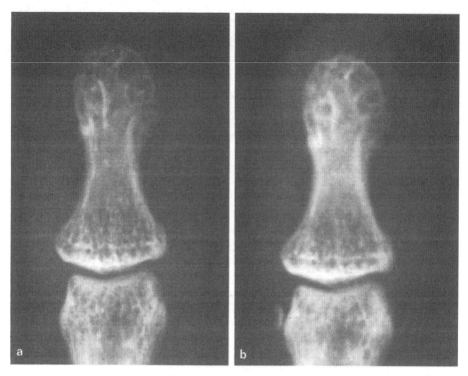

Fig. 11a,b. a Normal distal interphalangeal joint in a 35-year-old woman with lupus arthropathy. **b** four years later, capsular calcification appears at the same joint

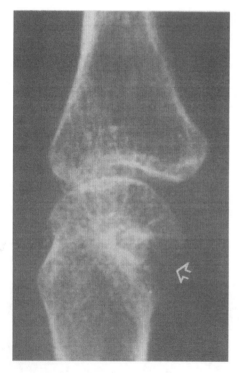

Fig. 12. Occasionally, articular erosions are seen. Note marked marginal defect at the radial aspect of the metacarpal head *(arrow)*

Bony Proliferations

Isolated small proliferations at the ulnar styloids were observed in only 2 out of 62 patients (Fig. 13); such changes are generally characteristic of psoriatic arthropathy, ankylosing spondylitis, and subtypes of rheumatoid arthritis, and are uncommon in SLE.

Osteonecrosis

Osteonecrosis may complicate SLE. This abnormality may relate to immune-mediated vascular damage or may be a consequence of corticosteroid therapy. The incidence of osteonecrosis in SLE has been reported to be 5%—40% [19] with the most common site being the femoral head (Fig. 14); additional locations are the humeral head, metacarpal and metatarsal heads, and talus and navicular bones.

The radiographic changes of osteonecrosis have been well recorded. Long standing damage may lead to secondary degenerative changes of the joint. In non-weight-bearing articulations, e.g., the glenohumeral joint, patchy sclerosis and lucency may appear without significant subchondral collapse.

Lupus Nephritis

Clinically evident nephritis occurs in 40%—75% of patients [1]. Sonography may reveal kidneys with increased cortical echogenicity, while the pyramids are relatively sonolucent [20]. The renal size may be increased in the acute stage of nephritis. By contrast, small and shrunken kidneys are demonstrable in long-term nephritis (Fig. 15). These changes do not differ from other forms of glomeruloncaoritis or nephrosclerosis.

Salivary glands

Cellular infiltration of the parotid glands, as seen in SLE, contributes to the symptoms of secondary Sjögren's syndrome. The glands may show bilateral swelling. Sialography demonstrates ectasia of the ducts, which appear punctate (grade 1), globular (grade 2), cavitary (grade 3) or destructive (grade 4) (Fig. 16) [6, 30].

Sequential scintiscanning of the salivary glands is of diagnostic value, showing abnormally low uptake levels of 99mTc if Sjögren's syndrome is present (Fig. 17) [9].

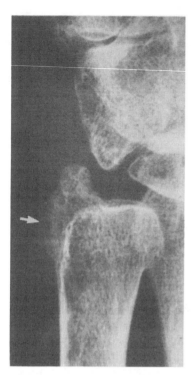

Fig. 13. Bony proliferation at the ulnar styloid *(arrow)*

Fig. 14. Osteonecrosis of femoral head depicted in axial projection. Note segmental depression *(arrows)* with linear subchondral radiolucency reflecting a fracture beneath the cartilage and sclerosis ▼

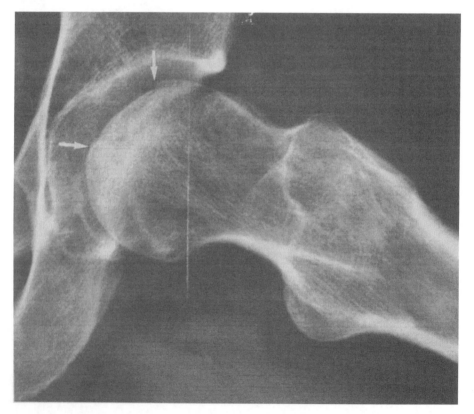

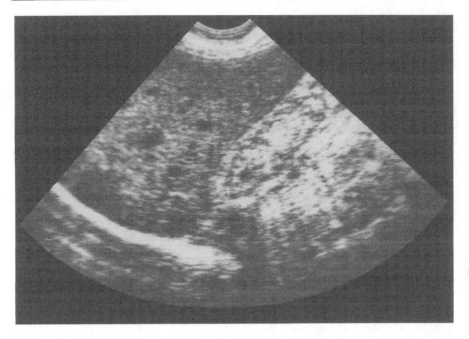

Fig. 15. Supine longitudinal sonogram of the right kidney in a patient with chronic lupus nephritis. Renal size is small. Note that the renal cortical echogeneicity is raised and is greater than that of the liver

Overlap Disorders

Clinical, laboratory, and radiological findings of SLE are usually distinctive and diagnostic. Occasionally, typical radiological features of other collagen diseases such as scleroderma, polymyositis, Sjögren's syndrome, or rheumatoid arthritis may coexist with SLE. Overlapping features of SLE, scleroderma, and polymyositis are seen together in mixed connective tissue disease, which is a separate, serologically defined entity [12, 26, 29].

In this paper, the author has attempted to show the value of various techniques, including conventional X-ray and isotope or ultrasound scanning, in the diagnosis of SLE and the differentiation of this disorder from other connective tissue diseases. In contrast to serologic techniques, radiographic changes in SLE are nonspecific, but can help the clinician in his effort to make the correct differential diagnosis and institute appropriate treatment.

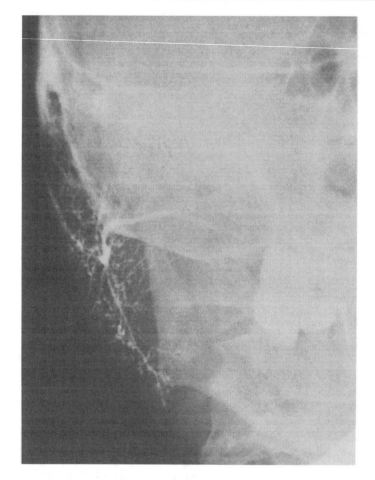

Fig. 16. Sialography of the parotid glands showing punctate sialectasia (grade 1) with a normal primary duct system in a patient with SLE and secondary Sjögren's syndrome (Courtesy of the Central Institute for Radiodiagnostics, University of Vienna)

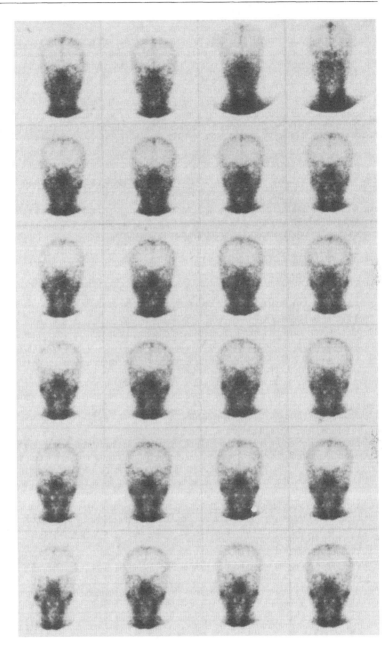

Fig. 17. Sequential scintiscanning showing late onset and diminution of uptake in the parotid and the submandibular glands. Note also the shrinkage of the glands (Courtesy of the Central Institute for Radiodiagnostics, University of Vienna)

288 G. Seidl

References

1. Adu D, Cameron JS (1982) Lupus nephritis. In: Clinics in rheumatic diseases, vol. 8 Saunders, Philadelphia, pp 153—182
2. Bleifeld CJ, Inglis AE (1974) The hand in systemic lupus erythematosus. J Bone Joint Surg 56A:1207—1215
3. Braunstein EM, Weissmann BN, Sosmann JL, Schur PH (1983) Radiologic findings in late-onset systemic lupus erythematosus. Am J Roentgenol 140:587—589
4. Budin JA, Feldman F (1975) Soft tissue calcifications in systemic lupus erythematosus. Am J Roentgenol 124:358—364
5. Castaneda-Zuniga WR, Hogan MT (1976) Cavitary pulmonary nodules in systemic lupus erythematosus. Radiology 118:45—48
6. Chisholm DM (1973) Salivary gland function in Sjögren's syndrome. Br Dent J 135 (9):393—399
7. Deak P (1958) Die Akroosteosklerose. ROFO 89:59—66
8. Evans JA, Hastings DE, Urowitz MB (1977) The fixed lupus hand deformity and its surgical correction. J Rheumatol 4:170
9. Feine U, zum Winkel K (1980) Nuklearmedizin-Szintigraphische Diagnostik. Thieme, Stuttgart, pp 163—171
10. Foad BSI, Sheon RP, Kirsner AB (1972) Systemic lupus erythematosus in the elderly. Arch Intern Med 130:743—746
11. Fraser RG, Pare JA (1978) Diagnoses of diseases of the chest, vol 2, Saunders, Philadelphia, pp 894—900
12. Herman PG, Balikian JP, Seltzer St E, Ehrie M (1978) The pulmonary-renal syndrome Am J Roentgenol 130:1141—1148
13. Hunninghake GW, Fauci AS 1979. Pulmonary involvement in the collagen vascular diseases. Am. Rev. Resp. Dis. 119:471—503
14. Kelley WN, Harris ED, Ruddy S, Sledge CB (1981) Textbook of rheumatology, vol 1, Saunders, Philadelphia, pp 1115—1132
15. Labowitz R, Schumacher HR Jr (1971) Articular manifestations of systemic lupus erythematosus. Ann Intern Med 74:911—921
16. Matthay RA, Schwarz MI, Petty TL, Stanford RE, Gupta RC, Sahn SA, Steigerwald JC (1974) Pulmonary manifestations of systemic lupus erythematosus: review of twelve cases of acute lupus pneumonitis. Medicine (Baltimore) 54:397—409
17. Noonan CD, Odone DT, Engleman EP, Splitter St. D (1963) Roentgenographic manifestations of joint disease in systemic lupus erythematosus. Radiology 80:837—843
18. Resnick D, Niwayama G (1981) Diagnosis of bone and joint disorders, vol 2, Saunders, Philadelphia, pp 1204—1229
19. Resnick D, Niwayama G (1981) Diagnosis of bone and joint disorders, vol. 2. Saunders, Philadelphia, pp 1180—1203
20. Rosenfield AT, Taylor KJW, Siegel NS (1979) Ultrasound in renal parenchymal disease. Am J Roentgenol 132:1031
21. Russell AS, Percy JS, Rigal WM, Wilson GL (1974) Deforming arthropathy in sytemic lupus erythematosus. Ann Rheum Dis 33:204
22. Scherak O, Hofner W, Haber P, Kummer F, Kolarz G, Seidl G (1979) Zur Diagnose und Differentialdiagnose pulmonaler Manifestationen bei Kollagenosen. Praxis der Pneumologie 33:1168—1177
23. Scherak O, Hofner W, Haber P, Kummer F, Kolarz G, Seidl G (1980) Systemic lupus erythematosus and pulmonary manifestation. Ann Rheum Dis 414—415
24. Seidl G, Smolen J (1986) Röntgenologische Veränderungen an den Händen bei systemischem Lupus erythematosus. (Submitted for publication)
25. Sergent JS, Lockshin MD (1973) Primary pulmonary hypertension and SLE. N Engl J Med 288:1078

Radiographic Features 289

26. Silver TM, Farber StJ, Bole GG, Martel W (1976) Radiological features of mixed connective tissue disease and scleroderma-systemic lupus erythematous overlap. Radiology 120:269—275
27. Taylor TL, Ostrum H (1959) The roentgen evaluation of systemic lupus erythematosus. Am J Roentgenol 82:95—107
28. Turner-Stokes L, Turner-Warwick M (1982) Intrathoracic manifestation of SLE. In: Clinics in rheumatic diseases Vol. 8, Saunders, Philadelphia, pp 229—242
29. Udoff EJ, Genant HK, Kozin F, Ginsberg M (1977) Mixed connective tissue disease: the spectrum of radiographic manifestations. Radiology 124:613—618
30. Valvassori GE, Potter GD, Hanafee WN, Carter BL, Buckingham RA (1982) Radiology of the ear, nose and throat. Thieme, Stuttgart
31. Webb RW, Gamsu G (1981) Cavitary pulmonary nodules with systemic lupus erythematosus: differential diagnosis Am J Roentgenol 136:27—31
32. Weissman BN, Rappoport AS, Sosman JL, Schur PH (1978) Radiographic findings in the hands in patients with systemic lupus erythematosus. Radiology 126:313—317
33. Winkler P, Baenkler HW, Pfuhl E, Gutmann W (1980) Die Bedeutung der Röntgendiagnostik der Hände beim systemischen Lupus erythematodes: aus einer retrospektiven klinisch-röntgenologischen Studie von 124 Patienten mit Kollagenosen. Acta Rheumatol 5:255—272

The Lupus Subset Idea*

J. S. Smolen, A. D. Steinberg, and T. M. Chused

The broad clinical spectrum of systemic lupus erythematosus (SLE) has always been an enigma to clinicians: in contrast to the majority of autoimmune diseases, SLE does not have a single "target organ"; rather, a variety of organ systems may be involved. Nevertheless, individual patients tend to present with a limited number of clinical features and not the whole spectrum of possible ones. (The small sample of patients shown in Table 1 illustrates this point.) Moreover, in the course of flares, patients tend to present with the same symptoms manifested previously, and a small number of "new" features may or may not be present in addition.

Table 1. Some clinical and serologic features in a small sample of SLE patients

Patient	REN[a]	TP	LP	CNS	MY	LUNG	SIC	DNA	Sm	Ro	COOM
A (17)[b]	−	−	−	−	−	−	−	+	−	+	−
B (1)	−	−	−	−	−	−	+	+	−	−	−
C (12)	−	−	−	+	−	−	−	+	−	−	−
D (41)	−	−	−	+	−	−	−	+	−	−	−
E (2)	−	−	−	+	+	−	+	+	−	−	−
F (145)	−	−	−	+	−	+	−	+	−	−	−
G (24)	−	−	−	+	+	+	+	+	−	−	−
H (27)	−	−	+	−	−	+	−	+	−	+	−
I (96)	+	+	+	−	−	−	−	+	−	−	+
J (91)	+	+	+	−	−	−	−	+	−	−	−
K (93)	+	+	+	−	−	−	−	+	+	+	−
L (85)	+	+	+	+	−	−	−	+	−	−	−
M (88)	+	+	+	+	−	−	−	+	−	−	−
N (61)	+	+	−	+	−	−	−	+	−	−	−
O (191)	+	+	−	+	+	+	−	+	ND	ND	+
P (135)	+	−	+	+	−	−	−	+	−	−	−

[a] REN, severe nephritis; TP, thrombocytopenia; LP, leukopenia; CNS, CNS-involvement; MY, muscle involvement; SIC, sicca syndrome, LUNG, pulmonary involvement (excluding pleuritis); DNA, Sm, Ro, antibodies to the respective nuclear antigens; COOM, antierythrocyte antibodies

[b] The numbers in parentheses refers to the number of the patient studied, whose complete analyses are shown in other tables and in reference [36]. These patients were selected to emphasize differences between individuals

---

* Supported in part by Fonds zur Förderung der wissenschaftlichen Forschung and Medizinisch-wissenschaftlicher Fonds des Bürgermeisters der Stadt Wien.

Although antinuclear antibodies are characteristic of patients with SLE, serologic features also vary from patient to patient. Thus, some patients have antibodies to Sm and others do not, although they may have antibodies to DNA. Contrariwise, antibodies to double-stranded DNA, a hallmark of the disease, may be absent in a small number of patients. Antibodies to additional nuclear antigens (see pp. 105—123 and 88—104) may be present in a large number of patients, and, interestingly, once present, these patterns usually persist and the patient does not acquire antibodies to other specificities.

Tissue typing has also revealed differences in HLA associations in different countries [31, 32], indicating some diversity of the genetic background of the disease.

Finally, therapeutic responses vary from patient to patient; in some, symptomatic therapy or low doses of corticosteroids are sufficient to control the disease, while others require administration of higher doses of steroids. In a third group, lupus only responds to immunosuppressive agents, and there are a few patients whose diseases progress despite vigorous therapy.

Numerous studies of thousands of patients with SLE indicate that SLE disease in one patient may differ from SLE disease in another patient. This conclusion is bolstered by our knowledge of the genetic and phenotypic diversity of genetically determined murine lupus, in which different strains of mice with SLE-like diseases have different clinical and serologic manifestations, but with antinuclear antibodies as the connecting link [4, 40 and pp. 22—86].

Studies of SLE in twins suggest a strong genetic component in the human disease. The concordance for SLE is about 70% in identical twins compared with ‹10% in fraternal twins and siblings [5, 8]. Several investigators have also commented on the similarity of clinical and serologic features in twin SLE patients [5, 8, 9], raising the possibility that clinical and serologic manifestations of SLE patients might be genetically predetermined.

Thus, the question arises: Is human SLE a single entity, or does it rather represent a number of syndromes with overlapping clinical features? The answer to this question is important for several reasons: (a) for the understanding of pathogenetic mechanisms; (b) for prediction of major organ involvement and thus for prognostic reasons; (c) for optimization of therapeutic approaches; and (d) for rationalization of clinical research on SLE.

Analysis of the major T cell subsets in SLE patients has recently revealed that the distribution of Leu 3a and Leu 2a T cells correlates to some extent with clinical features of SLE [6, 35, 36] (Table 2). However, these investigations were performed in patients who have had SLE for several years and the vast majority of these patients had been treated with corticosteroids and/or immunosuppressive agents, at least in the past. Therefore, a prospective investigation is needed to validate the results obtained. Due to the difficulties in obtaining large numbers of newly diagnosed and untreated SLE patients and the need for follow-up for several years, such a prospective study will not soon be forthcoming.

Fries and Holman have investigated individual clinical and serologic variables by computer analysis for prediction of future events or influence upon disease progression [18]. We have taken a different approach — the use of cumulative clinical and serologic features — to delineate disease patterns [35, 36]. The main

292   J. S. Smolen et al.

Table 2. Correlation of clinical features with T cell subset distribution[a,b]

Feature	Low R_T	Normal R_T	High R_T
Severe nephritis	+++	++	+/−
Leukopenia	++	++	+
Thrombocytopenia	+	+/−	−
CNS disease	+/−	++	++
Muscle involvement	+/−	+	++
Lung involvement	−	+/−	+
Sicca syndrome	−	+/−	++
False-positive STS	−	+/−	++

[a]   −, 0%—10%; +/−, 11%—25%; +, 26%—40%; ++, 41%—60%; +++, >60% of the patients of a given group affected; distribution among all SLE patients was 23%, 54%, and 23% for low, normal, and high R_T, respectively [5, 7]. R_T=T4 (Leu 3a)/T8 (Leu 2a) cells

[b]   Features not shown did not differ with regard to distribution; however, DNA binding was significantly higher in patients with a low ratio when compared with the other patients [36]

reasons for this "cumulative approach" are as follows: (a) at a given time, patients do not present with the whole spectrum of clinical features they might suffer from in the course of their disease; (b) in some patients, certain organs are never involved; (c) clinical symptoms not seen during the first 3—5 years only occasionally develop in later years [17 and our own observations]. Thus, the cumulative approach, in our opinion, provides the best measure of an individual patient's spectrum of clinical manifestations. This should facilitate the detection of potential associations between clinical features and their relation to serologic features and genetic factors.

Table 3 shows a simple analysis using such cumulative data; in this table, the incidence of a variety of features in patients with a given abnormality has been determined. Clearly, some features occur more frequently than expected in association with others.

These associations are more easily perceived graphically (Fig. 1) and indicate that there are at least two clusters of symptoms. Within each cluster there are a variety of features associated with each other; between the clusters there are negative associations of the respective manifestations. There are also associations between certain serologic and certain clinical features (Fig. 1), further supporting the notion of heterogeneity. Moreover, it is these clinical features which have been found associated with the distribution of the major T cell subpopulations in previous investigations [Table 1 and 6, 35, 36].

The lupus subset idea is not new. Aside from the analyses of Fries and Holman and those provided herein, several other attempts have been made recently. Thus, SLE in elderly individuals is often oligosymptomatic and frequently has a relatively benign course [13]. Subdivisions have also been attempted on the basis of serologic characteristics, especially antinuclear antibody specificities. Thus one group of patients with SLE has been named "ANA-negative" lupus [15, 27], and these patients have a few characteristic clinical and serologic features (see pp. 170—196). Another group of lupus patients has been termed subacute cutaneous lupus erythematosus [37 and p. 227—250). Interestingly, there is a high inci-

Table 3. Correlation of clinical and serologic features in SLE patients

	SIGREN +	SIGREN −	TP +	TP −	LP +	LP −	CNS +	CNS −	RAY +	RAY −	LAD +	LAD −	MY +	MY −	SIC +	SIC −	LUNG +	LUNG −	SERO +	SERO −	HYPERT +	HYPERT −	All SLE
SIGREN	—	—	67	46**	60	40**	48	51	32	58§§	48	52	36	58**	33	57**	37	54*	57	40*	70	38§§	50
TP	26	13**	—	—	29	8§§	18	19	21	16	21	18	17	19	17	20	20	19	20	16	26	20	19
LP	61	41**	78	44§§	—	—	51	49	46	49	56	47	40	55	51	46	49	50	54	44	52	48	50
CNS	43	46	38	40	44	42	—	—	45	36	52	37*	52	39	39	44	67	36§§	40	47	46	41	40
RAY	26	52§§	42	34	37	40	41	32	—	—	37	39	39	38	49	33	50	36	32	47	40	38	36
LAD	43	48	48	44	49	41	53	37*	45	47	—	—	54	40	49	44	54	42	44	45	40	46	45
MYA	29	50**	38	41	33	47	47	35	40	39	47	34	—	—	53	32**	70	32§§	47	33	40	42	40
SIC	22	44**	30	34	36	31	31	35	41	27	36	31	45	25**	—	—	38	33	30	37	37	31	33
LUNG	19	31*	26	24	24	25	37	14§§	28	18	30	21	37	10§§	22	19	—	—	33	13§	25	26	25
SERO	61	43*	62	56	62	51	52	59	44	59	55	56	62	47	46	55	76	50§	—	—	58	56	57
HYPERT	50	21§§	37	35	37	34	39	34	35	34	32	38	33	36	38	33	35	36	37	34	—	—	36
Ro	26	46**	42	37	35	41	22	52§§	45	32	35	40	44	33	52	28**	58	32**	43	32	43	34	37
La	4	9	11	5	7	5	6	7	3	9	0	5	8	6	6	7	12	5	10	2	8	6	6
Sm	8	11	11	9	9	9	8	10	13	8	15	4**	15	6	9	10	12	9	12	6*	3	13	9
RNP	15	19	16	16	20	13	16	17	29	11**	19	14	28	11**	21	15	15	17	20	12	14	19	16
COOM	34	25	44	26*	37	22*	28	30	27	30	38	22**	31	29	31	27	35	28	31	27	29	29	30
STS	10	17	7	15	14	13	12	15	12	16	14	13	8	19	12	17	6	16	11	16	10	16	13

* $0.1 > P < 0.05$; ** $P < 0.05$; § $0.1 > Pc > 0.05$ (i.e., $P < 0.01$); §§ $Pc < 0.05$

[a] Indicated are the percentages of patients with (+) or without (−) a given clinical feature who have the clinical or serologic variables shown in the left-hand column. Statistical analysis was performed using the χ^2-test; Pc denotes P corrected (multiplied) by the number of clinical features analyzed. Note that there is either positive or negative association. It is obvious that in these 2×2 analyses it is difficult to appreciate multiple associations. Those are shown in Fig. 1

[b] SIGREN, significant renal disease; TP, thrombocytopenia; LP, leukopenia; CNS, central nervous system involvement; RAY, Raynaud's phenomenon; LAD, lymphadenopathy; MYA, muscle involvement; SIC, sicca syndrome; LUNG, lung involvement; SERO, serositis; HYPERT, hypertension; Ro, La, Sm, RNP, antibodies to the particular nuclear antigen; COOM, positive Coombs' test; STS, false-positive serologic test for syphilis. Total number of patients studied was 194; further details can be obtained from reference [36]

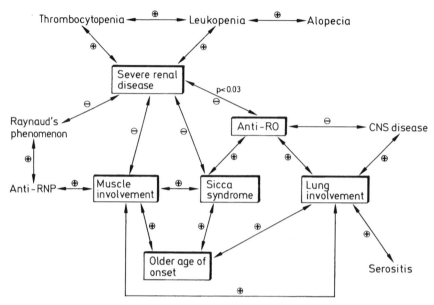

Fig. 1. Association between certain clinical and serologic features of sle. ⊕ denotes significant (p <0.05) positive correlation (association), ⊖ denotes significant negative relationship (dissociation) of the respective features (Kendall Tau B analysis). (Adapted from [36])

dence of anti-SSA (Ro) in patients constituting the last three subsets mentioned. Moreover, if one examines Fig. 1, the negative associations between anti-Ro and both severe Kidney and CNS disease indicate that anti-Ro is associated with a relatively benign course in SLE. It should be noted, however, that this conclusion — just as all other statements made herein — is based upon the statistical analyses presented and does not imply that anti-Ro could not be associated with severe organ involvement in some of the patients; in fact, severe nephritis has been observed in anti-Ro positive SLE patients (see Table 3), and participation of Ro-anti-Ro immune complexes in lupus nephritis has been reported [26].

How can we account for the differences in clinical manifestations among patients with SLE?

First of all, it is well known that, for example, patients with renal disease have higher titers of anti-ds-DNA antibodies than those without [30]. Thus, one factor may be the quantity of antibodies produced. The avidity of such autoantibodies also may be critical for the development of nephritis; in addition, the immunoglobulin isotype and the size of immune complexes formed are important for their capacity to activate complement [1, 19, 24, 31, 42] and their deposition in different organs [11, 22, 25, 41]. Thus, the presence of different autoantibody systems and immune complex characteristics may be responsible for different clinical manifestations. Moreover, immune complex clearing [16] may also be important in this context.

Secondly, the qualities of the autoantibodies produced are influenced genetically and/or by the function and interactions of regulatory T cells [3, 7, 23, 33,

The Lupus Subset Idea **295**

38]. Thus, a certain genetic background or lack of an important regulatory subset in one but not another group of patients [21, 28, 29, 35 and SF Schlossman, pers. comm.] may lead to differences in expression of certain antibodies. Moreover, the presence of autoantibodies directed against regulatory intracellular proteins [20] in subpopulations of patients may perturb the functions of subsets of immunocompetent cells [2] in the subgroups of patients concerned.

And finally, the genetic backgrounds may differ among individual patients as they do among individual strains of inbred autoimmune mice (see pp. 22—49) and may be a major determinant of the immune abnormalities underlying the clinical features of our patients. Aside from the genetic implications of the immunoglobulin studies [21, 29], the negative association between anti-Ro and both kidney and CNS involvement might indicate that in the majority of patients with anti-Ro (SSA) the genetic background does not include genes predisposing to severe kidney or CNS disease. Alternatively, their genes might protect against such major organ involvement.

Well, how does one approach our patients in the light of this heterogeneity? We believe that the approach to a patient with SLE is twofold: One, we have to recognize that an SLE patient does not have to conform to strict clinical rules (even the revised ARA classification criteria allow for more than 10000 different clinical and serologic combinations) and therefore his disease is his individual SLE which we must try to understand and treat. Two, we have to regard our patients as our teachers; their disease teaches us about its diversity; if we will have the privilege of performing additional investigations our awareness of this diversity may help us to understand discrepant results in previous studies [10, 12, 14] and, thereby, to move forward. Obviously, we will have to concentrate not only on further immunologic investigations, but also on studies of the genetic and environmental contributions to the diseases.

In conclusion, there is compelling evidence that human SLE does not constitute a single disease entity; however, it is not clear at present how many lupus syndromes exist. Since lupus is a polygenic disease and since a variety of environmental insults may participate in its pathogenesis [see 8, 9, 34], it must be assumed that the number of such syndromes is large. Therefore, in order to facilitate recognition and definition of lupus subsets, very large populations of patients must be studied. Only collaborative efforts by several centers will achieve such goals. Thus, further clarification of the heterogeneity of SLE awaits additional clinical and basic scientific studies which represent a challenge for the near future.

References

1. Aarden L, Lakmaker F, DeGroot E, Feltkamp TEW (1979) Avidity of antibodies to DNA in relation to SLE. Behring Inst Mitt 64
2. Alarcon-Segovia D, Llorente L, Fishbein E, Diaz-Jouanen E (1982) Abnormalities in the content of nucleic acids of peripheral blood mononuclear cells from patients with systemic lupus erythematosus: relationship to DNA-antibodies. Arthritis Rheum 25:304—317
3. Alpers JH, Steward MW, Soothill JF (1972) Differences in immune elimination in inbred mice. The role of low affinity antibody. Clin Exp Immunol 12:121

4. Andrews BS, Eisenberg RA, Theofilopoulos AN, Izui S, Wilson CB, McConahey PJ, Murphy ED, Roths JB, Dixon FJ (1978) Spontaneous lupus-like syndromes. Clinical and immunopathological manifestations in several strains. J Exp Med 148:1198—1215
5. Arnett FC, Shulman LE (1976) Studies in familial systemic lupus erythematosus. Medicine (Baltimore) 55:313—322
6. Bakke AC, Kirkland PA, Kitridou RC, Horwitz DA (1983) Lymphocyte subsets in systemic lupus erythematosus. Arthritis Rheum 26:745—750
7. Berzofsky JA, Richman LK, Killion DJ (1979) Distinct H-2-linked Ir genes control both antibody and T cell responses to different determinants on the same antigen, myoglobin. Proc Natl Acad Sci USA 76:4046—5050
8. Block SR, Winfield JB, Lockshin MD, D'Angelo WA, Christian CL (1975) Studies of twins with systemic lupus erythematosus: a review of the literature and presentation of 12 additional sets. Am J Med 59:533—552
9. Block SR, Lockshin MD, Winfield JB, Christian CL (1976) Immunologic observations on 9 sets of twins either concordant or discordant for SLE. Arthritis Rheum 19:545—554
10. Bresnihan B, Jasin HE (1977) Suppressor function of peripheral blood mononuclear cells in normal individuals and in patients with systemic lupus erythematosus. J Clin Invest 59:106—116
11. Cochrane CG, Hawkins D (1968) Studies on circulating immune complexes. III. Factors governing the ability of circulating immune complexes to localize in blood vessels. J Exp Med 127:137
12. Delfraissy JF, Segond P, Gelanaud P, Wallon C, Massias P, Dormont J (1980) Deprived primary in vitro antibody response in untreated systemic lupus erythematosus. T helper cell defect and lack of defective suppressor cell function. J Clin Invest 66:141—148
13. Dimant J, Ginzler EM, Schlesinger M, Diamond HS, Kaplan D (1979) Systemic lupus erythematosus in the older age group: computer analysis. J Am Ger Soc 27:58—61
14. Fauci AS, Steinberg AD, Haynes BF, Whalen G (1978) Immunoregulatory aberrations in systemic lupus erythematosus. J Immunol 121:1473—1479
15. Fessel WJ (1977) ANA-negative systemic lupus erythematosus. Am J Med 64:80—86
16. Frank MM, Hamburger MI, Lawley TJ, Kimberly RP, Plotz PH (1979) Defective reticuloendothelial system Fc-receptor function in systemic lupus erythematosus. N Engl J Med 300:524—530
17. Fries JF, Weyl S, Holman HR (1974) Estimating prognosis in systemic lupus erythematosus. Am J Med 57:561—565
18. Fries JF, Holman HR (1975) Sytemic lupus erythematosus: a clinical analysis. In: Smith LH Jr (ed) Major problems in internal medicine, vol 6. Saunders, Philadelphia
19. Gershwin ME, Steinberg AD (1974) Qualitative characteristics of anti-DNA antibodies in lupus nephritis. Arthritis Rheum 17:947—954
20. Hardin JA, Rahn DR, Shen C, Lerner EM, Steitz JA (1982) Antibodies from patients with connective tissue diseases bind specific subsets of cellular RNA-protein particles. J Clin Invest 70:141—147
21. Isenberg DA, Shoenfield Y, Madalo MP, Rauch J, Reichlin M, Stollar DB, Schwartz RS (1984) Anti-DNA idiotypes in systemic lupus erythematosus. Lancet 2:418—421
22. Johnson KJ, Ward PA (1982) Biology of disease: newer concepts in the pathogenesis of immune complex-induced tissue injury. Lab Invest 17:218—226
23. Kappler JW, Marrack P (1978) Role of H-2 linked genes in helper T cell function. IV. Importance of T-cell genotype and host environment in I-region and Ir gene expression. J Exp Med 148:1510—1522
24. Leon SA, Green A, Ehrlich GE, Poland M, Shapiro B (1977) Avidity of antibodies in SLE: relationship to severity of renal involvement. Arthritis Rheum 20:23—29
25. Levinsky RJ, Cameron JS, Soothill JF (1977) Serum immune complexes and disease activity in lupus nephritis. Lancet 1:564
26. Maddison PJ, Reichlin M (1979) Deposition of antibodies to a soluble cytoplasmic antigen in the kidneys of patients with systemic lupus erythematosus. Arthritis Rheum 22:858—863
27. Maddison PJ (1982) ANA-negative SLE. Clin Rheum Dis 8:105—119

The Lupus Subset Idea 297

28. Manohar V, Brown E, Leiserson WM, Chused TM (1982) Expression of Lyt-1 by a subset of B-lymphocytes. J Immunol 129:532—536
29. Moutsopoulos HM, Steinberg AD, Fauci AS, Lane HC, Papadopoulos NM (1983) High incidence of free monoclonal lambda chains in the sera of patients with Sjögren's syndrome. J Immunol 130:2663—2665
30. Pennebaker JB, Gilliam JN, Ziff M (1977) Immunoglobulin classes of DNA-binding activity in serum and skin in systemic lupus erythematosus. J Clin Invest 60:1331—1338
31. Reinertsen JL, Klippel JH, Johnson AH, Decker JL, Steinberg AD, Mann DL (1978) B-lymphocyte alloantigens associated with systemic lupus erythematosus. N Engl J Med 299:515—518
32. Scherak O, Smolen JS, Mayr WR (1980) HLA-DRw3 and systemic lupus erythematosus. Arthritis Rheum 23:954—957
33. Singer A, Hathcock KS, Hodes RJ (1979) Cellular and genetic control of antibody responses. V. Helper T-cell recognition of H-2 determinants on accessory but not B cells. J Exp Med 149:1208—1226
34. Smolen JS, Steinberg AD (1981) Systemic lupus erythematosus and pregnancy: clinical, immunological, and theoretical aspects. In: Gleicher N (ed) Reproductive immunology. Liss, New York, pp 283—302 (Progress in Biological research, vol 67)
35. Smolen JS, Chused TM, Leiserson WM, Reeves JP, Alling D, Steinberg AD (1982) Heterogeneity of immunoregulatory T cell subsets in systemic lupus erythematosus. Correlation with clinical features. Am J Med 72:783—790
36. Smolen JS, Morimoto Ch, Steinberg AD, Wolf A, Schlossman SF, Steinberg RT, Penner E, Reinherz E, Reichlin M, Chused TM (1985) Systemic lupus erythematosus: delineation of subpopulations by clinical, serologic, and T cell subset analysis. Am J Med Sci 289:139—147
37. Sontheimer RD, Thomas JR, Gilliam JN (1979) Subacute cutaneous lupus erythematosus. A cutaneous marker for a distinct lupus erythematosus subset. Arch Dermatol 115:1409—1415
38. Soothill JF, Steward MW (1971) The immunopathological significance of the heterogeneity of antibody affinity. Clin Exp Immunol 9:193
39. Stanworth DR, Turner MW (1978) Immunochemical analysis of immunoglobulins and their subunits. In: Weir DM (ed) Handbook of experimental immunology, 3rd edn, vol 1. Blackwell, Oxford, pp 61—6102
40. Steinberg AD, Huston DP, Taurog JD, Cowdery JS, Raveche ES (1981) The cellular and genetic basis of murine lupus. Immunol Rev 55:121—154
41. Weigle WO, Maurer PH (1957) The molecular ratios of soluble rabbit antigen-antibody complexes. J Immunol 79:223
42. Winfield JB, Faiferman I, Koffler D (1977) Avidity of anti-DNA antibodies in serum and IgG glomerular eluates from patients with systemic lupus erythematosus. Association of high-avidity anti-native DNA antibody with glomerulonephritis. J Clin Invest 59:90

Part V:
Therapeutic Aspects of SLE

An Experimental Therapeutic Approach: Clinical and Immunological Aspects of Plasmapheresis

C. C. ZIELINSKI

Introduction

The ancient Greek concept of health being the result of an equilibrium of fluids (initially corresponding to the four elements) in the human body has resulted in the application of techniques aimed at the restitution of a balance of liquids once it has been perturbed and therefore led to disease. Bloodletting was applied by such eminent physicians of the ancient Greek world as Hippocrates and Praxagoras, and received further support from the theories of Aristotle, whose impact on the ways of thinking in the Western hemishere can be traced far into the modern age [103]. Indeed, doctors practiced the art of bloodletting well into the nineteenth century despite deplorable results, some of which have been reported [25, 148]. With the advent of better, though still incomplete, knowledge of serologic mechanisms and the resulting localization of some pathogenic substances in the fluid phase, bloodletting gained a completely new theroretical background, becoming more sophisticated by virtue of the new ability to remove plasma only. The technique of plasmapheresis (PP), first introduced by Fleig [36] and Abel et al. [2] at the beginning of the twentieth century, was hampered, however, by the lack of technologic means of avoiding side-effects which resulted from rapid volume changes. The first clear indication for the performance of PP was reported by Schwab et al. [121], who showed a PP-induced improvement of hyperviscosity in Waldenström's macroglobulinemia [78]. Finally in the 1970s, new technologic and electronic means led to the production of sophisticated cell separators which allowed for the selective removal of blood components and which could be used for the continuous replacement of plasma removed either by centrifugation or filtration. This, combined with the quickly expanding knowledge in clinical immunology and the ability to produce safely administrable plasma substitution fluids which rendered the procedure relatively harmless, led to an explosion in the use of PP [47] in a variety of diseases with scattered and anecdotal reports of improvement in individual patients. Controlled trials were mor difficult to perform, as the procedure of PP is very expensive and time consuming [49] and consequently sufficient patient numbers were difficult to recruit [43]. Moreover, due to specific problems stemming from the procedure itself, appropriate controls for a study on the efficacy of PP in a given disease are very difficult to find.

In this chapter, the effects of PP will be described in the context of immune-mediated disorders, leaving aside all other forms of application of plasma exchange technology. The aim is to give an overview of the therapeutic concepts involving PP at which we have arrived by reporting a study in which patients with active severe systemic lupus erythematosus (SLE) underwent different PP schedules. Furthermore, the effect of PP upon various immunologic systems and circuits will be described. It is not this chapter's goal, however, to deal with therapeutic concepts of SLE extending beyond the scope of plasma exchange technology.

Basic Considerations

Two considerations can underlie the decision to perform PP:

1. That PP removes pathologic factors circulating in the patient's plasma which are either pathogenic themselves or which sustain the pathologic process or aggravate symptoms: Such a removal can be either unselective, as in routine centrifugal PP, or selective with the help of membranes [81, 125, 145] or columns filled with adsorbants [9, 10, 97, 131, 138, 139].
2. That PP can substitute factors in which the patient's plasma is deficient (reviewed in refs. 51, 98, 137): Patients with deficits in coagulation factors have, for example been successfully treated by PP using appropriate substances for plasma substitution [134].

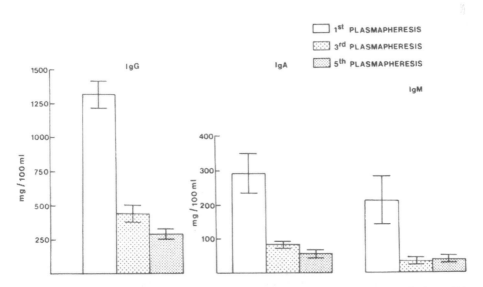

Fig. 1. Course of immunoglobulin concentrations under plasmapheresis (plasma substitute: 5% human albumin)

302   C. C. Zielinski

With these two basic principles in mind, the following variables have to be considered:

1. The substitution fluid and the complications arising from its use (Table 1)
2. The "marker substance" as an indicator of response to treatment [123]
3. The decision as to how often PP should be performed
4. Additional therapy

Plasma Substitution Fluid

The decision as to which substitution fluid should be used will mainly depend on evaluation of the risk—benefit ratio. With the two substances mainly used for plasma substitution being fresh frozen plasma (FFP) and 5% human albumen (5% HA), the evaluation of risk will have to consider on the one hand the possible transfer of hepatitis virus and other infectious agents such as the human T-cell lymphotrophic virus III [21] and the danger of allergic reactions, and on the other a depletion of plasma proteins (Table 1). We have experience in using both HA and FFP in our patient population. As shown in Fig. 1, the depletion of serum immunoglobulins was alsmost complete during a coures of consecutive PPs in which 5% HA was used for substitution. Moreover in a further analysis of the effect of plasma replacement with 5% HA on humoral immunologic parameters, we have found, in accordance with other authors, a very pronounced drop in the serum concentrations of complement components C3 and C4 [61, 63, 113]. These plasma protein depletions did not occur when FFP was used for plasma substitution (Table 2). Although we observed neither an anaphylactic reaction to the infusion of FFP nor associated infectious complications, 5% HA is used routinely in our patient population because of its easy availability and the advantage provided by a defined substance. To date, no adverse effects of the substitution of plasma with 5% HA have been seen in our unit in over 500 PPs.

Being confronted with a patient population which was immunocompromised owing to either the unterlying disease or immunosuppression, we did experience, however, intercurrent infectious episodes due to gram-negative microorganisms, herpes zoster and cytomegalovirus in three patients (from a total of 45 patients).

Table 1. Substances used for plasma substitution and their complications

Substance	Complications
Fresh frozen plasma	Transfer of viruses, e.g., hepatitis virus, human T-cell lymphotropic virus III
	Allergic reactions
	(Hypocalcemia)
5% Human albumin	Depletion of immunoglobulins, complement, coagulation factors, and other plasma proteins
	Hypocalcemia
	Complications due to electrolyte imbalances

Table 2. Serum immunoglobulin and complement concentrations under plasmapheresis using different substitution fluids

Substitution fluid		IgG[a]	IgA	IgM	C3	C4
Fresh frozen plasma	Before PP	1283.0 ± 134.6	173.3 ± 15.5	122.5 ± 20.7	186.4 ± 13.7	37.7 ± 3.9
(exchange volume: 82.4% ± 5.7%)	After PP	1010.5 ± 70.8	164.4 ± 10.3	111.6 ± 10.9	154.2 ± 7.1	21.4 ± 1.9
5% Human albumin	Before PP	1074.2 ± 107.1	168.6 ± 20.6	103.1 ± 28.6	163.4 ± 19.2	27.0 ± 2.8
(exchange volume: 80.4% ± 3.4%)	After PP	412.9 ± 62.9	70.0 ± 10.0	52.9 ± 18.9	68.6 ± 7.7	12.2 ± 1.6

[a] mg/100 ml; data are given as mean ± standard error

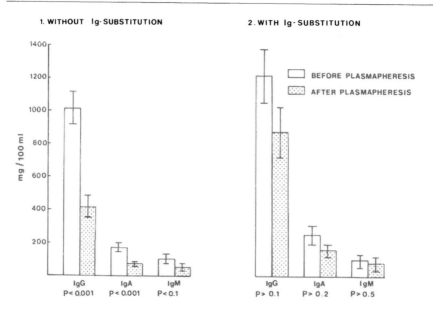

Fig. 2. Immunoglobulin substitution in plasma exchange with 5% human albumin: influence upon immunoglobulin concentrations

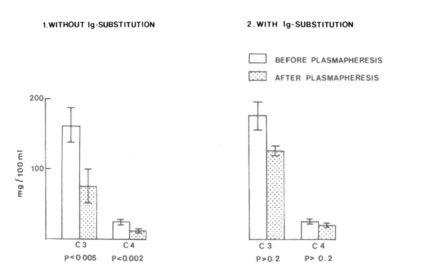

Fig. 3. Immunoglobulin substitution in plasma exchange with 5% human albumin: influence upon complement concentrations

An Experimental Therapeutic Approach   **305**

Therefore, ways had to be sought to circumvent the problem of Ig depletion occuring as a consequence of plasma exchange with 5% HA. By infusing 5 g immunoglobulin concentrate (Endobulin; Immuno AG, Vienna, Austria) together with the regular substitution fluid (5% HA; Immuno) into the patient during PP, not only Ig depletion (Fig. 2) but also the drop in the serum concentrations of C3 and C4 could be counteracted (Fig. 3) [165]. Whereas the effect on serum Ig concentrations can be interpreted as simply one of substitution, the resulting stability of complement levels cannot be explained in such a way, as no significant concentrations of complement were found to be present in the immunoglobulin concentrate. One conceivable mechanism could be, however, the prevention of complement activation by the tubing [160] as a consequence of immunoglobulin substitution. In the context of Ig depletion, 5% HA thus became in our hands a substance which can safely be used as a plasma substitute even in immunocompromised patients.

However, the possibility of reinfusing substances which are bound to the substitution substance must also be considered. We have found, for example, that the substitution fluid used routinely in our laboratory contained large amounts of dehydroepiandrosterone sulfate (DHEA-S). Further investigations have shown that not only the preparation of one company but also five other products contained similar amounts of DHEA-S. Although the role of DHEA-S in the circuit of endocrine regulatory mechanisms has not yet been completely clarified [60, 153], this observation is mentioned in order to draw the reader's attention to the fact that various substances can be present even in defined plasma substitution fluids.

The "Marker Substance"

Together with a "marker lesion" (e.g., palpable purpura, lupus erythema, Raynaud's syndrome, pruritus, histologic changes observed in biopsy material, etc.), the "marker substance" forms an indicator of response to treatment. The exis-

Table 3. Removal of antibodies by plasmapheresis

Disease	Antibody
Autoimmune hemolytic anemia	Antierythrocyte antibodies
Posttransfusion purpura	Antithrombocyte antibodies
Alloimmunization to Rh(D) antibody	Antibody to Rh(D) antigen
Unresponsiveness to factor VIII concentrates in factor VIII deficiency	Anti-factor VIII antibodies
Myasthenia gravis	Anti-acetylcholine receptor antibodies
Pemphigus	Anti-epidermal cell membrane glycoprotein antibodies
Systemic lupus erythematosus	Anti-DNA antibodies, anti-T8 lymphocyte antibodies, anti-NK cell antibodies, antineutrophil antibodies, circulating immune complexes

306 C. C. Zielinski

tence of substances which have been blamed for the propagation of autoimmune disease and the serum concentrations of which can be measured has been used as a rationale for the performance of PP in certain states of disease. In immune-mediated diseases, the "marker substance" is usually a pathologic antibody produced in the course of the autoimmune process, e. g., anti-DNA antibodies and other autoantibodies as well as circulating immune complexes (CISs) in SLE [41], antiacetylcholine receptor antibodies in myasthenia gravis [24, 96], antierythrocyte antibodies in autoimmune anemia [16], and antithyroglobulin, antimicrosomal antibodies as well as thyroglobulin binding inhibiting immunoglobulin in autoimmune thyroid disorders [132]. Although the assessment of these antibody levels during the course of PP treatment must be considered a sine qua non for the objective evaluation of the success of treatment, clinical observations do not necessarily always support this assumption. While the measurement of serum antibody concentrations in certain groups of diseases can be used very conveniently for the assessment of the effect induced by plasma exchange therapy (Table 3), other autoimmune diseases can prove refractory to serologic monitoring. For example, in a study on the effect of PP performed together with immunosuppression by azathioprin in patients with endocrine orbitopathy, neither an immediate nor a long-term effect on the levels of possibly relevant autoantibodies was found by us to be induced by the therapeutic intervention. Clinically, however, an objective ophthalmic improvement in three of the six patients had occured [166]. In studies performed by other investigators, too, the clinical response could not be correlated with immunologic monitoring methods [22, 64]. Thus, although the longing for a "marker substance" is legitimate and such a substance often seems to be at hand, not enough insights have yet been gained into the immunopathology of autoimmune diseases to supply laboratory methods sufficiently sensitive to achieve a better understanding of the clinical processes induced by PP either with or without the addition of immunosuppressive drugs.

Alternatively, in immune-mediated diseases the monitoring of the kinetics of other unspecific substances, e. g., Ig and complement component concentrations, CICs, etc., can help in gaining objective insights into the course of various diseases under PP. As certain immune-mediated diseases are characterized by an increase in serum Ig levels or by the formation of immune complexes leading to hypocomplementemia, assessment of the aforementioned parameters might very well contribute to the evidence of improvement achieved by the application of plasma exchange methodology. Moreover, the reduction of CICs by PP maintain organ function [75]. Following the course of yet another group of substances, acute phase proteins, makes possible observation of immediate effects of PP upon the inflammatory or tissue destructive process (see below). Thus, in autoimmune disease, monitoring of the kinetics of serum concentrations of such substances as Ig, complement components, and CICs and of acute phase proteins might at present constitute the best means of controlling the therapeutic effect reached by PP.

Finally — as with other therapies — attention should be paid to the changes in blood chemistry profiles which, of course, also in the case of plasma exchange procedures can supply evidence of improved function of certain organ systems, although it must be kept in mind that PP reduces the serum concentrations of certain substances included in the routinely performed blood chemistry profiles.

Frequency of Performance

To our knowledge, no definitive controlled data have yet been accumulated concerning the required number of plasma exchanges in a given disease [15]. At times, the disappearance of the "marker substance" or the "marker lesion" can give a clue as to when PP therapy can be discontinued. It must remembered, however, that a single PP reduces the amount of pathogenic factors only partially [113]. In order to gain insights into the amount of certain substances removed by a single PP and to provide tools for the assessment of the efficacy of plasma exchange, a series of studies have dealt with mathematical models for the evaluation of the rate of removal of palsma proteins in context with the equilibrium between the extra- and the intravascular compartments [6, 11, 41, 63, 99, 104]. Although the analysis of such studies may be tedious for nonmathematicians, it is necessary for the physician who performs PP in a certain patient population to be able to evaluate the ability of this treatment to remove those plasma components condidered of interest. In our population, we have applied the following formula: $R = ((V-S)/V)n$, where R is the percentage of the original plasma factor following plasma exchanges, V is the plasma volume, S is the quantitiy of plasma removed per pass, and n is the number of passes [99], and have modified it for continuous plasma exchange procedures in that n was calculated accordingly. Selected results of this study concerning some plasma proteins are shown in Fig. 4. It is evident that the complement component C3 was removed to a similar degree as predicted, while acid glycoprotein, α-antitrypsin,

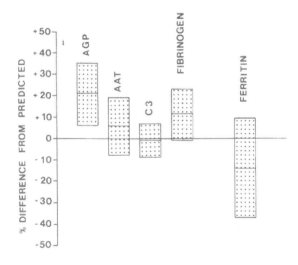

Fig. 4. Removal characteristics of plasma constituents

308 C. C. Zielinski

and fibrinogen were removed to a higher and ferritin to a lesser degree than expected [105], which may be due to the high rate of resynthesis of the latter protein or to a divergent pattern of redistribution of the various substances.

Although — in accordance with the data of Orlin and Berkman [99] — mathematical evidence clearly showed the ability of PP also to remove such plasma proteins as cholinesterase and alkaline phosphatase (both removed as predicted according to the mathematical model) as well as other plasma components, e. g., cortisol, ACTH (both removed as predicted), DHEA-S, and prolactin (both removed less than predicted; ref. 104), not enough data have been generated as to the number of PPs needed for an adequate clinical and serologic effect. Thus the number of applied PP protocols has ranged from 6—10 performed in 2—3 weeks [55, 101, 119, 141, 152] to 20 or more procedures carried out over a prolonged period and at greater intervals [18, 19, 44, 59]. Staring in 1982, our study covers experience of PP treatment during more than 2 years, during which time three different schedules were applied in the treatment of patients with active SLE, finally resulting in controlled data on these three approaches.

Additional Therapy

Therapy administered in addition to the performance of PP is mainly aimed at the suppression of renewed synthesis of substances previously removed by plasma exchange (reviewed in ref. [57]). As pointed out in detail below, the initial concept of the application of PP in immune-mediated disorders in which no synchronized immunosuppression was attempted [19, 55, 59, 119] resulted in serious complications, including a rebound of disease activity [55, 119]. It is, therefore, the accepted belief that patients with active immune-mediated disorders undergoing PP should receive additional immunosuppressive medication [41, 55, 56, 57, 119].

Current Status of the Application of PP in SLE

The Rationale for the Performance of PP:
Autoantibodies and Circulating Immune Complexes

Recent years have witnessed a vast expansion of insights into the pathogenesis of SLE. As reviewed in previous chapters, the main immunologic disturbances in SLE lie in the hyperactivity of B cells as well as in an imbalance of T cell-mediated mechanisms involved in immunoregulation (reviewed in ref. [143]). Moreover, lymphokines [135, 156], intracellular defects [58], and obviously also genetic components [83, 111, 117, 122] contribute to the pathogenesis of the disease. The ultimate effect of immunologic disturbances in SLE is manifested by the formation of autoantibodies directed against an almost unlimited number of structures of the human body, but primarily against DNA which represents an ubiquitous antigen [122]. Other autoantibodies are directed against lymphocyte subclasses and are able to lyse mainly T cells with suppressor function, with the result of disturbed immune equilibrium [89, 114, 115]. However, autoantibodies also directed against other types of white blood cell, including anti-natural killer cell (NK) antibodies [110] and anti-polymorphonuclear cell (PMN) antibodies [30, 107, 129] have been described. The presence of anti-NK cell antibodies can be of particular importance in autoimmune disease, as this cell population has been shown to have the ability to terminate an ongoing immune process [4]. Moreover, the occurrence of antithrombocyte and antierythrocyte antibodies can constitute a serious clinical problem.

The emergence of autoantibodies leads in turn to the formation of CICs, the concentration of which ultimately becomes so high that it results in paralysis of the reticuloendothelial system and thus inability of the latter to fulfill its phagocytic function [76]. CICs are then deposited in various organs, impairing their function.

According to these immunopathologic concepts, steroids and — more recently — immunosuppressive drugs have been introduced into the treatment of active severe forms of SLE [8, 28, 130] with the aim of suppressing autoantibody production. Although most patients do well under this therapeutic regime in that remission can be achieved, the clinical management of patients with very active forms of disease can constitute a problem. This has led to a search for alternative therapeutic approaches to this group of patients, with probably the most prominent being plasma exchange [53]. It has been well accepted that PP can be of immediate benefit in patients with active forms of SLE [108] by eliminating "deleterious substances" the nature of which remained undefined at first [2]. Data accumulated subsequently suggested that these substances were CICs [53, 75, 76] the removal of which might have led to remission via the normalization of the function of immunocompetent cells [86, 88] and of the reticuloendothelial system, resulting in restoration of phagocytosis [76]. These insights were brought into question by clinical observations demonstrating that the improvement of SLE achieved by PP did not necessarily depend on the presence of CICs [20]. Therefore, it must be assumed that the PP-associated removal of the kind of autoantibodies mentioned above most probably also played a role in the induction of remission. This could have been achieved by the normalization of cellular immunoregulatory function, thus aiming at very basic mechanisms in the immunopathogenesis of SLE.

The State of the Art

The efficacy of PP in the management of SLE is difficult to evaluate due to the lack of controlled studies and the varying degree of severity of the disease. The first study on the effect of PP in SLE published by Verrier Jones et al. in 1976 [53] suggested that patients with SLE with high amounts of CIC responded better to PP treatment than patients who had no evidence for the presence of CICs. This and a subsequent study by the same group [54] showed in 8 of 14 patients a clinical or serologic improvement induced by the application of plasma exchange technology. A further analysis of the PP-associated kinetics of serologic and immunologic changes connected with SLE demonstrated the basic ability of PP to lower anti-DNA-antibodies and CICs [55]. In the same study, patients who were under no additional immunosuppressive treatment showed a rebound of both clinical and serologic manifestations of disease activity once PP was discontinued. Similarly, patients under corticosteroid treatment showed only a transient response to PP, whereas patients who also received cyclophosphamide experienced sustained benefit. These results were corroborated by the study of Schlansky et al. [119] on patients with SLE under sole treatment with PP; they found a dramatic deterioration after the discontinuation of PP, although a transient improvement of symptoms had occured during the course of plasma exchanges. The performance of different PP schedules, including multiple treatments performed over a short period [55, 101, 119, 141, 152] as well as prolonged PP therapy [18, 19, 44, 59], did not achieve the desired remission, either. Thus, the sole treatment of SLE by PP has to be judged as an inefficient and perhaps even hazardous form of treatment.

However, the strategy of connecting PP with additional immunosuppression with corticosteroids and cyclophosphamide sheds a different light on the complex situation: In a compilation of the relevant literature, the application of corticosteroids in patients with SLE under PP has been demonstrated to result in a clinical and serologic improvement in a high percentage of cases (81%; ref. [57]), with no rebound having been described [1, 54, 55, 59, 119]. Even better results have been obtained by the addition of cyclophosphamide to the previous therapeutic strategy of PP plus corticosteroids [1, 46, 54, 55. 87. 101, 118], in that prolonged remission lasting up to several years [118] has been achieved. Finally, very recent trials have applied high-dose cyclophosphamide together with PP in patients with very active severe forms of SLE, with very promising results [37, 45]. Thus, the current state of the art of the applications of PP in SLE makes the simultaneous administration of immunosuppressive drugs mandatory. These can consist of either corticosteroids or corticosteroids plus cyclophosphamide. This insight is hampered, however, by lack of information about the ideal PP schedule to be chosen and the form and amount of immunosuppressive drugs necessary to gain control over the activity of severe forms of SLE, which can constitute a life-threatening condition and, moreover, often prove resistant to the usual form of immunosuppressive treatment. Therefore, trials on the value of PP combined with various immunosuppressive drugs in patients with severe SLE, are currently in progress [37, 123].

Objectives of the Present Study

The aim of the study presented here was to establish the best form of treatment involving PP for patients with highly active forms of SLE, whereby the following criteria had to be fulfilled:

1. In order to be entered into the study, patients were required to suffer from highly active forms of SLE which had to be refractory to conventional treatment with high doses of corticosteroids and immunosuppressive drugs.
2. Improvement had to be demonstrated clinically (in patients with "marker lesions") and by serologic methods.
3. In order to rule out immediate effects of plasma exchange treatment, remissions of both clinical and serologic changes had to be sustained for at least 4 weeks after PP treatment had been terminated.

In the light of the aforementioned phenomenon of autoantibody formation in SLE, it was also attempted to establish the effect of PP upon various humoral and cellular immune functions.

Methods

Patient Selection

Ten patients (nine females, one male; mean age: 29.2 ± 3.1 yrs.; mean duration of disease: 10.6 ± 3.7 months) with active severe forms of SLE according to the criteria of the American Rheumatism Association [34] were included in the study. The patients' symptoms and manifestations of disease had been refractory to treatment with corticosteroids and immunosuppressive drugs (cyclophosphamide or azathioprine). All patients also had persisting serologic signs of disease activity, such as high titers of antinuclear antibodies (ANA), including their subfractions (Sm, nRNP, Ro and La; ref. [136]), high binding capacity of anti-DNA antibodies, severe hypocomplementemia, circulating immune complexes, and high serum concentrations of acute phase proteins, including α_1-antitrypsin (AAT) and α_1-acid glycoprotein (AGP). Clinically, vasculitis (seven patients), palpable purpure (six patients), arthralgia (nine patients), Raynaud's disease (eight patients), and serositis (four patients) including pleurisy and pericarditis constituted accompanying symptoms. Leukopenia was present in four, anemia in six, and thrombocytopenia in three. Nephritis and involvement of the central nervous system were each found in three patients. A summary of the patients' symptoms is shown in Table 4.

Previous treatment had consisted of corticosteroids (50—100 mg prednisolone/day) and immunosuppressive drugs, including azathioprin (150 mg/day) and cyclosphamids (100 mg/day), for at least 8 weeks, but no clinical or sero-

312 C. C. Zielinski

logic remission was achieved. In order to avoid the deleterious effects of PP earlier reported in patients with SLE [55, 119], only patients under appropriate immunosuppressive therapy were studied.

Table 4. Course of symptoms in patients with severe active SLE under various plasmapheresis schedules

Symptom	No. of patients	Continuous[a] (n = 10)		Chronic intermittent[a] (n = 6)		PP + high-dose cyclo-phosphamide[a] (n = 6)	
		Improve-ment	Relapse	Improve-ment	Relapse	Improve-ment	Relapse
Raynaud's phenomenon	8	8	4	4	3	4	0
Vasculitis	7	6	6	1	0	4	0
Palpable purpura	6	4	4	2	0	3	0
Arthralgia	9	9	7	5	4	6	1
Serositis	4	0		0		4	(1)
Leukopenia	4	1	0	0		3	0
Anemia	6	1	0	0		3	0
Thrombocytopenia	3	1	0	0		3	0
Nephritis	3	1	0	0		2	0
CNS involvement	3	0		0		3	0

[a] Treatment schedule (see the section on methods). The number of patients with improvement and relapse (occurring within 4—8 weeks) of symptoms are given

Plasmapheresis Schedules

After the patients had failed to respond to conventional treatment with corticosteroids and immunosuppressive drugs for at least 8 weeks, as shown by the persistence of both marker lesions and substances, they were included in the PP program. This consisted of the following schedules, the evaluation of which finally resulted in controlled data on the efficacy of each approach (Fig. 5):

1. Six to eight consecutive PPs performed in 2—3 weeks.
2. Chronic intermittent PP (weekly plasma exchange procedures) after the patients from group 1 had failed to respond to the initial PP treatment, as judged by the persistence of clinical and serologic alterations.

The administration of both corticosteroids and immunosuppressive drugs was continued under the performance of schedules 1 and 2.

3. One or two PPs followed by a bolus of high-dose (750—1000 mg) cyclophosphamide. When patients received this form of therpy, only oral corticosteroids, no further immunosuppressive drugs, were continued.

A flow chart summarizing the therapeutic schedule is shown in Fig. 5. Ten patients were treated according to schedule 1 ("consecutive PP treatment"). Of these, six also underwent schedules 2 ("chronic intermittent PP treatment") and 3 ("PP plus high-dose cyclophosphamide") because signs of high disease activity had persisted. Two patients did not participate in schedules 2 and 3 for technical reasons.

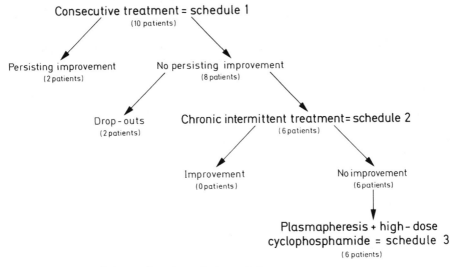

Fig. 5. Flow chart of plasmapheresis methods applied

Plasmapheresis was performed on a continuous IBM 2997 blood cell separator with 75%–125% of the patients' total plasma being exchanged with 5% human albumin (Immuno AG; Vienna, Austria), whereby ACD-B served as anticoagulant (full blood: ACD-B = 15:1).

Laboratory Monitoring

Blood was drawn before and after PP and in schedule 3 on the day after the administration of high-dose cyclophosphamide. Tests were repeated after intervals of 4 and 8 weeks after the treatment concerned had been terminated. Data on serology relevant to SLE were obtained by the assessment of ANA titers by immunofluorescence on rat liver sections, of anti-DNA antibody binding capacity by radioimmunoassay (The Radiochemical Center, Amersham, UK), and of concentrations of immunoglobins G, A, and M, complement components C3 and C4, and acute phase proteins AGP, AAT, and C-reactive protein (CRP) by nephelometry. The concentrations of CIC were established by the solid phase C1q-binding method [48]. Additional data pertaining to routine parameters were obtained from the general hospital laboratory.

Experimental Immunologic Investigations

Data on lymphocyte stimulations by mitogens and the influence of the patients' inactived (56°C, 30 min) sera upon the stimulation of control lymphocytes with various concentrations of pokeweed mitogen (PWM, used in three dilution) and concanavalin A (Con A, two dilutions) were acquired by routine methods [161]. Natural killer cell (NK) assay of both the patients' lymphocytes and control lymphocytes in the presence of the patients' inactivated sera were performed with 51Cr-labelled K562 target cells [67] in the presence of three concentrations (100:1, 50:1, 25:1) of effectors, as described previously [162].

Moreover, the patients' sera were also tested for their ability to influence leukocyte functions of locomotion (LL) and the production of oxygen radicals triggered by phorbol myristate acetate (PMA). All procedures, including the isolation of polymorphonuclear leukocytes, were performed as previously described [13, 158]. For the assessment of LL, the leading front method was applied [95] in which 1.25×10^6 leukocytes were incubated at 37°C in an atmosphere containing 5% CO_2 for 90 min. 0.5% casein (Merck, Darmstadt, West Germany) diluted in phosphate-buffered saline (PBS) served as a chemotaxigen, whereas random mobility was estimated with PBS only [158]. Results were obtained by measuring the distance of migration of cells into 3-μm pore filters (Millipore Corp,; Bedford, Mass.) by using the micrometer on the fine-focus knob on the microscope. Oxygen radical production was assessed by a luminal-amplified chemoluminescence (CL) assay using either sera derived from patients with SLE of phorbol myristate acetate as stimulants, as described previously [29, 164].

Both assessments of leukocyte function, LL and CL, were done with the patients' own cells and with control leukocytes in the presence of SLE serum derived from patients before each PP. In order to characterize the factors influencing various cell functions, sere were used in the native form as well as treated by threefold heating (56°C, 30 min) and freezing (-20°C) and, finally, after dialysis through a membrane with a molecular cut-off range of 8000–12000 daltons [5].

Statistics

Statistical evaluation of the results was performed by Student's t-test for paired samples. Data are given as mean ± standard error (SEM).

The Effect of Various Plasmapheresis Schedules upon the Achievement of Remission

Consecutive Treatment (Schedule 1)

While continuing previous treatment with corticosteroids and immunosuppressive drugs (cyclophosphamide or azathioprin), all patients presented herein underwent six to eight consecutive PPs in a time course of 2—3 weeks (i. e., two or three PPs at 24-h intervals, the rest at 48-h intervals). The patients were monitored continuously during treatment for the manifestation of their clinical symptoms and for the course of serologic markers of SLE activity. The following clinical and serological observations were made during the treatment or shortly thereafter.

Clinical Symptomatology

Symptoms from Raynaud's syndrome, vasculitis, palpable purpura, and arthralgia disappeared either during or shortly after the termination of the treatment schedule. However, the symptoms from these accompanying disorders relapsed mostly within 4 weeks after PP treatment had been discontnued. In general, five of ten patients had an overall — although transient — benefit from the procedure. A detailed analysis of the effect of consecutive PP upon various symptoms is shown in Table 4 (p. 311).

One patient had a sustained improvement in kidney function demonstrated by a decrease in serum creatinine levels (from 6.3 mg/100 ml before PP treatment to 2.7 mg/100 ml afterward), an increase in creatinine clearance (from 15 to 45 ml/min), and a decrease in proteinuria (from 5.5 to 2.9 g/24 h). This is not surprising, as other forms of glomerulonephritis have been shown to be responsive to similar therapeutic interventions [12, 65, 75, 77, 151, 168]. One additional patient had a remarkable sustained improvement in both arthralgia and symptoms from Raynaud's phenomenon. Hematologic problems, including leukopenia and anemia, improved in one patient, while thrombocytopenia was ameliorated in another.

In the majority of our patient population, nevertheless, the concept of numerous PPs performed within a short period under the additional administration of immunosuppressive drugs was disappointing and did not bring about the success described by other authors [1, 46, 54, 55, 87, 101, 118], when judged on an intermediate- or long-term basis. Rather, we share the experience of Wei et al. [152], whose controlled trial of PP in mild active SLE showed no clear-cut benefit. Other authors have reported almost identical protocols, although they did not use immunosuppressive drugs in addition to corticosteroids [1, 54, 55, 59, 119]. Our patients, however, were all on combined immunosuppressive therapy which — according to the experience reported in the literature [1, 46, 54, 55, 87, 101, 118] — should have influenced positively the results of PP, yet failed to do so. A possible explanation might be the prolonged and exceptional disease activity in our patients and the fact that they were selected for PP treatment only after therapeutic regimes with immunosuppressive drugs had been of no benefit. Thus, what might have very well been true for patients with mild or intermediate active disease could not be reproduced in severe active SLE.

Serologic Findings

Concecutive plasma exchange treatments did not achieve the desired long-lasting effect of a reduction in disease activity, as assessed by serologic and immunologic means. Although titers of ANA dropped and anti-DNA binding capacity became substantially lower immediately after an individual PP treatment (Fig. 6), Figs. 7–10 demonstrate that neither the titers of ANA nor the concentrations of anti-DNA-antibodies nor the decrease in serum C3 levels were influenced by a series of consecutive PPs when the time points before the start of PP treatment and 1 month after its termination were compared (Figs. 1–10; $P > 0.1$ in each case). The titers of ANA subfractions did not show any changes, either, when followed throughout the course of PP treatment. As can be seen from the behavior of serum concentrations of C3 and C4, hypocomplementia as one of the manifestations of the presence of immune complexes also persisted despite treatment, wehen judged on an intermediate-term basis of 4 weeks. Similarly, acute phase proteins AAT and AGP did not show any decrease in serum concentra-

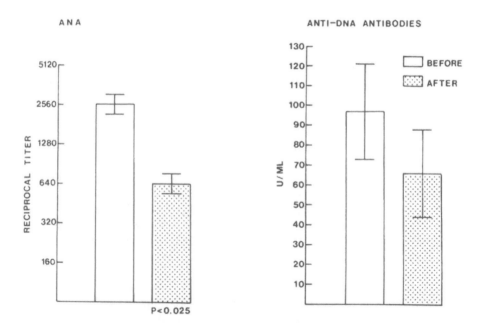

Fig. 6. ANA titers and anti-DNA antibodies before and after one PP

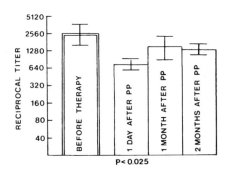
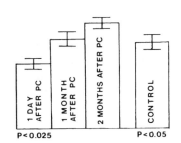

Fig. 7. Kinetics of antinuclear antibodies. "Control" signifies the time of testing after the end of a treatment course by plasmapheresis and high-dose cyclophosphamide *(PC)*. Differences between serum concentrations found at a given point in time and the levels before the initiation of therapy were analyzed by Student's *t*-test (*P* values are shown)

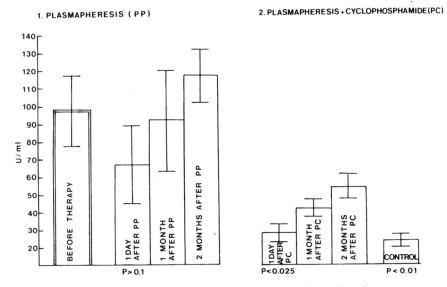

Fig. 8. Course of anti-DNA antibodies (see legend to Fig. 7 for explanation)

tions, which would have signaled a decrease in disease activity ($P > 0.1$, respectively; Fig. 10). However, after a longer period of observation no rebound in the production of ANA, anti DNA antibodies and of CICs was found, as has been reported in patients under PP without additional immunosuppression [55, 119], although anti-DNA antibody concentrations in the patients' sera did show a tendency to increase when assessed 1 and 2 months after the conclusion of PP therapy (Fig. 8). This pattern should not be interpreted as a real rebound but rather

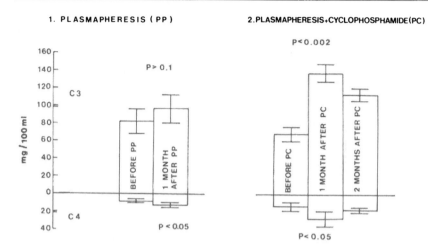

Fig. 9. Course of serum concentrations of C3 and C4 (see legend to Fig. 7)

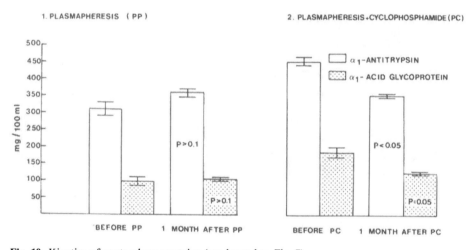

Fig. 10. Kinetics of acute phase proteins (see legend to Fig. 7)

as continued and increasing activity of the disease. This assumption is further substantiated by the increase in serum concentrations of AAT (Fig. 10) found 4 weeks after the termination of therapy.

In summary, the performance of a course of PP treatments combined with the oral adminstration of corticosteroids and immunosuppressants led to only a transient improvement of symptoms which relapsed after PP therapy had been discontinued. Analogously, no long-lasting improvement in immunologic parameters of SLE activity was found. Thus, this form of therapy did not fulfill expectations as to its ability to control the underlying disease for a prolonged

An Experimental Therapeutic Approach **319**

period. The serologic markers indicating a renewed increase in disease activity led us to initiate the next PP schedule (chronic intermittent treatment), which will be discussed in the following section.

Chronic Intermittent Treatment (Schedule 2)

Of the ten patients who entered the study and who had undergone treatment schedule 1, six had to be continued on the chronic intermittent PP regime due to the recurrence of symptoms and clinical as well as serologic signs of disease activity once schedule 1 had been discontinued (Table 4). A mean of 13.9 ± 2.1 plasma exchanges was performed in this group of patients over 5.5 ± 0.9 months.

After the symptoms of SLE had recurred, mostly within 4—8 weeks — an interval also observed by other investigators [57] — the patients received plasma exchange treatment twice or thrice at 24-h intervals and were re-plasmapheresed at weekly intervals. While on this schedule, the patients were kept on the immunosuppressive regime consisting of corticosteroids and cyclophosphamide. As previously, the patients were observed closely for their clinical course and for the kinetics of their serologic markers.

Clinical Symptomatology

Table 4 (p. 311) shows our experience with this treatment modality concerning the patients' individual symptoms. Three of the six patients experienced an improvement of their symptoms while on the protocol. They relapsed, however, once the treatment was discontinued. In contrast, the symptoms of the other three patients were not influenced at all. As in the part of the investigation presented before, symptoms from Raynaud's disease and arthralgia were the fastest to disappear under renewed treatment (Table 4), as observed by other investigators [55, 135a], although, especially in the case of joint pain, a placebo effect cannot be completely excluded [32]. Hematologic alterations were not influenced by this form of treatment at all. As the rest of symptoms also showed only moderate or no reactions to PP therapy, we believe that the presented approach did not truly contribute to a reversal of disease activity. However, no clinical exacerbation of disease was found under this protocol, either. The clinical impression was rather that the disorder was kept at a certain level of activity without further influencing its course.

Serologic Findings

The serologic findings in patients with SLE undergoing chromic intermittent PP treatment not only further substantiated the clinical impression of continued disease, but in addition actually indicated a progression of SLE. Thus, titers of ANA (median before treatment: 1:640; after treatment: 1:640) and of anti-DNA antibody binding capacity (mean ± SEM before treatment: 64.9 ± 12.2 U/ml; after treatment: 66.6 ± 23.4 U/ml; $P > 0.1$) were practically unchanged after treatment when compared with pre-PP levels. Similarly, levels of acute phase proteins AAT and AGP not only failed to signal a decrease in disease activity but rather indicated a progression. Thus, AAT levels increased significantly from 362.5 ± 24.5 mg/100 ml before the chronic intermittent schedule was started to 452.9 ± 23.3 mg/100 ml at the time of discontinuation of this treatment ($P <$ 0.05), and the serum soncentrations of AGP (before treatment: 109.8 ± 14.1 mg/100 ml; after treatment: 185.6 ± 32.1 mg/100 ml) and of C-reactive protein (before treatment: 1.67 ± 0.2 mg/100 ml; after treatment: 5.7 ± 2.9 mg/100 ml) showed a similar tendency. C3 and C4 remained sharply decreased after this kind of PP treatment, as they had been before (*C3:* before: 97 ± 17 mg/100 ml; after: 68.7 ± 7.8 mg/100 ml; *C4:* before: $13,5 \pm 2.5$ mg/100 ml; after: 13.1 ± 4.2 mg/100 ml). However, no signs of a rebound of immunologic parameters were observed, which was most probably achieved by the concomitant administration of immunosuppressive drugs.

In summary, chronic intermittent PP performed simultaneously with the administrations of immunosuppressive drugs did not lead to a reduction in the activity of severe SLE. Rather, serologic markers pointed to an increase in disease activity which necessitated the application of schedule 3 (PP combined with a bolus of high-dose cyclophosphamide). Taking into account the relatively long duration of treatment by chronic intermittent PP, the increasing concentrations of acute phase proteins as indicators of disease activity could point to the fact that this form of treatment is detrimental in patients whose disease requires quick intervention and relief of symptoms.

Plasmapheresis Plus High-Dose Cyclophosphamide (Schedule 3)

Prompted by earlier studies of patients with SLE whose disease recurred after the termination of a series of PPs and whose serologic parameters indicated a rebound in the formation of autoantibodies and CICs [55, 119], several investigators have speculated that the administration of high-dose immunosuppressive drugs after PP might suppress autoantibody production by B cells [37, 45]. Lacking another from of immunopharmacologic intervention, it is tempting to try to suppress this process by the administration of immunosuppressive drugs. As the patients reported in this chapter had received continuous immunosuppressive treatment with cyclophosphamide, it was decided to administer an intravenous bolus of high-dose cyclosphamide 6—8 hours after the last PP out of a series of two plasma exchange treatments which were performed at 24-h intervals. Applying this protocol, the following observations were made:

Clinical Symptomatology

All six patients treated according to this protocol showed persisting benefit covering subjective symptoms, organ dysfunction, and hematologic disorders. Although, as can be seen in Table 4 (p. 311), symptoms and clinical signs of disease activity had disappeared after the first combined treatment, a subsequent increase in serologic markers suggested repetition of the treatment to maintain remission. This was done three times in three patients and four times in two, at intervals of approximately 2 months. After completion of this schedule, remission has now lasted for 1 year in three patients and for 6 months in two (with the sixth patient no longer under our observation for geographic reasons).

Serologic Findings

Figures 6—9 demonstrate that the clinical impression of achievement of remission was also supported by serologic and immunologic means. Figure 7 shows that ANA titers had dropped significantly ($P < 0.025$) 24 hrs. after PP (i. e., 16 hrs. after the administration of cyclophosphamide) and remained low for 4 weeks, whereupon a renewed — although much less pronounced — increase was found. After completion of the treatment series, ANA titers were significantly lower ($P < 0.05$) than at the start of PP therapy. The levels of anti-DNA antibodies showed an even more pronounced response, demonstrated by a sharp drop in anti-DNA antibody binding capacity after treatment ($P < 0.025$; Fig. 8), and had reached almost normal concentrations (22.9 $\pm$ 3.4 u/ml) at the time of termination of treatment, indicating that a decrease in disease activity had finally been achieved [68, 106, 120]. Although anti-DNA antibody concentrations increased slightly 1 and 2 months thereafter, they never reached pre-PP treatment levels, and remained low during the entire observation period.

The effect of PP plus high-dose cyclophosphamide upon serum concentrations of C3 and C4 is shown in Fig 9. When assessed 1 month after therapy, both C3 and C4 serum concentrations had increased significantly ($P < 0.002$ and $P < 0.05$, respectively) to normal levels, which can be taken as an indication of decreased formation of immune complexes. The effect of a stabilization of complement concentrations was seen not only at 2 months after treatment but also on a long-term basis.

Finally, acute phase proteins also showed a decrease in serum concentrations (Fig. 10). Both AAT and AGP concentrations showed a significant and stable decline ($P < 0.05$ and $P = 0.05$, respectively) once therapy had been instituted. This is the more remarkable as these two compounds had shown a constant increase throughout treatment and observation (Fig. 10), starting at the time of the first of the consecutive PPs (schedule 1) right through the course of chronic intermittent PP up to the first PP followed by a bolus of cyclophosphamide. Assuming that the constant increase in serum concentrations of acute phase proteins reflects a permanent increase in disease activity despite various schedules of PP therapy and the administration of immunosuppressive drugs, the increase in SLE activity could be interrupted only by schedule 3.

In summary, the ongoing process of SLE activity in patients with a severe form of disease could be stopped only by a combined regimen of PP and high-dose cyclophosphamide. The question remains, however, as to the importance of the various components (i. e., PP and cyclophosphamide) in the system. In other words: Would the sole administration of a bolus of cyclophosphamide in the same concentration as that used suffice to achieve a similar clinical and serologic effect or is the additional performance of plasma exchange a sine qua non

322   C. C. Zielinski

for the effect of the regimen. Data gathered during the patients' maintenance therapy indicate that the sole administration of high-dose cyclophosphamide keeps anti-DNA antibodies at a certain, admittedly low, level without eradicating them any further or even completely. This might serve as circumstantial evidence that the reduction of mainly autoantibody formation to the degree demonstrated in Fig. 8 is probably only achievable by the mechanistic strategy of removal of autoantibodies by PP combined with suppression of renewed synthesis by a large dose of an immunosuppressive agent. Although it can be envisaged that high-dose cyclophosphamide might ultimately lead to a decrease in autoantibody concentrations similar to that reported in this section, it can nevertheless be of value in severe life-threatening forms of SLE to achieve a depletion of autoantibodies as quickly as possible in an attempt to remove several factors, including CICs, and to manipulate immunologic mechanisms in order to maintain the function of vital organs. The latter assumption is corroborated by data of other authors who have used similar therapeutic approaches [45].

Complications of Plasma Exchange Treatment

The high costs of plasma exchange technology make the performance of PP in disease in which the benefit of such a procedure is not clearly evident prohibitive for many centers which cannot afford merely experimental therapies. Fear of possible side-effects either during or after plasma exchange also militates against PP. Experience drawn from a number of publications show that this fear is indeed justified. PP treatment can be hampered by a series of clinical side-effects ranging from minor difficulties such as orthostasis, chills, and symptoms arising from citrate toxicity like light headedness, nausea, and paresthesias [15, 23, 33, 133], to major problems, including changes in left ventricular function [39] and an imbalance in electrolyte levels causing cardias arrhytmias and even cardiac arrests (the latter have occured mainly after large volume plasma exchanges) [7, 133]. Moreover, pulmonary failure and disturbances of the central nervous system have been reported [7]. When 5% HA has been used as plasma substitution fluid, laboratory investigations have shown a very pronounced drop in certain plasma protein concentrations, including immunoglobulins and complement components (Figs. 1—3; ref. 61), as well as in coagulation factors [38, 62]. The depletion of immunoglobulins may lead to an increase in the number of infectious episodes following PP [109, 133, 155].

Some of the side-effects resulting from an imbalance of electrolytes can be avoided by the substitution of potassium and calcium during or immediately after the plasma exchange [17] and by avoiding the removal of large plasma volumes. Following this route, we have observed side-effects in only 11.3% or our procedures (Table 5), with infections occuring in 3 of 45 patients. It must be stressed, however, that according to our protocols only relatively low volumes of the patients' plasma are being exchanged and that close monitoring of the patients' cardiac function is of utmost importance. Nevertheless, it must be kept in

Table 5. Complications of plasmapheresis observed in connection with 390 plasma exchanges performed in a total of 45 patients in our unit

Complication	Incidence	
	Absolute number	Percentage
Venous access problems[a]	20	5.1
Hypocalcemia	14	3.6
Hypercoagulability	5	1.3
Orthostasis	5	1.3
Total number of procedures with complications	44	11.3
Infections	3 patients	

[a] Requiring discontinuation of the procedure

mind that PP is a potentially dangerous intervention which should be used as strictly as possible and performed only in experienced centers where trained staff is available.

Results of Experimental Immunologic Investigations

The knowledge of alterations in humoral and cellular immunity in SLE, reviewed above, has prompted us to perform a series if experimental immunologic investigations in order to gain insight into the effect of PP upon the presence of autoantibodies, CICs, and the modulatory behavior of the serum upon various cellular functions. The results of these experiments will be presented below.

Humoral Immunity

Immunoglobulins

Whereas the kinetics of ANA titers, including their subfractions, of anti-DNA antibody serum concentrations, and of levels of C3 and C4 have been presented in previous sections, the course of immunoglobulin (Ig) concentrations has remained unmentioned. It deserves to be reported, however, because it further adds to the evidence that SLE is a disease in which control over B cell functions has been lost (reviewed in [143]). Observation of the kinetics of immunoglobulin isotypes under PP as one of the means of expression of polyclonal activation of B cells might provide additional in vivo information regarding the immunopathology of SLE.

Patients with various diseases who are being treated by a regimen of immunosuppressive drugs combined with plasma exchange in which 5% HA is used for plasma substitution tend to become depleted of Ig (Fig. 1). In an assessment of

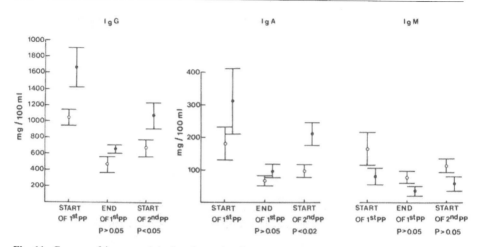

Fig. 11. Course of immunoglobulins from the first to the second plasmapheresis. ●, patients with SLE; ○, controls. The differences in serum immunoglobulin levels in control patients and patients with SLE at a given point in time were analyzed by Student's *t*-test (*P* values are shown)

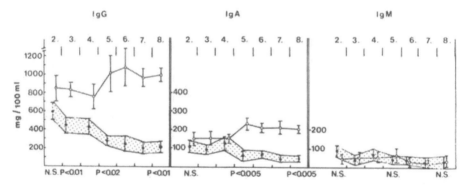

Fig. 12. Kinetics of immunoglobulins in patients with SLE on plasmapheresis. ●, SLE patients; ○, controls. *Nos. 2—8* stand for the number of plasma exchanges. The differences in serum immunoglobulin concentrations in control patients and patients with SLE found before the performance of a certain plasma exchange number were analyzed by Student's *t*-test (*P* values are shown)

the kinetics of Ig in patients with SLE we have found another pattern of behavior: As reported earlier [167], serum concentrations of IgG, IgA, and IgM were reduced by the first PP in patients with SLE and in control patients (Fig. 11). However, serum concentrations of IgG and IgA increased again significantly ($P < 0.05$ and $P < 0.02$, respectively) in patients with SLE during the interval between the termination of the first PP and the beginning of the next one 24 hrs. later, while no such increase was found in the control group (Fig. 11). This kind of an increase in serum IgG and IgA concentrations in patients with SLE treated by PP according to schedule 1 as compared with serum Ig levels of control persons turned out not to be a singular phenomenon following one plasma exchange, but persisted throughout the course of the entire protocol (Fig. 12). Thus, it was not possible to lower serum IgG and IgA concentrations by a course of consecutive PPs, although the patients received immunosuppressive drugs. In contrast, patients with glomerulonephritis undergoing an identical treatment protocol had a very pronounced drop in their serum Ig concentrations, as shown in previous studies [168]. In summary, the behavior of Ig under PP and conventional immunosuppressive treatment supplies further evidence of the increased and uncontrolled synthetic activity of B cells in SLE.

Whereas there was a parallelism in the behavior of autoantibodies and serum Ig concentrations in patients on schedule 1, this was lost when schedule 3 was applied; Although anti-DNA antibodies were substantially lowered by the latter approach (Fig. 8), Ig concentrations remained stable at 24-hr. intervals and also when assessed 6—8 weeks after the performance of the last PP which was part of the combined treatment.

Anti-DNA Antibodies

Almost all investigators agree that serum concentrations of anti-DNA antibodies can be lowered by plasma exchange [53, 55, 152]. There can be no doubt that the removal of anti-DNA antibodies is a welcome achievement since, among other parameters, the activity of SLE has been correlated with the level of serum concentrations of anti-DNA antibodies [68, 106, 120]. However, mere PP without additional therapeutic measures such as the administration of immunosuppressive agents can result in a rebound of anti-DNA antibody concentrations once PP has been discontinued, leading in turn to deleterious clinical effects [55, 119]. In order to counteract this phenomenon, the current trend is to administer immunosuppressive therapy to plasmapheresed patients with high serum concentrations of anti-DNA antibodies [37, 45, 57]. In doing so in a modified form, i.e., by the use of high doses of cyclohosphamide, not only could a rebound of anti-DNA antibody concentrations be prevented, but their levels were permanently reduced to almost normal values in the current study.

Circulating Immune Complexes (CICs)

Like anti-DNA antibodies, CICs are also removed by PP [53, 55, 152] but show a rebound when patients on plasma exchange treatment are not being immunosuppressed [55, 119]. Some investigators have demonstrated a correlation be-

326 C. C. Zielinski

tween the presence of CICs and the degree of SLE activity [3], giving clinical importance to the assessment of serum concentrations of CICs. The detection of CICs can be achieved in many ways including, to name but a few, various C1q-binding assays, the Raji cell test, and conglutinin-binding methods (reviewed in [154]), with the degree of hypocomplementemia in the patients' sera providing additional indirect evidence for the presence of immune complexes [154]. However, no single method is yet considered ideal for the detection and estimation of CICs [154]. In the population presented here, solid phase C1q-binding assays demonstrated the presence of CICs in only four patients, although all patients were severely hypocomplementemic at the time of inclusion in the PP program (Fig. 9), indicating that in the majority of patients CICs probably went undetected by the C1q-binding assay. Although hypocomplementemia was ameliorated by the performance of treatment schedule 1, it was ultimatley normalized only by schedule 3. CICs detected by the C1q-binding method had disappeared much earlier, i.e., during schedules 1 or 2. The normalization of hypocomplementemia coincided, however, with the lowering or the disappearance of anti-DNA antibody concentrations, with a decrease in serum levels of acute phase proteins, and, finally, with the sustained clinical improvement, which suggests that the parameter of serum concentrations of C3 and C4 might have really corresponded with the presence of CICs and with disease activity.

The disappearance of CICs in the course of SLE has important implications for the immunopathology of the disease: Soluble antigen—antibody complexes are known to impair suppressor T cell function [88] as well as to induce activation of B cells in the murine system [86]. Also, phagocyte function has been shown to be ameliorated by the removal of CICs, resulting in an improvement of the activity of the reticuloendothelial system [76]. All these factors could thus have been the underlying reasons for the clinical improvement in our patients, which is further emphasized by the fact that neither CICs nor hypocomplementemia reappeared once remission had been achieved. Additional data on the presence and disappearance of CICs will also be presented in the section on polymorphonuclear leukocytes (see below).

Additional Means of Assessing Disease Activity

The concentrations of anti-DNA antibodies, of other autoantibodies, of CICs, and of C3 and C4 as well as of the lytic complex CH50 are the object of routinely and widely applied techniques for the evaluation of SLE activity. As an additional means serving the same purpose we would like to draw the reader's attention to the measurement of acute phase proteins, such as CRP, AAT, and AGP, in the patients' sera and report our experience in this area. Whereas in the past only a qualitative estimation of the presence of CRP was feasible, recent advances have also made quantitative assessments possible, allowing for more exact statements about the significance of the presence of this acute phase protein [70]. CRP as well as other acute phase proteins have some properties which can be taken advantage of in the setting of SLE under PP:

- The serum concentration of CRP is known to be a parameter of activity of various disorders, including SLE (reviewed in [90, 91]).
- Although CRP as well as other acute phase proteins are removed by PP, CRP quickly returns to previous concentrations due to its swift rate of resynthesis [169].
- Thus, CRP concentrations remain fairly untouched by the plasma exchange procedure itself, even when 5% HA is used for plasma substitution, while other parameters, including the erythrocyte sedimentation rate and the concentration of complement components, cannot be used properly due to depletion (Fig. 3) and the relatively long latency needed for resynthesis.

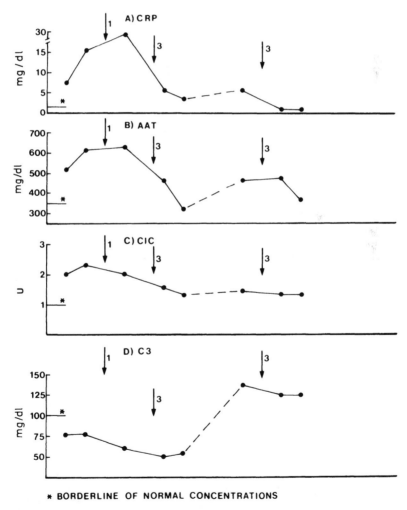

* BORDERLINE OF NORMAL CONCENTRATIONS

Fig. 13. Course of various parameters of disease activity in SLE. *CRP*, C-reactive protein; *AAT*, α-antitrypsin; *CIC*, circulating immune complexes. See the section on "methods" for a detailed description of the method of assessing serum concentrations

In view of these considerations, we have measured serum concentrations of CRP, AAT, and AGP in our entire population of SLE patients under PP, and our findings are summarized in Fig. 13, which shows the course of CRP, AAT, and AGP in correlation with C3 concentrations and CIC levels in a representative patient undergoing first, consecutive PP treatment and later, PP plus high-dose cyclophosphamide. Although the illustration shows only one case, the same experience was gained in other patients with SLE, proving the exceptional usefulness of assessment of acute phase protein concentrations in the serologic evaluation of disease activity. This method gains even more importance in the context of PP, where a perturbance of plasma proteins occurs which in turn makes the use of traditional parameters of SLE activity difficult.

Peripheral Blood Mononuclear Cells

As shown in the preceding chapters of this book, different parts of the cellular immunologic system are heavily deranged in SLE. It exceeds the frame and purpose of this chapter to again review these disturbances in detail. Here, we want to concentrate mainly on the changes in cellular immunity pertinent to or achieved by PP as well as our own experience and the results of other authors regarding the influence of the patients' sera upon mitogen-induced functions of mononuclear cells (MNCs).

B and T Cells

Knowledge of the disturbed immunoregulation in SLE has prompted many investigators to study the effects of PP and its potential to induce a normalization of immune circuits. In the search for an answer to this question, both functional assays using mitogens as well as phenotypic characterizations with monoclonal antibodies for the assessment of membrane antigens of T cells have been applied, but despite these sophisticated techniques no clear conclusions have been reached as yet. Thus, Tsokos et al., who have studied a series of in vitro immune functions in a double-blind controlled study on patients with SLE on real or sham PP, did not find any changes in the percentage of cells forming rosettes with sheep red blood cells (SRBC), in T cell function (assessed by stimulation of peripheral MNCs with a series of mitogens and alloantigens), in the degree of allogeneic cell-mediated lympholysis, or, finally, in the number of cells secreting immunoglobulins either spontaneously or after induction with pokeweed mitogen (PWM), when data from before and after a series of plasma exchange procedures were compared [141]. Bonomini et al., in contrast, did detect increases in SRBC rosette-forming cells and in Con A-induced suppressor activity after only a few PPs, together with a decrease in inhibition of rosette formation of control MNCs by the patients' sera [14]. Finally, Abdou et al. [1] have reported a PP-associated normalization of Con A-induced suppressor activity upon Ig synthesis.

Studies on the effect of PP upon phenotypic characteristics of T cells using monoclonal antibodies which subdivide this cell population into various groups with different functional properties (reviewed in [109]) have also produced disappointing and controversial results. While Bonomini et al. failed to show a PP-induced change in T cell phenotypes [14], Kiprov [66] as well as Fiorini et al. [35] have reported a decrease in T4/T8 ratios after PP of patients with SLE under additional immunosuppressive therapy. These latter findings are the more remarkable as a pronounced disequilibrium between helper and suppressor T cells — known to be present in SLE — could have been corrected by the application of PP and immunosuppression, thus leading to maintained remission. Although such an outlook is very attractive, the underlying cause is most probably the PP-related removal of lymphocytotoxic antibodies directed mainly against the T8+ subset which are associated with this particular autoimmune disorder [74, 89, 114, 115]. A decrease of these autoantibodies could result in an increase of T8+ cells and normalization of the T4+/T8+ ratio and, finally, in a shift away from the previous T cell subset patterns [127].

How can we reconcile such divergent findings in patients with the same disease? The most likely answers are the varying degree of disease activity, nonuniform PP schedules, and the kind and dosage of drugs used for additional treatment. There can be no doubt that with the advent of more and more monoclonal antibodies directed against increasing numbers of T cell membrane antigens and with the expanding knowledge of the structures they identify [109], the picture will become even more intricate before the effect of PP upon immunologic circuits is understood. As for the present, however, PP appears to have an unclear effect upon the disequilibrium within the T cell population of patients suffering from SLE.

Influence of SLE Sera upon Blastogenesis

Expanding knowledge of the presence of autoantibodies directed against lymphocyte subpopulations in the sera derived from patients with SLE [74, 89, 114, 115] has initiated investigations on blastogenic responses of MNCs in the presence of SLE serum [114, 115, 116]. We have therefore studied the influence of the

Table 6. Influence of SLE sera upon responses to mitogens of control lymphocytes

Serum added[a]	Mitogen	Dilution/concentration	dpm[b]
Control	Pokeweed mitogen	100:1	43372±6445
		50:1	40057±5535
		25:1	50810±3790
SLE		100:1	53466±4971
		50:1	44477±6261
		25:1	41361±5687
Control	Concanavalin A	60 µg	20635±4658
SLE			32933±5391

[a] Heat inactivated (56°C, 30 min) sera, diluted 1:10
[b] Mean ± standard error

330 C. C. Zielinski

patients' sera upon mitogenic responses to PWM and Con A. Inactivated sera derived from patients before each PP performed during the course of schedule 1 were diluted 1:10 and added to control MNCs which were stimulated with either PWM or Con A. Table 6 shows that the sera had not modified the response of control MNCs to the two mitogens even before the initiation of the PP schedule, when compared with sera derived from healthy control individuals. This might correspond with the failure to demonstrate the presence of both cold-[115] and warm-reactive [74] autoantibodies directed against lymphocytes in our patients' sera (data not shown). Although this is surprising in view of the high percentage of patients with SLE and their relatives whose sera contain antilymphocytic antibodies [26, 82], it can be explained easily by the fact that our patients were all heavily pretreated with steroids and additional immunosuppressive agents. This should also be kept in mind when reviewing our data presented in the following sections.

Natural Killer Cells

The natural killer cell (NK) activity of patients with SLE has been shown rather uniformly to be impaired [40, 52, 100, 124, 142], and the decrease was found to be more pronounced in patients with active than in those with inactive disease [52, 126, 142], although the latter results have been disputed [40]. Similar to the presence of autoantibodies directed against suppressor T cells, the sera of patients with SLE also have been found to contain autoantibodies directed against NK cells [110]. All these data are of potential importance when one considers the results of Abruzzo and Rawley, who have recently shown that NK cells are able to terminate an ongoing immune response [4]. Such a role in the immune network could move NK cells to the center of interest as regulatory components in autoimmune diseases.

Although the NK cell activity of the few patients tested was slightly decreased before the initiation of schedule 1, as compared with the NK activity of healthy controls, SLE sera obtained at various time points of the PP treatment during schedule 1 did not modify the NK activity of control persons (Table 7). These results might again reflect the fact that our patients had all been treated before

Table 7. Influence of SLE sera upon natural killer cell activity

Serum origin[a]	Effector : target ratio		
	100:1	50:1	25:1
0 (*n* = 18)	52.0±3.9[b]	40.9±3.7	38.4±3.4
Control (*n* = 17)	47.7±5.2	43.4±6.1	36.6±5.6
SLE	57.1±8.1	45.7±6.1	32.3±6.1

[a] Heat inactivated (56°C, 30 min) sera, diluted 1:10
[b] Data are given as mean of % lysis ± standard error

they had undergone PP and that pretreatment might modulate a series of cellular phenomena despite serologic and clinical evidence of disease activity. This possibility gains additional weight given that although preformed immune complexes have been shown to inhibit NK cell activity in vitro, no correlation has been found between the presence of CICs in SLE sera and the decrease in NK activity [42].

Natural killer cell activity in both human and murine systems can be enhanced by interferon [27, 140]. Recent data on the effects of interferon on NK cell activity in patients with SLE have suggested that two groups of patients might exist: one comprising patients with decreased NK activity and defective NK responses to interferon (i.e., no increase in activity), the other comprising patients with normal NK activity and normal responses to interferon (reviewed in [143]). Unfortunately, very little is known about the ability of PP to induce or alter the production of lymphokines. This should be studied, however, because, together with the recent evidence of the potential importance of NK cell activity in autoimmune disorders, it could provide an additional justification for the performance of PP in autoimmune diseases.

Polymorphonuclear Leukocytes

The function of polymorphonuclear leukocytes (PMNs) in SLE has been much less investigated than that of other peripheral blood cells. The place of PMNs in the first row of antimicrobial defense mechanisms and the highly increased rate of infections in SLE [31, 102, 128, 144] make this cell population and its function very interesting. Due to an increased rate of infections as a possible complication of PP [109, 133, 155], we feel that PMNs and their function must be mentioned and considered when reviewing the subject.

As scattered studies have reported a disfunction of PMNs in patients with SLE [71], we will report our own data mainly concerning two mechanisms, i.e., leukocyte locomotion (LL) and oxygen radical production assessed by a chemoluminescence assay (CL).

Leukocyte Locomotion

Defects in LL can be ascribed to cell-inherent defects [50, 84, 92, 159], the presence of cell-directed LL-inhibiting serum factors [72, 80, 146, 147, 157, 159], or the inability to activate serum to produce chemotactic factors [79, 112, 149, 150, 158]. Whereas a study testing LL in untreated patients with SLE has clearly demonstrated a defect in the PMN cell population concerning this ability [71], we did not find any such defect in three of our heavily pretreated patients when they had reached remission after schedule 3 (depth of migration into the filter by the leading front method: 100 ± 2.7 µm, 96.8 ± 1.8 µm, 73 ± 6.6 µm; values in 16 healthy control persons tested simultaneously: 97.3 ± 2.4 µm). These discrepant findings suggest that the decrease in LL in untreated patients might be due to several factors, including CICs, which are known to inhibit LL in a variety of disorders [73, 93, 94], anti-PMN antibodies [30, 107, 129], or other factors such as

332 C. C. Zielinski

the chemotactic factor inactivator which emerges as an acute phase reactant [69]. Serum-associated LL inhibition (SALLI) has been found in a variety of disorders, including immune-mediated diseases [72, 102] and malignancies [80, 147, 157, 159]. Although serum factors responsible for the effect of SALLI have been isolated and characterized [80], the phenomenon of LL inhibition is often mediated by CICs [73, 93, 94]. The influence of sera of patients with SLE — as a prototype of diseases in which CICs play an eminent role — upon LL should therefore result in a pronounced inhibition of this PMN function. In order to test this assumption, we have performed a series of experiments which are summarized in Table 8. As can be seen, very pronounced inhibition of locomotion of control PMNs (between 27% and 69%) was accomplished by SLE sera (diluted 1:10) derived from six of eight patients, whereas sera derived from control persons never inhibited LL by more than 20%. Only further dilution of the patients' sera to 1:25 and 1:50, treatment by heating (30 min at 56°C), and freeze-thawing abrogated SALLI and in the majority of cases reduced the degree of inhibition to below 20%. In contrast, dialysis of the patients' sera through a membrane with a molecular cut-off range between 8000 and 12000 daltons did not influence SALLI, in that a persistent inhibition of LL was detected.

Next, the ability of PP to remove the factor responsible for the reduction of LL was studied. The data resulting from these investigations did not show any change of the LL inhibitory capacity of the respective patient's serum during the course of PP schedule 1. Moreover, SALLI persisted also when patients had reached remission following schedule 3. Thus, it must be assumed that a factor different from CICs must be responsible for serum-associated LL inhibition in SLE. This assumption is further emphasized by our observation that sera derived from patients with immune complex-mediated glomerulonephritis did not inhibit LL or that their LL-inhibitory capacity was lost during the course of PP. The discrepancy between LL inhibition and the presence of CICs is further illustrated by evidence obtained in CL assays which is shown below.

Table 8. Inhibition of leukocyte locomotion by sera derived from patients with SLE

Dilution of untreated serum			% Inhibition of leukocyte locomotion[a]		
1:10	1:25	1:50	Serum 1:10, 56°C, 30 min	Serum 1:10, freeze-thaw	Serum 1:10, dialyzed[b]
49.5	26	19	3	10	62
15	2	22	24	2	Not done
38	3	0	0	19	0
42	25	11	0	29	Not done
0	0	0	2	0	0
69	3	0	0	23	65
48	11	2	21	13	57
27	Not done	Not done	0	0	31

[a] Data are given as % inhibition of leukocyte locomotion by the serum added, as compared with assays performed without the addition of serum. Control sera never inhibited leukocyte locomotion by more than 20%
[b] See the section on methods

Oxygen Radical Production Assessed by Chemoluminescence

Two methods for the assessment of the production of oxygen radicals were applied: Control PMNs were incubated with SLE sera in a dilution of 1:10, whereupon the generation of oxygen radicals was tested either immediately or after the addition of PMA in order to exclude the presence of an inhibiting factor. Our results show that the sera of four out of seven patients with active SLE tested induced a very high oxygen radical production, which is in accordance with the reports of other authors [29]. In the course of PP schedule 1, CL decreased consecutively with the number of PPs, down to control levels after three to five PPs (Fig. 14). After the intermission between treatment schedules 1 and 2, the potency of oxygen radical production had again increased to pretreatment levels. No difference between control and SLE sera was found im PMA-triggered assays.

It is very likely that the induction of oxygen radical production by the patients' sera was due to the presence of CICs, which were removed by a series of PP treatments. An alternative explanation could be the presence of anti-PMN

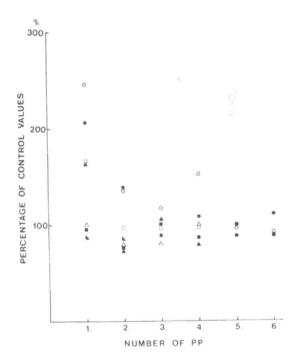

Fig. 14. Chemoluminescence assays with sera of SLE patients. Control values were obtained by the assessment of induction of oxygen radical production by sera derived from healthy control persons. The ability of SLE sera to increase further chemoluminescence in comparison with control sera is shown

autoantibodies in the patients' sera [30, 107, 129]. The findings in CL assays and the results obtained in LL experiments testing SALLI are discrepant. Therefore, a factor inhibiting the locomotion of PMNs which is different from CICs and could be an intricate part of the disease might be present in the patients' sera and be responsible for our findings. Further experiments are under way to shed more light on these questions.

Conclusions

The application of plasma exchange technology has gone a long way from its beginnings as adjuctive therapy in SLE, as first suggested by Verrier-Jones et al. [53], to a time when rather sceptical reports have emerged [123]. It is fair to assume that slowly we will acquire an attitude of sceptical approval and constructive criticism toward this method, as it is on its way to becoming more sophisticated through the application of new techniques which allow for selective removal of "deleterious substances" instead of the crude removal of total plasma.

From the very outset, the concept of PP has predisposed it for application in immune-mediated disorders, where immunopathologically relevant substances could be removed and the exchange of plasma thus contribute to the achievement of remission. PP therapy of SLE as a prototype of immune-mediated disorders which can result in a dysfunction of vital organs has been the topic of many trials (reviewed in [57]), but no clear-cut results have been obtained, although some controlled data have already been [141, 152] or are currently being [37, 123] accumulated. In the study presented here, we have investigated patients with severe active forms of SLE who have been resistant to immunosuppressive treatment. The aim of the study was the achievement of prolonged remission primarily covering a period of at least 4—8 weeks and, ultimately, a persistent decrease in disease activity. In contradiction to previous assumptions, we present evidence that only one to two PPs are enough in order to achieve remission, provided they are followed by the administration of high-dose cyclophosphamide. No other PP schedule — even if it involved a series of plasma exchange treatments performed over a long period — achieved similar success. Rather, SLE activity even progressed under other PP schedules.

These results have several interesting implications:

- Although other programs can achieve transient amelioration of symptoms and disease activity, prolonged remission is achieved only by PP plus high-dose cyclophosphamide.
- Remission achieved by this therapy is not only a clinical observation but can also be documented by serologic means.
- Besides producing the best results, PP plus high-dose cyclophosphamide is by far the most cost-effective procedure.

An Experimental Therapeutic Approach **335**

The good results obtained by this therapeutic approach should, however, be treated with caution, as side-effects — although not observed in the current trial — can include problems arising from both PP and cyclophosphamide. In contrast, maintenance therapy can consist of less severe measures than with other therapeutic regimes, as remission is achieved faster and to a more pronounced degree. It should be borne in mind that the concept of PP combined with high-dose cyclophosphamide is an intervention involving very serious measures. Therefore, its application should be restricted to patients with severe disease, while less active forms might be better treated by other means, including plasma exchange regimes, as has been suggested previously [85].

Recent data have demonstrated that patients with nephritis due to SLE have a better prognosis when treated with cyclophosphamide in due time [8]. It remains to be seen whether this finding will also hold true for patients treated by our protocol.

Our experimental immunologic data also have produced some novel insights into the pathology of severe SLE, with the most striking being (a) the lack of reduction of serum Ig levels despite their removal by PP in the presence of immunosuppressive drugs and (b) evidence for the existence of a serum factor different from CICs which was able to inhibit locomotion of PMNs, while CICs were definitely the reason for serum-associated induction of CL in PMNs. In contrast to investigations by other authors, we were not able to detect any PP-associated changes in serum-mediated influence upon the function of peripheral blood mononuclear cells. Therefore, it is tempting to speculate that the therapeutic interventions described in this report were able to reduce the activity of the disease, but did not result in a modification of SLE-associated underlying immunologic defects. Thus, the final conclusion to be drawn is that patients with severe SLE under PP plus high-dose cyclophosphamide treatment should be monitored very closely once they have reached remission in order to detect renewed signs of disease activity.

Summary

Plasmapheresis (PP) has been applied as an experimental therapeutic approach in various forms of SLE. In this chapter, three PP schedules (1. consecutive treatment consisting of six to eight PPs performed in 2—3 weeks; 2. chronic intermittent treatment with PPs performed at weekly intervals; 3. one or two PPs followed by high-dose cyclophosphamide) for the treatment of severe active SLE are presented, and the relevant literature is reviewed. Only the combined treatment consisting of PP and high-dose cyclophosphamide was able to induce long-lasting remission, the other schedules resulting in transient improvement. The achievement of remission was demonstrated by both clinical impression and serologic data, including a decrease in anti-DNA antibody binding capacity, an increase in serum concentrations of complement components C3 and C4, and a decrease in acute phase proteins.

Experimental immunologic data have produced evidence of increased IgG and IgA levels in patients with severe SLE on PP and immunosuppression, as compared with control patients treated with similar schedules. In addition, serum-associated inhibition of leukocyte locomotion turned out to be a mechanism uninfluenced by PP and probably not mediated by CICs alone. Serum-induced chemoluminescence, in contrast, depended on the presence of CICs in the patients' sera. However, no influence of SLE sera upon the function of mononuclear cells was found. We conclude that although the activity of SLE can be controlled by the introduced procedure, underlying disease-associated mechanisms remain uninfluenced.

Acknowledgments.
The author thanks Professors G. Geyer, C. Steffen, and M. M. Eibl for their suggestions, support, and encouragement. Without these the performance of the study described in this chapter would have been impossible. Dr. Joseph S. Smolen contributed ideas and suggestions to the design of the study and has referred patients, as did Drs. A. Wolf and J. Slany. Many thanks are also due to Doctors C. Müller, P. Preis, and C. Gisinger for their help in the laboratory, in the generation of experimental data, and in the Apheresis Unit. Further help was provided by Ms. W. Kalinowska and Ms. H. Hiesberger in performing expert technical assistance and by Ms. C. Schneider, R. N., in organizing the Apheresis Unit. This study was supported in part by the Anton Dreher Memorial Donation for Medical Research.

References

1. Abdou MI, Lindsley HB, Pollock A, Stechschulte DJ, Wood G (1981) Plasmapheresis in active systemic lupus erythematosus: effects on clinical, serum and cellular abnormalities. case report. Clin Immunol Immunopathol 19:54—55
2. Abel JJ, Rowntree LG, Turner BB (1914) Plasma removal with return of corpuscles (plasmapheresis). J Pharmacol Exp Ther 5:625—641
3. Abrass CK, Nies KM, Louie JS, Border WA, Glassock RJ (1980) Correlation and predictive accuracy of circulating immune complexes with disease activity in patients with systemic lupus erythematosus. Arthritis Rheum 23:273—282
4. Abruzzo LV, Rowley DA (1983) Homeostasis of the antibody response: Immunoregulation by NK cells. Science 222:581—585
5. Ahmad R, Zielinski CC, Mannhalter JW, Zlabinger G, Rockenschaub A, Eibl MM (1982) Plaque-forming cells in human cord blood: a soluble factor suppressing differentiation but not proliferation of B cells. Int. Arch. Allergy Appl. Immunol. 69:132—136
6. Apstein CS, Zilversmit DB, Lees RS, Georg PK (1978) Effect of intensive plasmapheresis on the plasma cholesterol concentration with familial hypercholesterolemia. Atherosclerosis 31:105—115
7. Aufeuvre JP, Morin-Hertel F, Cohan-Solal M, Lefloch A, Baudelot J (1980) Hazards of plasma exchange: A nation-wide study of 3431 exchanges in 592 patients. In: Sieberth HG (ed) Plasma exchange. Schattauer, Stuttgart, p 149
8. Balow JE, Austin HA, Muenz LR, Joyce KM, Antonovych TT, Klippel JH, Steinberg AD, Plotz PH, Decker JL (1984) Effect of treatment on the evolution of renal abnormalities in lupus nephritis. N Engl J Med 311:491—495

An Experimental Therapeutic Approach **337**

9. Bansal SC, Bansal BR, Thomas HL, Siegel PD, Rhoads JE, Cooper DR, Terman DS, Mark R (1978) Ex vivo removal of serum IgG in a patient with colon carcinoma. Cancer 42:1—18

10. Bensinger WI, Baker DA, Buchner D, Clift RA, Thomas ED (1981) Immunoadsorption for removal of A and B blood-group antibodies. N Engl J Med 304:160—162

11. Berkman EM, Orlin JB (1980) Use of plasmapheresis and partial plasma exchange in the management of patients with cryoglobulinemia. Transfusion 20:171—179

12. Blumenstein M, Samtleben W, Habersetzer R, Gurland HJ (1982) Plasma-Austausch bei Nierenerkrankungen. Dtsch Med Wochenschr 107:1854—1856

13. Böyum A (1968) Isolation of mononuclear cells and granulocytes from human blood. Scand J Clin Lab Invest 21 [Suppl 97]:77—104

14. Bonomini V, Vangelista A, Frasca GM, Nanni-Costa A, Borgnino LC (1984) Effect of plasmapheresis on cellular immunity abnormalities in patients with systemic lupus erythematosus. Clin Nephrol 22:121—126

15. Borberg H (1981) Problems of plasma exchange therapy. In: Gurland HJ, Heinze V, Lee HA (eds) Therapeutic plasma exchange. Springer, Berlin Heidelberg New York, p 191

16. Branda RF, Moldow CF, McCullough JJ, Jacob HS (1975) Plasma exchange in the treatment of immune disease. Transfusion 15:570—576

17. Buskard NA, Varghese Z, Wills MR (1976) Correction of hypocalcemic symptoms during plasma exchange. Lancet 2:344—345

18. Clark WF, Lindsay RM, Cattran DC, Chodirker WB, Barnes CC, Linton AL (1981) Monthly plasmapheresis for systemic lupus erythematosus with diffuse proliferative glomerulonephritis: a pilot study. Can Med Assoc J 125:171—174

19. Clark WF, Lindsay RM, Ulan RA, et al. (1981) Chronic plasma exchange therapy in systemic lupus erythematosus nephritis. Clin Nephrol 16:20—23

20. Cohen J, Lockwood CM, Calnan CD (1980) Plasma exchange in the treatment of leukocytoclastic vasculitis. J R Soc Med 73:457—460

21. Curran JW, Lawrence DN, Jaffe H, et al. (1984) Acquired immunodeficiency syndrome (AIDS) associated with transfuions. N Engl J Med 310:69—75

22. Dandona P, Marshall NJ, Bidey SP, Nathan A, Havard CWH (1979) Successful treatment of exophthalmos and pretibial myxedema with plasmapheresis. Br Med J 1:374—376

23. Das PC, Smit Sibinga CT (1983) Complications of therapeutic plasma exchange. Lancet 2:455—456

24. Dau PC, Lindstrom JM, Cassel CK, Denys EH, Shev EE, Spitler LE (1977) Plasmapheresis and immunosuppressive drug therapy in myasthenia gravis. N Engl J Med 297:1134—1140

25. Davies NE, Davies GH, Sanders ED (1983) William Cobbett, Benjamin Rusk, and the death of General Wiashington. JAMA 249:912—915

26. DeHoratius RJ, Messner RP (1975) Lymphocytotoxic antibodies in family members of patients with systemic lupus erythematosus. J Clin Invest 55:1254—1258

27. Djeu JY, Heinbaugh JA, Holden HJ, Herberman RB (1979) Augmentation of mouse NK cell activity by interferon and interferon inducers. J Immunol 122:175—179

28. Donadio JV (1984) Cytotoxic-drug treatment of lupus nephritis. N Engl J Med 311:528—529

29. D'Onofrio C, Maly FE, Fischer H, Maas D (984) Differential generation of chemiluminescence-detectable oxygen radicals by normal polymorphonuclear leukocytes challenged with sera from systemic lupus erythematosus and rheumatoid arthritis patients. Klin Wochenschr 62:710—716

30. Drew SI, Carter BM, Guidera DP, Terasaki PI (1977) Autoimmune cytotoxic granulocyte antibodies in health and disease. Transplant Proc 9:1887—1994

31. Dubois EL, Wierzchowiecki M, Cox MB, Weiner M (1974) Duration and death in systemic lupus erythematosus: an analysis of 249 cases. JAMA 227:1399—1402

32. Dwosh IL, Giles AR, Ford PM, Pater IL, Anastassiades TP, et al. (1983) Plasmapheresis therapy in rheumatoid arthritis. N Engl J Med 308:1124—1129

33. Editorial (1982) Hazards of apheresis. Lancet 2:1025—1026
34. Editorial (1984) Disease criteria for systemic lupus erythematosus. Arch Intern Med 144:252—253
35. Fiorini G, Paracchini ML, Fornasieri A, Sinico RA, Colasanti G, Gibelli A, D'Amico G (1982) Modifications in peripheral blood lymphocyte subpopulations induced by plasmapheresis and immunosuppressive drugs. Plasma Ther 3:389—393
36. Fleig C (1909) Autotransfusion of washed corpuscles as a blood washing procedure in toxinemia: heterotransfusion of washed particles in anemia. Bull Mens Acad Sci Lett. Montpellier 1:4—9
37. French Cooperative Group (1984) Randomized trial of plasma exchange in severe acute systemic lupus erythematosus: methodology. Ann Med Interne (Paris) [Suppl 22] (abstract # 85).
38. Gelabert A, Puig L, Maragall S, Monteagudo J, Castillo R (1980) Coagulative alterations during massive plasmapheresis. In: Sieberth HG (ed) Plasma exchange. Schattauer, Stuttgart, p 71
39. Gisinger C, Punzengruber C, Silberbauer K, Preis P, Zielinski CC (1985) Cardiac effects of plasmapheresis evaluated by echocardiography. Plasma Ther 6:547—550
40. Goto M, Tanimoto K, Horiuchi Y (1980) Natural cell-mediated cytotoxicity in systemic lupus erythematosus. Arthritis Rheum. 23:1274—1281
41. Gurland HJ, Samtleben W (1983) Klinische Einsatzmöglichkeiten und technische Durchführung der Plasmapherese. Internist 24:14—26
42. Haas H, Havel A, Lange A, Gross W, Flad HD, Schlaak M (1984) Circulating immune complexes and NK-activity in systemic lupus erythematosus. Immun Infect 12:109—110
43. Hakim RM, Merrill JP (1983) Plasmapheresis: prospects for expanded clinical trials. In: Nosé Y, Malchesky PS, Smith JW (eds) Plasmapheresis: new trends and therapeutic applications. Isao, Cleveland, p 21
44. Hamblin I, Smith D (1980) Plasma exchange as a long term treatment of systemic lupus erythematosus. In: Siebert HG (ed) Plasma exchange. Schattauer, Stuttgart, p 185
45. Hamburger MI, Kaell AT, Bennet RS (1984) Plasmapheresis and cyclophosphamide in systemic lupus erythematosus. Ann Med Interne (Paris) 135, [Suppl 21] (abstract # 83)
46. Hamilton WAP, Vergani D, Bevis L, Tee DEH, Zilkha KJ, Cotton LT (1980) Plasma exchange in systemic lupus erythematosus. Lancet 1:1249
47. Handley SL (1982) Therapeutic apheresis: industry research report. Unterberg and Towbin, New York
48. Hay FC, Nineham LJ, Roitt IM (1976) Routine assay for the detection of immune complexes of known immunoglobulin class using solid phase Clq. Clin Exp Immunol 24:396—400
49. Health technology case study 23 (June 1983) Safety, efficacy and cost effectiveness of therapeutic apheresis. Office of Technology Assessment, Washington, D. C.
50. Hill HR, Ochs HD, Quie PG, Pabst HF, Klebanoff SJ, Wedgwood RG (1974) Defect in neutrophil granulocyte chemotaxis in Job's syndrome of recurrent "cold" staphylococcal abscesses. Lancet 2:617—619
51. Höcker P, Pittermann E (1985) Die Plasmaaustauschbehandlung in der Hämatologie, Wien Klin Wochenschr 97:115—122
52. Hoffman T (1980) Natural killer function in systemic lupus erythematosus. Arthritis Rheum 23:30—35
53. Jones JV, Bucknall RC, Cumming RH, Asplin CM, Faser ID, Bothamley J, Davis P, Hamblin TJ (1976) Plasmapheresis in the management of systemic lupus erythematosus? Lancet 1:709—711
54. Jones JV, Cumming RH, Bacon PA, Evers J, Fraser ID, Bothamley J, Tribe CR, Davia PG, Hughes GRV (1979) Evidence for a therapeutic effect of plasmapheresis in patients with systemic lupus erythematosus. Q J Med 48:555—576
55. Jones JV, Robinson MF, Parciany RK, Layfer, McLeod B (1981) Therapeutic plasmapheresis in systemic lupus erythematosus. Arthritis Rheum 24:1113—1120

An Experimental Therapeutic Approach **339**

56. Jones JV (1982) Plasmapheresis in systemic lupus erythematosus. Clin Rheum Dis 8:243—260
57. Jones JV (1983) Plasmapheresis in rheumatology. In: Lysaght MJ, Gurland HJ (eds) Plasma separation and plasma fractionation. Karger, Basel, p 99
58. Kammer GM, Birch RE, Polmar SH (1983) Impaired immunoregulation in systemic lupus erythematosus: defective adenosine-induced suppressor T lymphocyte generation. J Immunol 130:1706—1712
59. Kater L, Derksen RHWM, Houwert FA, Hene RJ, Struyvenberg A, Gmelig-Meyling RJH, Verroust P (1981) Effect of plasmapheresis in active systemic lupus erythematosus. Netherlands J Med 24:209—216
60. Kauppila A, Ylikorkala O (1983) Stable prolactin level after enhanced estradiol production following dehydroepiandrosterone sulfate. Am J Obstet Gynecol 138:271—272
61. Keller AJ, Urbaniak SJ (1978) Intensive plasma exchange on the cell separator: effects on serum immunoglobulins and complement components. Br J Haematol 38:531—540
62. Keller AJ, Chirnside A, Urbaniak SJ (1979) Coagulation abnormalities produced by plasma exchange on the cell separator with special reference to fibrinogen and platelet levels. Br J Haematol 42:593—603
63. Keller F, Wagner K, Faber U, Scholle J, Neumayer HM, Maiga M, Schultze G, Offermann G, Molzahn M (1983) Elimination kinetics of plasma exchange. Klin Wochenschr 61:1115—1122
64. Kelly W, Longson W, Smithard D, Fawcitt R, Wensley R, Noble J, Keley J (1983) An evaluation of plasma exchange for Graves' ophthalmopathy. Clin Endocrinol 18:485—493
65. Kincaid-Smith P, d'Apice AJF (1978) Plasmapheresis in rapidly progressive glomerulonephritis. Am J Med 65:564—566
66. Kiprov DD (1983) Influence of plasmapheresis on cellular immunity. In: Lysaght MJ, Gurland HJ (eds) Plasma separation and plasma fractionation. Karger, Basel, p 48
67. Klein E, Ben-Bassat H, Newmann H (1976) Properties of the K562 cell line, derived from a patient with chronic myeloid leukemia. Int J Cancer 18:421—431
68. Koffler D, Carr R, Agnello V, Thoburn R, Kunkel HG (1971) Antibodies to human polynucleotides in human sera: antigenic specificity and relation to disease. J Exp Med 134:294—307
69. Kreutzer DL, Hupp JR, McCormick JR (1982) Elevation of serum chemotactic factor inactivator activity during acute inflammatory reactions in rabbits and humans. In: Kushner I, Volanakis JE, Gewurz H (eds) C-reactive protein and the plasma protein response to tissue injury. Ann NY Acad Sci 389:451—453
70. Kushner I (1982) The phenomenon of the acute phase response. In: Kushner I, Volanakis JE, Gewurz H (eds) C-reactive protein and the plasma protein response to tissue injury. Ann NY Acad Sci 389:39—48
71. Landry M (1977) Phagocyte function and cell-mediated immunity in systemic lupus erythematosus. Arch Dermatol 113:147—154
72. Lanzer G, Zielinski CC, Knapp W, Eberl R, Steffen C (1981) Leukocyte locomotion and regulative serum effects in rheumatoid arthritis. Z Rheumatol 40:66—71
73. Leung-Tack J, Maillard J, Voisin GA (1979) Chemotaxis inhibition induced in polymorphonuclear neutrophils by soluble immune complexes. Int Archs Allergy Appl Immunol 58:365—374
74. Litvin DA, Cohen PL, Winfield JB (1983) Characterization of warm-reactive IgG anti-lymphocyte antibodies in systemic lupus erythematosus: relative specificity for mitogen-activated T cells and their soluble products. J. Immunol. 130:181—186.
75. Lockwood CM, Rees AJ, Pinching AJ, Pussell B, Sweny P, Uff J (1977) Plasma-exchange and immunosuppression in the treatment of fulminating immune-complex crescentic nephritis. Lancet 1:63—67
76. Lockwood CM, Worlledge S, Nicholas A, Cotton C, Peters DK (1979) Reversal of impaired splenic function in patients with nephritis or vasculitis (or both) by plasma exchange. N Engl J Med 300:524—530

340 C. C. Zielinski

77. Lockwood CM, Pusey CD, Peters DK (1983) Indications for plasma exchange: renal diseases. In: Lysaght MJ, Gurland HJ (eds) Plasma separation and plasma fractionation. Karger, Basel, p 145
78. Ludwig H (1982) Multiples Myelom: Diagnose, Klinik und Therapie. Springer, Berlin Heidelberg New York
79. Maderazo EG, Ward PA, Woronick CL, Kubik J, DeGraff AC (1976) Leukotactic dysfunction in sarcoidosis. Ann Intern Med 84:414—419
80. Maderazo EG, Anton TE, Ward PA (1978) Serum-associated inhibition of leukotaxis in humans with cancer. Clin Immunol Immunopathol 9:166—167
81. Malchesky PS, Wojcicki J, Horiuchi T, Lee JM, Nosé Y (1983) Membrane separation processes for macromolecule removal. In: Nosé Y, Malchesky PS, Smith JW (eds) Plasmapheresis: new trends in therapeutic applications. Isao, Cleveland, p 51
82. Messner RP, DeHoratius RJ (1978) Epidemiology of antilymphocyte antibodies in systemic lupus erythematosus. Arthritis Rheum 21 [Suppl]:S167—S170
83. Miller KB, Schwartz RS (1979) Familial abnormalities of suppressor cell function in systemic lupus erythematosus. N Engl J Med 301:803—809
84. Miller ME, Oski EA, Harris MB (1971) Lazy leukocyte syndrome: A new disorder of neutrophil function. Lancet 1:665—669
85. Miller ML, Steinberg AD (1983) Systemic lupus erythematosus — immunoregulatory therapies. Clin Rheum Dis 9:617—628
86. Möller G (1969) Induction of DNA synthesis in normal human lymphocyte cultures by antigen—antibody complexes. Clin Exp Immunol 4:65—78
87. Moran CJ, Parry HF, Mowbray J, Richards DJM, Goldstone AH (1977) Plasmapheresis in systemic lupus erythematosus? Br Med J 1:1573—1574
88. Moretta L, Mingari MC, Romanzi CA (1978) Loss of Fc receptors for IgG from human T lymphocytes exposed to IgG immune complexes. Nature 272:618—620
89. Morimoto C, Reinherz EL, Distaso JA, Steinberg AD, Schlossman SF (1984) Relationship between SLE T cell subsets, anti-T cell antibodies, and T cell functions. J Clin Invest 73:689—700
90. Morley JJ, Kushner I (1982) Serum C-reactive protein levels in disease. In: Kushner I, Volanakis JE, Gewurz HJ (eds) C-reactive protein and the plasma protein response to tissue injury. Ann NY Acad Sci 389:39—48
91. Morrow W, Isenberg JWDA, Parry HF, Snaith ML (1981) C-reactive protein in sera from patients with systemic lupus erythematosus. J Rheum 8:599—604
92. Mowat AG, Baum J (1971) Chemotaxis of polymorphonuclear leukocytes from patients with diabetes mellitus. N Engl J Med 284:621—627
93. Mowat AG, Baum J (1971) Chemotaxis of polymorphonuclear leukocytes from patients with rheumatoid arthritis. J Clin Invest 50:2541—2549
94. Mowat AG (1976) Neutrophil chemotaxis in patients with rheumatoid arthritis: mechanisms responsible for impairment. Ann Rheum Dis 33:286
95. Müller C, Zielinski CC, Passl R, Eibl MM (1984) Divergent patterns of leukocyte locomotion in experimental posttraumatic osteomyelitis. 65:299—303
96. Newsom-Davis J, Pinching AJ, Vincent A, Wilson SG (1978) Function of circulating antibody to acetylcholine receptor in myastenia gravis: investigation by plasma exchange. Neurology 28:266—272
97. Nilsson IM, Jonsson S, Sundqvist SB, Ahlberg A, Bergentz SE (1981) A procedure for removing high titer antibodies by extracorporeal protein-A-sepharose adsorption in hemophilia: substitution therapy and surgery in a patient with hemophilia B and antibodies. Blood 58:38—44
98. Nydegger UE (1983) Choice of the replacement fluid during large volume plasma exchange. Res Clin Lab 13:103—109
99. Orlin JB, Berkman EM (1980) Partial plasma exchange using albumin replacement: removal and recovery of normal plasma constituents. Blood 56:1055—1059.
100. Oshimi K, Sumiya M, Gonda N, Kano S, Takaku F (1979) Natural killer cell activity in systemic lupus erythematosus. Lancet 2:1023—1025

101. Parry HF, Moran CJ, Snaith ML, Richards JDM, Goldstone AH, Nineham LJ, Hay FC, Morrow WJW, Roitt IM (1981) Plasma exchange in systemic lupus erythematosus. Ann Rheum Dis 40:224—228
102. Perez HD, Audron RI, Goldstein IM (1979) Infection in patients with systemic lupus erythematosus: association with a serum inhibitor of complement-derived chemotactic activity. Arthritis Rheum 22:1326—1333
103. Popper KR (1975) Die offene Gesellschaft und ihre Feinde, 4th edn, Francke, Munich
104. Preis P, Templ H, Kuzmits R, Zielinski CC (1984) Eliminationsraten bei Plasmapherese dargestellt andhand verschiedener Plasmaproteine, Hormone und Akutphasenproteine. Acta Med Austriaca [Suppl] 2:34
105. Preis P, Linkesch W, Eibl MM, Zielinski CC (1984) Shifts in ferritin and acute phase proteins under plasmapheresis. RIA '84, Milan, p 49
106. Reichlin M (1981) Current perspectives on serological reactions in SLE patients. Clin Exp Immunol 44:1—10
107. Rekvig OP, Hannestad K (1977) Certain polyclonal anti-nuclear antibodies cross-react with the surface membrane of human lymphocytes and granulocytes. Scand J Immunol 6:1041—1054
108. Recommendations of the Arthritis Foundation and the American Rheumatism Association on plasmapheresis in rheumatic diseases, Feb. 1981
109. Romain PL, Schlossman SF (1984) Human T lymphocyte subsets; functional heterogeneity and surface recognition structgures. J Clin Invest 74:1559—1565
110. Rook AH, Tsokos GC, Quinnan GV, Balow JE, Ramsey KM, Stocks N, Phelan MA, Djeu JY (1982) Cytotoxic antibodies to natural killer cells in systemic lupus erythematosus. Clin Immunol Immunopathol 24:179—185
111. Rose NR, Kong YC, Sundick RS (1980) The genetic lesions of autoimmunity. Clin Exp Immunol 39:545—550
112. Rosenfeld SL, Baum J, Steigbigel RT, Leddy JP (1976) Hereditary deficiency of the 5th component of complement in man. J Clin Invest 57:1635—1643
113. Rother K, Thies K (1983) Plasmapherese-Therapie. Internist 24:1—13
114. Sagawa A, Abdou NI (1979) Suppressor-cell antibody in systemic lupus erythematosus: possible mechanisms for suppressor-cell dysfunction. J Clin Invest 63:536—539
115. Sakane T, Steinberg AD, Reeves JP, Green I (1979) Studies of immune functions of patients with systemic lupus erythematosus. J Clin Invest 64:1260—1269
116. Sakane T, Steinberg AD, Reeves JP, Green I (1979) Studies of immune functions of patients with systemic lupus erythematosus: Complement-dependent IgM anti-thymus-derived cell antibodies preferentially inactive suppressor cells. J Clin Invest 63:954—965
117. Scherak O, Smolen JS, Mayr WR (1980) HLA-DRw3 and systemic lupus erythematosus. Arthritis Rheum 23:954—957
118. Schildermans F, Dequeker J, van de Putte I (1979) Plasmapheresis combined with corticosteroids and cyclophosphamide in uncontrolled active systemic lupus erythematosus. J Rheum 6:687—690
119. Schlansky R, DeHoratius RJ, Pincus T, Tung KSK (1981) Plasmapheresis in systemic lupus erythematosus. Arthritis Rheum 24:49—53
120. Schur PH, Sandson J (1968) Immunologic factors and clinical activity in systemic lupus erythematosus. N Engl J Med 278:533—538
121. Schwab PJ, Fahey JL (1960) Treatment of Waldenström's macroglobulinemia by plasmapheresis. N Engl J Med 263:574—579
122. Shoenfeld Y, Schwartz RS (1984) Immunologic and genetic factors in autoimmune disease. N Engl J Med 311:1019—1029
123. Shumack KH, Rock GA (1984) Therapeutic plasma exchange. N Engl J Med 310:762—771
124. Sibbitt WL, Mathews J, Bankhurst AD (1983) Natural killer cells in systemic lupus erythematosus: defects in effector lytic activity and response to interferon and interferon inducers. J Clin Invest 71:1230—1239

342 C. C. Zielinski

125. Sieberth HG, Glöckner WM, Kierdorf H (1983) Cascade filtration for macromolecular separation. In: Lysaght MJ, Gurland HJ (eds) Plasma separation and plasma fractionation. Karger, Basel, p 223

126. Silverman SL, Cathcart ES (1980) Natural killing in systemic lupus erythematosus: inhibitory effects of serum. Clin. Immunol. Immunopathol. 17:219—226

127. Smolen JS, Chused TM, Leiserson WM, Reeves JP, Alling DW, Steinberg AD (1982) Heterogeneity of immunoregulatory T cell subsets in systemic lupus erythematosus. Am J Med 72:783—790

128. Staples PJ, Gerding DN, Decker JL, Gordon RS (1974) Incidence of infection in systemic lupus erythematosus. Arthritis Rheum 17:1—10

129. Starkebaum G, Price TH, Lee MY, Arend WP (1978) Autoimmune neutropenia in systemic lupus erythematosus. Arthritis Rheum 21:504—512

130. Steinberg AD (1981) Management of systemic lupus erythematosus. In: Kelley WN, Harris ED, Ruddy S, Sledge CB (eds) Textbook of Rheumatology. Saunders, Philadelphia, p 1133

131. Stoffel W, Borberg H, Greve V (1981) Application of specific extracorporeal removal of low density lipoprotein in familial hypercholesterolemia. Lancet 2:1005—1007

132. Strakosch CR, Wenzel BE, Row VV, Volpé R (1982) Immunology of autoimmune thyroid disorders. N Engl J Med 307:1499—1507

133. Sutton DMC, Cardella CJ, Uldall PR, Deveber GA (1981) Complications of intensive plasma exchange. Plasma Ther 2:19—23

134. Taft EG (1979) Thrombotic thrombocytopenic purpura and dose of plasma exchange. Blood 54:842—849

135. Talal N, Dauphinee MJ, Wofsy D (1982) Interleukin-2 deficiency, genes and systemic lupus erythematosus. Arthritis Rheum 25:838—842

135a. Taplos G, White JM, Horrocks M, Cotton LT (1978) Plasmapheresis in Raynaud's disease. Lancet 1:416—417

136. Tan EM (1982) Autoantibodies to nuclear antigens (ANA): their immunobiology and medicine. Adv Immunol 33:167—182

137. Tani T, Oka T, Kosugi A, Tsunoda F, Nakane Y, Kodama M, Fujisawa A, Takada T, Toyoda Y (1972) Comparative study of replacement solutions in plasma exchange: their contents and clinical consequences. In: Oda T (ed) Therapeutic plasmapheresis II. Schattauer, Stuttgart, p 165

138. Terman DS, Buffaloe G, Mattioli C (1979) Extracorporeal immunoadsorption: initial experience in human systemic lupus erythematosus. Lancet 2:824—827

139. Terman DS, Yamamoto T, Mattioli M, Cook G, Tillquist R, Henry J, Poser R, Dashal Y (1980) Extensive necrosis of spontaneous canine mammary adenocarcinoma after extracorporeal perfusion over *Staphylococcus aureus* Cowans I. J Immunol 124:795—805

140. Trinchieri G, Santoli D (1978) Antiviral activity induced by culturing lymphocytes with tumor-derived or virus-transferred cells: enhancement of human natural killer cell activity by interferon and inhibition of susceptibility of target cells to lysis. J Exp Med 147:1314—1319

141. Tsokos GC, Balow JE, Huston DP, Wei N, Decker JL (1982) Effect of plasmapheresis on T and B lymphocyte functions in patients with systemic lupus erythematosus: a double blind study. Clin Exp Immunol 48:449—457

142. Tsokos GC, Rook AH, Djeu JY, Balow JE (1982) Natural killer cells and interferon responses in patients with systemic lupus erythematosus. Clin Exp Immunol 50:239—245

143. Tsokos GC, Balow JE (1984) Cellular immune responses in systemic lupus erythematosus. In: Schwartz RS (ed) Immunology of anergy and systemic lupus erythematosus. Karger, Basel, p 93 (Progress in Allergy 35)

144. Urowitz MB, Bookman AAM, Koehler BE, Gordon DA, Smythe HA, Ogryzlo MA (1976) The bimodal mortality pattern of systemic lupus erythematosus. Am J Med 60:221—225

145. Valbonesi M (1983) Cascade filtration in the management of paraproteinemic and immune complex disease. In: Lysaght MJ, Gurland HJ (eds) Plasma separation and plasma fractionation. Karger, Basel, p 245.

An Experimental Therapeutic Approach   **343**

146. VanEpps DE, Palmer DL, Williams RC (1974) Characterization of serum inhibitors of neutrophil chemotaxis associated with anergy. J Immunol 113:189—200
147. VanEpps DE, Williams RC (1976) Suppression of leukocyte chemotaxis by human IgA myeloma components. J Exp Med 114:1227—1242
148. Waldenström JG (1980) Plasmapheresis — bloodletting revived and refined. Acta Med Scand 208:1—4
149. Ward PA, Berenberg AJ (1974) Defective regulation of inflammatory mediators in Hodgkin's disease: supernormal levels of chemotactic factor inactivator. N Engl J Med 290:76—80
150. Ward PA, Goralnick S, Bullock WE (1976) Defective leukotaxis in patients with lepromatous leprosy. J Lab Clin Med 187:1025—1032
151. Warren SE, Mitas JA, Golbus SM, Swerdlin AR, Cohen IM, Cronin RE (1981) Recovery from rapidly progressive glomerulonephritis: improvement after plasmapheresis and immunosuppression. Arch Intern Med 141:175—180
152. Wei N, Klippel JH, Huston DP, Hall RP, Lawley TJ, Balow JE, Steinberg AD, Decker JL (1983) Randomised trial of plasma exchange in mild systemic lupus erythematosus. Lancet 1:17—21
153. Wiebe RH, Handwerger S (1983) Failure of acute changes in prolactin to affect DHEA-S secretion in the human. J Reprod. Med. 2:206—208
154. Williams RC (1980) Methods of detection (of immune complexes). In: Williams RC (ed) Immune complexes in clinical and experimental medicine, Harvard University Press, Cambridge, p 167
155. Wing EJ, Bruns FJ, Fraley DS, Segel DP, Adler S (1980) Infectious complications with plasmapheresis in rapidly progressive glomerulonephritis. JAMA 244:2423—2426
156. Ytterberg SR, Schnitzer TJ (1982) Serum interferon levels in patients with systemic lupus erythematosus. Arthritis Rheum 25:401—406
157. Zielinski CC, Pehamberger H, Endler AT, Knapp W (1979) Serum associated leukocyte locomotion inhibition and leukocyte motility in malignant melanoma: effect of BCG treatment. Clin Exp Immunol 38:92—98
158. Zielinski CC, Ahmad R, Endler AT, Eibl MM (1980) Mechanisms of leukocyte locomotion in hemophilia. J Med 11:65—78
159. Zielinski CC, Lanzer G, Ludwig HP (1982) Defects of leukocyte locomotion in multiple myeloma. J Clin Lab Immunol 7:111—114
160. Zielinski CC, Wolf A, Eibl MM (1983) Plasmapheresis for rheumatoid arthritis (letter). N Engl J Med 309:986—987
161. Zielinski CC, Mutschlechner R, Schwarz G, Eibl MM (1983) Transient immunoglobulin and antibody production: occurrence in two patients with common varied immunodeficiency. Arch Intern Med 143:1937—1940
162. Zielinski CC, Gisinger C, Binder C, Mannhalter JW, Eibl MM (1984) Regulation of NK cell activity by prostaglandin E2: the role of T cells. Cell Immunol 87:65—72
163. Zielinski CC, Weissel M, Schwarz HP, Till P, Eibl MM, Höfer R (1984) Plasmapherese and Immunsuppression bei endokriner Orbitopathie: Ergebnisse und als Komplikationen auftretende Infekte. Verh Dtsch Ges Inn Med 90:494—497
164. Zielinski CC, Dremsek PA, Ahmad R, Eibl MM (1984) Recurrent pyoderma in a family with a defect in leucocyte locomotion. Br Med J 289:1561—1563
165. Zielinski CC, Preis P, Eibl MM (1985) Effect of immunoglobulin substitution during plasmapheresis on serum immunoglobulin and complement concentrations. Nephron 40:253—254
166. Zielinski CC, Weissel M, Schwarz HP, Till P, Eibl MM, Höfer R (1985) Combined treatment of endocrine orbitopathy by plasmapheresis and immunosuppression: effects on immunologic and ophthalmologic parameters. In: Pickardt CR, Schleusener H, Weinheimer B (eds) Schilddrüse '83. Thieme, Stuttgart, pp 188—199
167. Zielinski CC, Smolen JS, Preis P, Penner E, Wolf A, Eibl MM (1984) Shifts in humoral immunologic parameters in patients with systemic lupus erythematosus under plasmapheresis and immunosuppression. In: Nosé Y (ed) Therapeutic apheresis: a critical look, ISAO, Cleveland, pp 221—224

168. Zielinski CC, Ulrich W, Syré G, Gisinger C, Preis P, Schwarz M, Balzar E, Eibl MM, Kovarik J (1985) Plasmapheresis and immunosuppression in the treatment of proliferative glomerulonephritis: Histologic evidence of improvement. Plasma Ther
169. Zielinski CC, Preis P, Aiginger P, Eibl MM (1985) Acute-phase-proteins and parameters of humoral immunity in patients with advanced Hogdkin's disease. J Cancer Res Clin Oncol

Future Immunotherapeutic Possibilities
in Autoimmunity

N. TALAL

Introduction

Autoimmune diseases are multifactorial and involve genetic, viral, hormonal, environmental, and emotional components. Any or all of these factors can contribute to a breakdown in normal immunologic control which is at the heart of the autoimmune problem. The chronic autoimmune and inflammatory diseases are fundamentally disorders of immunologic regulation in which the immune system makes mistakes and unleashes a series of inappropriate effector mechanisms resulting in target organ destruction. The target organ may be synovial tissue lining joint surfaces (as in rheumatoid arthritis), the brain (as in multiple sclerosis), or almost any organ in the body.

Genetic Predisposition

The immune system is governed by genetic factors residing both within but also outside of the major histocompatibility complex (MHC). A striking feature of the MHC antigens is their extraordinary polymorphism which has been conserved throughout evolution and is thought necessary for species survival. Because of natural selection, the risk of spread of infection is reduced in proportion to the heterogeneity of HLA-linked immune response genes. HLA antigens may cross-react with infectious agents, rendering the host tolerant to a particular pathogen, or they may serve as receptor for such pathogens. The multiple genes and two chain composition of HLA molecules (e.g., each of the three D-region loci, DP, DQ, and DR, contain several genes coding for α and β chains) make this enormous variation possible.

Recent studies have shown that the T cell antigen receptor is also composed of two chains (α and β) and is structurally homologous to both immunoglobulin and HLA. All three families of molecules are thought to derive from a single primordial gene product through an evolutionary process of gene duplication and mutation. The T cell receptor expresses idiotype and binds both Ia and antigen. The outcome of this interaction is probably the single most important discriminator between tolerance, immunity, and autoimmunity.

Normal individuals who are HLA-B8/DR3 have evidence of immunologic hyperresponsiveness as evidenced by studies of humoral and cellular immunity [1, 2]. Whether this IR gene effect is exerted at the level of the antigen presenting cell or at the level of the responding T cell is not yet known. In SLE, there is only a weak genetic association with HLA DR3 and DR2 [3], suggesting that we need to look for other genes that might also contribute to disease susceptibility.

These additional genes could involve other MHC loci (e.g., complement genes or genes regulating sex hormone metabolism), or genetic factors that may not even be known at present. Consider, for example, the status of oncogenes, which have just recently revolutionized our thinking about carcinogenesis. Oncogenes are genetic regions of DNA which exist in two forms called c-oncogenes (or proto-oncogenes) and v-oncogenes (or viral oncogenes). The c-oncogenes are normal cellular genes which are involved physiologically in growth and differentiation. They probably function normally in fetal development, regeneration and perhaps at other times. These genes are captured by tumor viruses, becoming v-oncogenes, in which form they contribute to tumorogenesis. Tumor viruses are retroviruses which can reinsert v-oncogenes into the host genome at sites and/or under circumstances where these genes are regulated and function differently than normal c-oncogenes. Over 20 oncogenes are now known and many of their products have been identified. Some oncogenes code for growth factors (e.g., platelet-derived growth factor), others for growth factor receptors or enzymes which function as thyrosine kinases (as do some growth factor receptors). Yet others code for DNA-binding proteins whose precise functions are unknown. Some oncogenes appear to function synergistically to induce malignancy.

Oncogenes are present in lymphocytes and can be induced by lymphocyte activators such as mitogens [4]. At least one oncogene *(myb)* is excessively expressed in the peripheral lymphoid organs of autoimmune MRL/*lpr* mice [5].

Viral Factors

Every attempt to isolate a virus or other etiologic agent from lupus patients has failed [6, 7]. Yet the feeling persists and grows stronger that both SLE and rheumatoid arthritis will in time be found to be caused by a virus.

The oncogene concept represents one mechanism by which viruses could contribute to the etiology of lupus. There may exist genes analogous to oncogenes (which might be called autogenes) that are involved in autoimmunity and perhaps also in the extensive lymphoproliferation and malignant lymphoma that can develop in some autoimmune patients [8].

Another strong argument implicating a virus comes from the recent experience with AIDS [9]. AIDS is the disorder of immune regulation par excellence. It is now firmly established that the human T cell leukemia virus type III, which is specifically cytopathic to OKT4 helper cells, is the cause of AIDS. There are many immunologic similarities between AIDS and SLE, including polyclonal B cell activation, serum immune complexes, increased serum β_2-microglobulin, acid-labile interferon, decreased AMLR, IL-2, and natural killer cell activity (Table 1). If AIDS, with all its immunologic abnormalities, is due to a virus, does it not seem likely that one or more viruses are involved in the etiology of lupus?

Table 1. Similarities between AIDS and autoimmunity

Polyclonal B cell activation
Immune complexes
Increased serum β_2-microglobulin
Acid labile interferon
Decreased autologous mixed lymphocyte response
Decreased interleukin-2
Decreased natural killer cells

Table 2. New therapeutic approaches to autoimmune disease

Specific deletion or suppression of autoreactive lymphocytes
Monoclonal anti-Ia antibodies (haplotype-specific immunosuppressive)
Monoclonal anti-idiotypic antibodies
Attenuation with T cell lines

General biologic approaches
Sex hormone modulation — androgen suppression
Dietary manipulation — calorie restriction
Total lymphoid irradiation

Future Therapeutic Possibilities

With such a complicated and multifactorial pathogenesis, it is difficult to know exactly what immunotherapeutic possibilities will turn out to be most successful. Therefore, the emphasis in this chapter is on the word future, for although immunorestorative therapy for autoimmune disease is now well established, with several important leads into therapeutic strategy, we are still far from any significant clinical impact.

In recent years, several new immunotherapeutic approaches of either a specific or a more general nature have been tried in autoimmune experimental models and in patients (Table 2). These include specific deletion or suppression of autoreactive lymphocytes using monoclonal anti-Ia antibodies, monoclonal anti-idiotypic antibodies to autoreactive clones such as anti-DNA in lupus, or attenuated T cell lines in experimentally induced autoimmune models like EAE. The more general approaches include sex hormone modulation, dietary manipulation, and total lymphoid irradiation.

Monoclonal Anti-Ia Antibodies

A variety of immunobiologic approaches are being undertaken in an attempt to achieve specific deletion or suppression of undesired immune responses in autoimmunity [10]. For example, both induced diseases such as experimental autoimmune myasthenia gravis (EAMG) and experimental allergic encephalomyelitis (EAE), and spontaneous disorders with features of systemic lupus erythematosus (SLE) developing in certain inbred murine strains, can be suppressed with monoclonal anti-Ia antibodies. In animal models like EAMG and EAE, it is possible to suppress the autoimmune process by administering specific monoclonal antibodies directed against the I-A molecules of the immune response gene region located in the MHC. This therapeutic strategy is based on the demonstrated ability of antibodies to class II MHC molecules to suppress the immune response to specific antigens under Ir gene control. This type of suppression of the immune response in F_1 mice using Anti-Ia directed against only one parenteral haplotype, termed haplotype-specific immunosuppression, is particularly relevant to the human situation, where heterozygosity at the Ir gene locus is the rule.

Monoclonal anti-I-A therapy both prevented induction of EAE and delayed onset of EAE following immunization of mice with spinal cord in adjuvant [10]. Only 5% of anti-I-A treated animals developed clinical symptoms, compared with nearly 60% of animals treated with an irrelevant monoclonal antibody (P<0.0001). These investigators believe that several mechanisms may explain their results, including a very interesting suggestion that alterations of Ia-positive cerebral capillary endothelial cells may modulate lymphocyte migration into the brain.

In EAMG, monoclonal anti-I-A antibody partially suppressed the cellular and humoral immune response to acetylcholine receptor, the inducing antigen. There was also a decrease in clinical manifestations [11].

Suppression of lupus nephritis was achieved in female B/W mice with monoclonal anti-I-A antibodies [12]. Treatment resulted in a highly significant improvement in proteinuria and survival in rats (P<0.0001) even after the onset of renal pathology.

Monoclonal anti-idiotypic Antibodies

Idiotypes are recognized in vivo, leading to physiologic anti-idiotypic responses that may normally act to prevent autoimmunity by limiting the expansion of autoreactive B or T cell clones or helpers for such clones. Theoretically, the administration of appropriately directed monoclonal anti-idiotypic antibody could be specifically immunosuppressive and therapeutically beneficial in autoimmunity.

Idiotypic antisera have been produced not only to B-lymphocyte receptors and their secreted Ig products, but now also to the antigen receptor on T cells. As a potential target in immunotherapy, shared idiotypes should exist for all, or at least the most relevant, autoreactive T cell clones.

The suppression of pathogenic antibodies to DNA was achieved by repeated inoculation of B/W mice with a monoclonal anti-idiotypic antibody directed against a major cross-reactive idiotype on B/W IgG antibodies to DNA [13]. One hundred micrograms of the anti-idiotype were inoculated i.p. every 2 weeks, beginning at 6 or 20 weeks of age. As controls, littermates received an IgG, non-DNA-binding myeloma or no treatment. In the young mice, nephritis and anti-DNA antibodies appeared at the same time in all groups, and their circulating antibodies to DNA did not bear the target idiotype. In the older mice, survival was significantly prolonged because of delay in the onset of nephritis; the total quantities of antibodies to DNA were diminished, and the target idiotype, initially present on circulating IgG, was deleted. However, these benefits were transient since the suppression of antibodies was followed by the appearance of large quantities of anti-DNA that did not bear the major idiotype. It seems likely that specific suppression of the major idiotype allowed the emergence of clones expressing more private idiotypes.

Attenuation Using T Cell Lines

Yet another approach to specific immunosuppression of EAE involves vaccination with T-lymphocyte cell lines specifically reactive with the inductive antigen, myelin basic protein. The cell line employed originated in rats that had developed EAE as a consequence of immunization with basic protein. This cell line was itself capable of inducing EAE after intravenous inoculation. However, attenuation of the cell line by irradiation or exposure to mitomycin C rendered it capable of transferring resistance to EAE following standard immunization with myelin basic protein [14]. Autoimmune arthritis has also recently been suppressed using attenuated T cell lines [15].

Other Immunologic Approaches

Although treatment with antibodies specific for lymphocytes is not new, recent work with monoclonal antibody reactive with the L3T4 molecule of mouse helper T cells (the equivalent of the human Leu-3 or T4 antigen) has shown therapeutic promise in B/W mice.

Autoimmune mice have decreased production of interleukin-2 (IL-2) as an important part of their immunoregulatory disorder. This raises the possibility of using natural or recombinant IL-2 as a therapeutic agent, as has been tried in AIDS. However, the short half-life of IL-2, deficient cell surface receptors for IL-2 in autoimmune mice, and the lack of success in AIDS suggest caution in this regard.

General Biologic Approaches to Therapy

Sex Hormone Modulation

In the B/W mouse model for lupus, female mice develop autoantibodies, immune complex glomerulonephritis, and die from renal failure several months earlier than males. This is related to the 10 times more frequent occurrence of SLE in females than in males. An accelerated disease indistinguishable from that in females develops in male B/W mice castrated prior to puberty. Although gonadectomy does not benefit female B/W mice, the administration of male hormone suppresses their disease and allows them to live a normal life span. Most importantly, this beneficial effect of androgen can be demonstrated as late as 6 months of age, a time when SLE is already well established in female B/W mice. Thus, androgen acts to suppress autoimmunity and estrogen to accelerate it [16—18].

As in human SLE, there is a delayed clearance of particulate immune complexes in B/W mice. Female B/W mice develop this abnormality earlier than males. Furthermore, this defect can be suppressed in female B/W mice by exposing them to sustained androgen. By contrast, defective clearance develops earlier in male B/W mice given sustained estrogen [19]. These results suggest an important influence of sex steroid hormones on the clearance of immune complexes in murine SLE, and offers an explanation for the clinical benefit achieved by androgen administration.

However, the RE system is not the only site of action for sex steroid hormones. There is a evidence for sex steroid hormone receptors in the lymphoid organs of both humans and mice. Moreover, sex hormones act to influence lymphocyte number and function. In recent studies from our own laboratory [20], Lyt-2$^+$ suppressor cells appeared to be the main target cells of hormonal modulation in normal and autoimmune mice. Both testosterone and estrogen significantly depleted these cells in the thymus but had differential effects in the peripheral lymphoid organs, particularly in the spleen. In general, estrogen depleted Lyt-2$^+$ cells, whereas testosterone increased or maintained this subpopulation of cells in spleen and lymph nodes. Similarly, the suppressor cell activity and IL-2 production on a per cell basis in estrogen-treated animals was diminished, whereas testosterone-treated animals had normal or enhanced activity.

The therapeutic effect of androgen on spontaneous autoimmunity can also be demonstrated in another lupus model, the MRL/*lpr* mouse [19, 21]. Autoantibody levels, renal function, and survival are all improved even in this very aggressive disease.

In patients, MG occurs three times more commonly in women than in men. In EAMG, AChR-specific lymphocyte proliferative and autoantibody responses were suppressed by ovariectomy and enhanced by orchidectomy. Moreover, testosterone-implanted animals demonstrated lower lymphocyte and autoantibody response to AChR as compared with sham-implanted animals.

Chronic thyroiditis occurs 4 times more frequently in women, but only after puberty. Experimental autoimmune thyroiditis can be induced in mice by administration of mouse thyroglobulin emulsified in complete Freund's adjuvant followed by injection of lipopolysaccharide. Evidence for the suppressive effect of androgen on autoimmunity was also obtained using this experimental thyroiditis model [22]. Similar results have been obtained studying spontaneous autoimmune thyroiditis in rats. Castration of male rats increased both autoantibodies and thyroiditis lesions so that their disease was now equivalent to females [23].

The female/male sex ratio in rheumatoid arthritis (RA) is 4/1. Cell wall peptidoglycan-polysaccharide fragments derived from many bacteria, e.g., group A streptococci, induce chronic polyarthritis in rats which resembles RA clinically, histologically, and radiologically. An interesting sex difference is demonstrated when group A streptococcal cell wall fragments are injected into LEW/N rats. LEW/N female rats are highly susceptible to arthritis whereas LEW/N males are resistant. Castrated LEW/N males, or β-estradiol-treated males whether or not castrated, developed an arthritis as severe as that seen in LEW/N females.

In SLE patients, there is a deviation in the normal metabolism of estradiol, resulting in an elevation of 16-hydroxylated metabolites [24]. These products bind to estrogen receptors and retain estrogenic activity. This metabolic abnormality could contribute to exacerbations of disease following the ingestion of oral contraceptives containing estrogen. There is also evidence for decreased total androgens in SLE.

In summary, sex steroid hormones greatly influence normal immune mechanisms and autoimmune disease, with androgens suppressing and estrogens augmenting. Androgens can suppress several autoimmune models, including lupus in B/W and MRL/*lpr* mice, MG, thyroiditis, and polyarthritis. The effects of sex hormones on autoimmunity probably represent physiologic actions being expressed on aberrant systems of immunoregulation. The possible utilization of these effects in the treatment of human autoimmune disease is being studied in several laboratories.

Dietary Manipulation

Calorie restriction of NZB and B/W mice had a profound influence on the development of autoimmunity and immune dysregulation. Dietary restriction of NZB mice inhibited early thymic involution, reduced the development of splenomegaly, and resulted in the prolonged maintenance of T cell immune function. Restriction of total calorie intake in B/W mice more than doubled the life span and decreased immune complex deposition in the kidneys. Well-fed B/W mice showed earlier thymic involution, disorganization, and dysfunction of T cell system, and the earlier onset of renal disease, accelerated autoimmunity, and death.

Dietary restriction also retarded the lymphoproliferative disease and autoimmunity that occurs in MRL/*lpr* mice. Dietary restriction more than doubled the life span of these mice and inhibited the development of both lymphoproliferation and autoimmunity.

Studies on the mechanism of these effects are currently under way. Whether specific nutrients or total calorie manipulation can ultimately be employed for patients with autoimmune disorders is uncertain at this time.

Total Lymphoid Irradiation

Another general biologic approach that has been tried in autoimmunity is total lymphoid irradiation (TLI). Initially developed for the treatment of Hodgkin's disease, TLI has been studied both in experimental models and in patients with SLE and RA [25].

Although the future clinical role of TLI in autoimmune diseases remains unclear, results thus far indicate that TLI is a unique immunosuppressive regimen when compared with currently used immunosuppressive drugs, which are relatively nonselective and have short-lived effects. TLI is thought to produce a more selective and long-lasting reduction in the number and function of helper T cells. TLI also is associated with the appearance of antigen-nonspecific suppressor cells.

New Pharmacologic Approaches to Therapy

In recent years, a number of thymic hormone peptides have been isolated from the serum and the thymus. They tend to be reduced in the serum of NZB and B/W mice and restored by thymic transplants. Recent clinical trials in rheumatoid arthritis with thymopoietin and thymulin used in high doses suggest some modest clinical improvement.

Levamisole (2, 3, 4, 6-tetrahydro-6-phenylimidazo[2, 1-*b*]thiazole) has been tried with some success in RA but has significant side-effects, particularly its ability to induce agranulocytosis. It is now generally no longer used in patient management.

Diethyl dithiocarbamate (DTC) or imuthiol has been developed as a less toxic sulfur-containing compound. Imuthiol has a thymic hormone-like effect and augments T cell properties.

Isoprinosine, a complex of *p*-acetamidobenzoic acid, *N,N*-dimethylamino-2-propanol, and inosine (molar ratio 3:1), is an antiviral and immunopotentiating drug. Isoprinosine is virtually nontoxic, with only hyperuricemia reported consistently as a side-effect. We have found that isoprinosine can correct the IL-2 abnormalities in the *lpr* gene model of murine lupus. Furthermore, isoprinosine in vitro enhanced mitogen responses and decreased elevated Ig production in SLE.

Cyclosporin has proved itself extremely valuable in the prevention of graft rejection and is beginning to receive attention in autoimmune disease. It is still too early to tell what its therapeutic role will be for these diseases.

Autoimmune diseases are multifactorial in origin and immunoregulatory in nature, in a way very similar to AIDS. Some type of unusual interactions between immune and viral mechanisms probably induce these diseases. Indeed, there are well documented examples in which immunodeficiency and autoimmunity occur together in the same patient and numerous immunologic similarities exist between AIDS and autoimmunity. In a sense, AIDS is a challenge and a testing ground for new forms of immunorestorative therapy that, if found, should prove useful also in the treatment of autoimmune diseases.

Acknowledgment.
These studies were supported in part by the General Medical Research Service of the Veterans Administration and by the RGK Foundation.

References

1. Ambinder JM, Chiorazzi N, Gibofsky A, Fotino M, Kunkel HG (1982) Special characteristics of cellular immune function in normal individuals of the HLA-DR3 type. Clin Immunol Immunopathol 23:269
2. Kallenberg CGM, Klaassen RJL, Beelen JM, The Hauw T (1985) HLA-B8/DR3 phenotype and the primary immune response. Clin Immunol Immunopathol 34:135—140
3. Reinertsen JL, et al. (1982) Family studies of B lymphocyte alloantigens in systemic lupus erythematosus. J Rheumatol 9:253
4. Kelly K, Cochran BH, Stiles CD, Leder P (1983) Cell-specific regulation of the *c-myc* gene by lymphocyte mitogens and platelet-derived growth factor. Cell 35:603—610
5. Mountz JD, Steinberg AD, Klinman DM, Smith HR, Mushinski JF (1984) Autoimmunity and increased *c-myb* transcription. Science 226:1087—1089
6. Christian CL (1982) Role of viruses in etiology of systemic lupus erythematosus. Am J Kidney Dis 2:114—118
7. Norden CW, Kuller LH (1984) Identifying infectious etiologies of chronic disease. Rev Infect Dis 6(2):200—213
8. Talal N (1984) The biological significance of lymphoproliferation in Sjögren's syndrome. Proceedings of the XVIth international congress of rheumatology, Sydney, Australia. Elsevier Science, The Netherlands
9. Talal N (1983) A clinician and a scientist look at acquired immune-deficiency syndrome (AIDS). A validation of immunology's theoretical foundation. Immunology Today 4(7):180—183
10. Steinman L, Trotter J, Waldor M, Sriram S (1985) New approaches to therapy of autoimmune disease. Concepts Immunopathol 1:85—95
11. Waldor M, Sriram S, McDevitt HO, Steinman L (1983) In vivo therapy with monoclonal anti-I-A antibody suppresses immune responses to acetylcholine receptor. Proc Natl Acad Sci USA 80:2713—2717
12. Adelman NE, Watling DL, McDevitt HO (1983) Treatment of (NZB X NZW)F$_1$ disease with anti-I-A monoclonal antibodies. J Exp Med 158:1350—1355
13. Hahn BH, Ebling FM (1984) Suppression of murine lupus nephritis by administration of an anti-idiotypic antibody to anti-DNA. J Immunol 132:187—190
14. Ben-Nun A, Wekerle H, Cohen IR (1981) Vaccination against autoimmune encephalomyelitis using attenuated cells of a T lymphocyte line reactive against myelin basic protein. Nature 292:160
15. Holoshitz J, Naparstek Y, Ben Nun A, Cohen I (1983) Lines of T lymphocytes induce or vaccinate against autoimmune arthritis. Science 219:56
16. Roubinian JR, Papoian R, Talal N (1977) Androgenic hormones modulate autoantibody responses and improve survival in murine lupus. J Clin Invest 59:1066—1070
17. Roubinian JR, Talal N, Greenspan JS, Goodman JR, Siiteri PK (1978) Effect of castration and sex hormone treatment on survival, antinucleic acid antibodies, and glomerulonephritis in NZB/NZW F$_1$ mice. J Exp Med 147:1568—1583
18. Roubinian JR, Talal N, Greenspan JS, Goodman JR, Siiteri PK (1979) Delayed androgen treatment prolongs survival in murine lupus. J Clin Invest 63:902—911
19. Shear HL, Wofsy D, Talal N (1983) Effects of castration and sex hormones on immune clearance and autoimmune disease in MRL/Mp-*lpr/lpr* and MRL/Mp-+/+ mice. Clin Immunol Immunopathol 26:361—369
20. Ahmed SA, Dauphinee MJ, Talal N (1985) Effects of short term administration of sex hormones on normal and autoimmune mice. J Immunol 134(5):204—210
21. Steinberg AD, Roths JB, Murphy ED, Steinberg RT, Raveche ES (1980) Effects of thymectomy or androgen administration upon the autoimmune disease of MRL/Mp-*lpr/lpr* mice. J Immunol 125:871
22. Okayasu I, Kon YM, Rose NR (1981) Effect of castration and sex hormones on experimental autoimmune thyroiditis. Clin Immunol Immunopathol 20:240

23. Ahmed SA, Penhale WJ (1982) Influence of testosterone on the development of autoimmune thyroiditis in thymectomized and irradiated rats. Clin Exp Immunol 48:367
24. Lahita RG, Bradlow HL, Fishman J, Kunkel HG (1982) Abnormal estrogen and androgen metabolism in the human with systemic lupus erythematosus. Am J Kidney Dis 2:206
25. Kotzin BL, Strober S (1985) Total lymphoid irradiation. In: Talal N, Gupta S (eds) Immunology of rheumatic diseases. Plenum, New York

Subject Index

Abortion 117, 181
Activity 108, 153, 155, 187, 189, 190
AIDS 347, 352
Allergic encephalomyelitis 347
Alopecia 171, 185, 187, 242
Amyloidosis 255
ANA-negative SLE (see also lupus subsets) 292
Androgens (see also sex hormones) 349
Anemia (see also Coombs test) 175, 187, 309
-, hemolytic in NZB mice 50, 66
Animal models (see also mouse strains) 73, 148, 155, 291, 295
Antibodies (see also the respective name) antiviral 61
-, monoclonal 88
Anticoagulant 176, 181, 189
Anti DNA antibodies 3, 7, 28, 29, 50, 61, 64, 65, 89, 237, 238
-, in CSF 263
-, removal by plasma exchange 303, 306
-, cross reactive 90
-, dissociation from NTA 63
-, monoclonal 89
-, in nephritis 220
-, ss-DNA 73, 75, 78, 184
-, ds-DNA 105, 108, 153, 171, 180, 182, 185, 187, 188, 196, 281, 290, 294
Anti Ia antibodies in therapy 347
Antiidiotypic antibodies 65, 94
-, in therapy 348
Antinuclear antibodies (see also indiv. ANA subsets) 3, 182, 293
-, patterns 73, 109, 112, 182
Antitrypsin 307, 312
ARA criteria 108, 185, 295
Arthralgia 312
Arthritis 76, 172, 187, 189, 224, 276
Aseptic necrosis 172, 283
Autoantibodies (see also the respective name) antierythrocyte 64, 309
-, antiglycolipid 252
-, antihistone 91
-, antilymphocyte 74, 79, 101

-, antineuronal 183, 252
-, anti NK cell 309
-, antiphospholipid 89
-, anti PMN cell 309
-, antipolynucleotide 89
-, anti T cell 309
-, antithrombocyte 309
-, lymphocytotoxic 252
-, removal by plasma exchange 305, 308
-, thymocytotoxic, in mice 63
Autoimmune myasthenia gravis 347
Autologous mixed lymphocyte react. 10, 11, 148
Azathioprine 99

B cell 74, 78, 81, 146, 156, 157, 158, 199
-, hyperactivity 9, 37, 50, 60, 64, 308
-, growth factor 156
-, oncogene expression 37
-, polyclonal activators 73, 76, 81, 156, 200
Bacteria, cell wall antigens 93
Blood-brain-barrier 252, 262
Brain scan, static and dynamic 262
Bullous pemphigoid 233
-, treatment 233
Butterfly rash 2
BXSB-Y gene 27, 35, 37, 60

Cardiolipin 89, 105, 117
Carditis, endocarditis 173
-, myocarditis 173
-, pericarditis 173, 187, 272
Carpal tunnel syndrome 256
Cerebrospinal fluid, examination 262
Chilblain lupus 232
Chorea 254
Choroid plexus, immune complexes in 220
Chronic cutaneous discoid LE 227
-, treatment 229
CNS involvement 117, 171, 183, 189, 290, 293
Complement 74, 78, 112, 184, 187, 189
-, alternative pathway 124, 125
-, biologic activity 126
-, Cl inhibitor deficiency 124, 129, 131

356 Subject Index

-, C3   302
-, C3b inactivator deficiency   127, 129, 137
-, C3 nephritic factor   126, 139
-, C4   302
-, CH 50   129
-, classical pathway   124, 125
-, deficiencies   98, 124, 128, 137, 233
-, in CSF   264
-, in serum   302
Computerized tomography   262
Coombs test   74, 78, 171, 175, 183, 290, 293
Corticosteroids (see also therapy)   3, 99, 310
C-reactive protein   147, 148, 185
Cutaneous lupus erythematosus, acute   237
-, subacute   234
Cyclosporin   352
Cyclophosphamide (see also therapy)   32,
   99, 310

Dermatitis herpetiformis   233
Dermatomyositis (see also muscle involve-
   ment)   272, 280
Diaphragm   276
Diet   349
DNA (see also anti-DNA)   115
Drug-induced lupus syndrome   12, 114

Electroencephalography   261
Electromyography   260, 261
Electroneurography   261
ENA   106
Endocarditis   221, 222
Endocrinium   9, 350
Environment   12, 228
-, factors   81
Epilepsy   254
Erythema multiforme   2, 233
Estrogen (see also hormones)   350

Familial SLE   291
Fatigue   171, 189
Fibrinogen   147
Fresh frozen plasma, for plasma exchange
   302

Genetic factors (see also familial SLE,
   HLA)   8, 346
-, Klinefelter syndrome   80
-, lpr gene   75, 79
-, lupus in males (see also Klinefelter syndrome, sex hormones)   77
-, xid gene   74, 78
-, Y chromosome   77, 80
gld gene   27, 35, 37, 79

Glomerulonephritis   74, 76, 108, 155, 171,
   179, 189, 283, 290, 293
-, classification in SLE   204
-, diffuse endocapillary   214
-, diffuse global   214
-, diffuse segmentally accentuated   211, 214,
   216
-, membraneous   214, 215
-, membranoproliferative   214
-, minimal glomerular change   205
-, nonlupus   219
gp 70   50, 61, 70, 73, 81
-, immune complexes   62
-, development of nephritis   67
Guillain-Barré syndrome   253, 261

Headache   254
Hematuria   214, 215
Hemorrhage, cerebral   272
Hepatitis   177, 224
Heterogeneity of SLE   82, 291, 295
Histone   105, 114, 184
HLA   346
-, B7   228
-, B8   233
-, B8/DR3   237, 346
-, DR3   237
HLA antigens   198, 291
Human albumen, for plasma exchange   302
Hydralazine   2
Hypergammaglobulinemia   112, 156, 185
Hypertension   173, 180, 189, 214, 215
-, pulmonary   222
Hypocomplementia (see complement)

Idiopathic thrombocytopenic purpura   117,
   175
Idiotypes   65, 94
Immune complexes   6, 74, 77, 170, 180, 184,
   294
-, cerebrospinal fluid   252
-, choroid plexus   252
-, circulating   3, 204
-, in glomeruli   218
-, peripheral nerves   253
-, removal by plasma exchange   306, 309
Immunoglobulins, genes   76
-, in CSF   263
-, isotopes (see also H cell)   294
Immunoregulation   10
Immunosuppression (see also therapy)   3,
   99, 310
Immunotherapy   344
Imuthiol   352
Infections   12
Interferon   152
Interleukin 1   146

Subject Index 357

Interleukin 2   36, 148, 149
Interleukin 3   156
Interstitial Jaccoud's arthropathy   180, 278
Ir gene   346
–, recognition of DNA   51
Irradiation, total lymphoid   351
Isoprinosine   352

Klinefelter syndrome (see genetic factors)

La   239, 310
La/SSB   105, 110, 171, 182, 198, 293
LE cell   186
–, phenomenon   3
LE hypertrophicus   232
LE panniculitis   231
–, treatment   232
Leukopenia   11, 171, 175, 189, 290, 293, 312
Levamisole   352
Lichen planus   242
lpr gene   27, 29, 32, 35, 36, 37, 60
lung involvement   76, 174, 271
–, pneumonitis (see also serositis/pleuritis)
    117, 171, 174, 189, 271, 290, 293
Lupus anticoagulant   89
Ly1 B cells   78
Ly5 T cells   76
Lymphadenopathy   11, 74, 177, 189
Lymph nodes   224
Lymphocyte, function   51
–, phenotype   51, 56
Lymphokines (see also individual lympho-
    kines)   81, 145

Macrophages/monocytes   146, 153
Major histocompatibility complex   346
–, recognition of DNA   51
Meningitis   254
Mesangiopathy   208
Methotrexate   99
Mice, BXSB   60, 89, 94
–, MRL   60, 75, 80, 82, 94, 107, 156, 350
–, NZB   50, 60
–, (NZB × B10.D2)   55
–, (NZB × BXSB)F1   27
–, (NZB × NFS)F1   53, 56
–, (NZB × NZW)F1   60, 80, 89, 94, 350
–, (NZB × SWR)F1   50, 60
–, (NZB × ZWD)F1   51
–, NZW   50, 61
–, Palmerstone North   79
–, Swan Mice   79
Mitogens   147, 149, 154, 200
Mixed connective tissue dis. (see also over-
    lap syndrome)   108, 109, 241
Muscle involvement (see also dermatomyosi-
    tis)   170, 189, 290, 293

Myasthenia gravis   181
Myelitis   254
Myopathy   222, 253
–, steroid-induced   260

Natural killer cells   150, 153, 155
Neonatal LE   240
Nephritis   312
–, in humans   204
–, in MRL   60
–, in NZB   66, 74, 81
–, in NZW   50, 61
–, tubulointerstitial   215
–, vasculitis   216
Nephrotic syndrome   214, 215
Nervous system, CNS   251, 312
–, peripheral nerves   251
Neuropathology   251
nRNP   98, 239, 312
Nzv 1, 2 genes   62

Oncogenes   31, 34, 38, 39
–, c-bas   38
–, c-myb   31, 34, 35, 38
–, c-myc   34, 37, 38
–, c-onc   31
–, c-raf   36, 38
–, v-onc   31
–, in BXSB   37
–, in NZB   37
Osteoporosis   276
Overlap syndrome (see also mixed connec-
    tive tissue)   115, 197, 285

Palpable purpura   309
Peritonitis   177
Phosphodiester   92
Phospholipids   92
Photosensitivity (see also subacute cutaneous
    lupus)   81, 171
Plasmapheresis   99, 302
Plasma proteins, removal by plasma ex-
    change   307
Pleuritis   174, 271
Pneumonitis   222
Pneumonia, chronic interstitial   222
Polyclonal B cell activators poly (I) (see B
    cells)   89
poly (dT)   89
Polymyositis   253
Polyneuritis   254, 261
Polyneuropathy   253
Polynucleotides   92
Porphyria cutanea tarda   243
Positron emission tomography   262
Pregnancy   12, 182
Progressive systemic sclerosis (see scleroder-
    ma)

358 Subject Index

Proteinuria 208, 214
Psoriasis 243
Psychiatric disorders 254

Raynaud phenomenon 171, 173, 234, 312
Reticuloendothelial system 309
Retroviruses 60
–, ecotropic 61
–, xenotropic 61
Rheumatoid arthritis 76, 115, 172, 197, 278, 280
Rheumatoid factor 76, 91, 112, 185, 198
RNA 106, 114
RNP 105, 171
Ro 7, 236, 312
–, photosensitivity 240
Rowell syndrome 233
Russel's bodies 224

Scleroderma 115
Serositis 171, 189, 221, 269, 312
Sex hormones 74, 80, 349
Sjögren's syndrome 110, 171, 177, 179, 181, 197, 285, 290, 293
Sm 3, 29, 64, 91, 98, 238, 312
Splenomegaly 224
SSA, SSB (see Ro/SSA)
Stroke 254
Subacute cutaneous LE 110, 292
Sun exposure 12, 228, 231, 238, 240
Synovitis 224

T cell 10, 149, 199
–, antigen receptor 346
–, helper 155
–, immunoregulation by 308
–, in NZB and crosses 63

–, lines in therapy 349
–, subsets 74f., 81, 158, 200, 294
–, suppressor 76, 150, 291
Therapy, azathioprine 99
–, corticosteroids 3, 99, 172, 175, 181, 188, 310
–, cyclophosphamide 32, 76, 99, 172, 174, 178, 310
–, immunosuppressive 3, 99, 172, 174, 178, 310
–, nonsteroidal antiinflammatory 175, 182
Thrombocytopenia 111, 117, 171, 175, 187, 290, 312
Thrombosis, CNS 254
–, thrombophlebitis 117, 173, 187, 271
Thymopoetin 352
Thymulin 352
Thymus 178, 181
Tolerance 73, 80
Tolerance resistance 51, 55
Twins 74, 77, 173

Vasculitis 76, 172, 176, 187, 222, 271, 312
–, necrotizing 236
–, in CNS 222
–, in lung vessels 222
–, in nephritis 216
Vimentin 91
Viruses 60

Wasserman reagin test 2

xid gene (see also genetic factors) 53, 56, 64
–, and oncogene expression 38

Y chromosome 77, 80

Printed by Publishers' Graphics LLC
DBT130520.15.20.125 20130520